D0526604

Elements of Research in Physical Therapy

THIRD EDITION

The First Century 1890-1990

SANS TACHE

Withdrawn from
Queen Margaret University Library
QUEEN MARGARET COLLEGE LIBRARY

Elements of Research in Physical Therapy

THIRD EDITION

Dean P. Currier, Ph.D.

Professor of Physical Therapy
Division of Physical Therapy
University of Kentucky
Lexington, Kentucky

WILLIAMS & WILKINS
Baltimore • Hong Kong • London • Sydney

Editor: John P. Butler
Associate Editor: Linda Napora
Copy Editor: Patricia Grayson
Designer: Joanne Janowiak
Illustration Planner: Ray Lowman
Production Coordinator: Adèle Boyd

Copyright © 1990
Williams & Wilkins
428 E. Preston Street
Baltimore, Md. 21202, U.S.A.

All rights reserved. This book is protected by copyright. No part of this book may be reproduced in any form or by any means, including photocopying, or utilized by any information storage and retrieval system without written permission from the copyright owner.

Accurate indications, adverse reactions, and dosage schedules for drugs are provided in this book, but it is possible that they may change. The reader is urged to review the package information data of the manufacturers of the medications mentioned.

Made in the United States of America

First Edition, 1979

Library of Congress Cataloging-in-Publication Data

Currier, Dean P.
  Elements of research in physical therapy/Dean P. Currier.—3rd ed.

     p.   cm.
  Includes bibliographical references.
  ISBN 0-683-02248-2
  1. Physical therapy—Research. I. Title.
RM708.C87   1990   89-22695
615.8′2′072—dc20   CIP

                              90 91 92 93 94
                   1   2   3   4   5   6   7   8   9   10

To Joan
Wendy
Tracey
Brad

Preface to the Third Edition

As physical therapy continues to develop new programs and improve its curricular standards, the updating of textbooks must also keep pace with the developmental changes. Nearly every chapter of this edition has received changes that will improve its usefulness to students taking courses in research methods. Instructors who teach the research process will find the contents are inclusive and presented with added clarity.

This edition includes new library tools, further explanation of the workings of the internal review board, a discussion on intrarater reliability and group-comparisons experimental design, and the addition of the one-way repeated measures analysis of variance. Especially noteworthy is the exemplary proposal (Appendix A), which reflects several changes in the regulations for investigations of human subjects.

The purpose of this book remains the same: to inform readers about the elements of research. While assisting physical therapy students and practitioners in understanding the research process, the book will promote an appreciation of clinical research and enhance the ability to utilize the research literature effectively. As physical therapy research gains in vigor and respect, this book, hopefully, will nurture research appetites. The ultimate result of physical therapy research is the improved care of patients.

I wish to thank my colleagues who have offered suggestions for improving the book. They use the book in their courses of research and have provided me guidance in features and approaches of the research process. Their input has been invaluable and will always be gratefully received.

Preface to the
First Edition

Physical therapy in North America has grown out of a need to service patients having disease or injury affecting mobility of their bodies, and it has developed sound educational techniques for teaching that body of knowledge which has evolved through the years. Only recently has proper experimentation and the nucleus of a synthetic rationale emerged to relate clinical procedures with scientific bases. Instruction in research methods has been included in the curricula for the initial preparation of physical therapists, but textbooks for research methods in physical therapy remain scarce.

The purpose of this book is to inform readers about the elements of research. The book was designed for a one–term course and must necessarily omit many aspects of research. For the undergraduate, the book can reduce barriers of fear caused by lack of understanding of research and can shape favorable attitudes toward it. The book can assist the graduate student in developing the thesis. For the practitioner uninstructed in research methods, the book will provide an understandable review of various research methods and procedures. The contents provide a basis for appreciating clinical research, for interpreting the research literature, and for exposing the reader to techniques that have immediate application to clinical investigations. The contents reflect the author's experience in teaching research methods as well as student critique of that instruction.

The first part of the book calls attention to the what, why, who, and where of research; developing a research problem; and searching the literature. The discussion on the proposal serves as a guide to the neophyte investigator for planning the research project. Because of recent emphasis on the rights of subjects in research, the consent of research subjects is discussed. The second part of the book establishes the roots of research; that is, the basics of data and measurement, as well as the methods and instrumentation used in the research process. The third part discusses several statistical procedures for analyzing data on which inferences and conclusions are based. The statistical procedures do not require prior knowledge of algebra. Theorems and derivation of statistical formulas have been omitted. The final part of the book completes the process by discussing methods of reporting research.

I would like to express my appreciation to the American Physical Therapy Association for permission to reprint some material. I am grateful to Professor Barrie Pickles for paving the way for physical therapy research at the University of Alberta and to Donna McTavish for her patience and efficiency in preparing trial copies of the manuscript. A very special thanks to colleagues who contributed time freely to review parts of the manuscript: Donna C. Boone, Elizabeth Davies Carruth, Carmella Gonnella, James E. Griffin, Don Lehmkuhl, Gary Holdgrafer, Shrawan Kumar, Mary Moffroid, James Vargo, and Steven Wolf.

Many of the quotations introducing the chapters are from Bartlett J: Familiar Quotations, ed 14. Boston, Little, Brown and Co, 1968, and Straus MB (ed): Familiar Medical Quotations. Boston, Little, Brown and Co, 1968.

I am grateful to the Literary Executor of the late Sir Ronald A. Fisher, F.R.S., to Dr. Frank Yates, F.R.S., to Longman Group Ltd., London, for permission to reprint Table C, Appendix, from their book *Statistical Tables for Biological, Agricultural and Medical Research,* ed 6, 1974, and to the *Biometrika* Trustees for permission to use Tables D and E, Appendix.

A bad book is generally a very easy book, having been composed by its author with no labour of mind what-ever; whereas a good book, though it be not necessarily a hard one, yet, since it contains important facts, duly arranged, and reasoned upon with care, must require from the reader some portion of the same attention and study to comprehend and profit by it, as it required from the writer to compose it.

PETER MERE LATHAM
(1789–1875)

Contents

Part One

DEVELOPING RESEARCH

1

Research and Physical Therapy

I keep six honest serving-men
(They taught me all I knew);
Their names are What and Why, and
When
And How and Where and Who.
Kipling
Just So Stories (1902)

Physical therapy is an expanding profession comprising art and science components. The growth and development of physical therapy depends on science to uncover, modify, and accommodate new information. Art is the skill that takes place in the practice of physical therapy.

Techniques, procedures, and methods to achieve movement, function, and improved health comprise art, not science. Art and science are sometimes said to be one and the same. Although related, the student must keep in mind that a fundamental difference exists between the two. The difference between art and science is that art is concerned with methods or ways of effecting certain outcomes, whereas science is concerned with theoretical truth.[1] Science can be defined as a body of knowledge gained through diligent and systematic study with concern for facts and principles.[2] Research is a method of science that supplies pieces of knowledge by finding answers to questions, hypotheses, theories, principles; research is an attempt to find the theoretical truth or answer the question "why?"

Peat[3] has identified the art component of physical therapy as that of human relationships, the occurrence of vested interest, tradition, and the placebo effect. The intensive, caring relationship that practitioners establish with their patients results in the patient gaining confidence in the physical therapist. Techniques are sometimes taught through therapist–therapist interaction by a process analogous to "ecclesiastical succession", in which the leader of a particular therapeutic approach teaches a few practitioners who, in turn, become qualified to instruct others. The

3

relation tends to justify the therapeutic approach through personal observation, "anecdotal justification." Vested interest occurs when practitioners cling to a belief that certain techniques are valuable although no objective evidence is available to support such faith. Tradition may occur in some clinical situations where technique is the primary factor, whereas teaching and learning are technical events without benefit of the underlying physiological bases. The placebo effect takes place when the physical therapist convinces the patient that his or her therapy is of value, although no objective support is available.

Science in physical therapy eliminates bias and enables reproducibility of results. It allows for universal communication by using terms that have a specific meaning and are used for all. Science permits accurate quantitative measurements of existing phenomena. Therapeutic approaches can be scientifically tested to validate their effectiveness, which adds credibility to physical therapy. Scientific achievement of physical therapists can be judged by disseminating results of research through publication.[3]

Some professions claim to be scientific and, therefore, must develop their bodies of knowledge through research.[4] Is a profession a science? an art? must it encourage research? Perhaps defining a profession may help to answer the questions. A profession is an occupation whose members possess a body of knowledge which is both identifiable and different from that of others, and the members assume responsibility for adding to that body of knowledge.

According to Greenwood[5], a profession possesses certain elements distinct from those of a nonprofession. The major distinction is the body of knowledge that has been organized into an internally compatible system on which the skills that characterize the profession are formed. The body of knowledge is a system of abstract propositions that focus on the uniqueness of the profession. The body of knowledge (theory) forms the basis on which the professional rationalizes his or her (clinical) practice. Mastery of the theory is essential before acquiring the skill to practice, and preparation for the profession must be an intellectual as well as a practical experience. The value and emphasis placed on the theory precipitates an activity that is usually not a part of a nonprofessional occupation; namely, formation of theory through systematic research. Research is required to develop valid theory which provides a firm base for the techniques and procedures used by the professional. In a technological profession, a researcher–theoretician is a class of labor that gradually develops between the theory–oriented and the practice–oriented members.[5] Physical therapy has a body of knowledge and a clinical science which has been called pathokinesiology.[6] The knowledge and principles of physical therapy must be developed, however, through research; and students of physical therapy must be aware of the whats, whos, whys, wheres and hows of research. Understanding how research is performed is considered essential for interpretation of the literature, for being identified as a professional.

WHAT IS RESEARCH?

Research has been defined as a method of science, but it needs clarification. Research is a diligent and systematic study that uses scientific inquiry or methods to compile or uncover facts, test hypotheses, and show relations. Kerlinger[7] has defined scientific research as systematic, controlled, empirical, and critical investigations about the presumed relations among natural phenomena. He further defined research by its use of hypothetical propositions.[7] Research provides "sight" or truth, uncovers facts and causes, improves reasoning, and adds knowledge. Research is the process permitting description of individual attributes or events. Research is the process of asking and answering questions, as well as the process of abstracting answers from observations.[8] It is "an activity designed to test a hypothesis and permit conclusions to be drawn."[9] Although no simple definition really tells what research is about or is agreed on by all disciplines, the following definition describes research as it is presented in this book.

> Research is the studying of a problem in pursuit of a definite objective through employing precise methods, with due consideration to the adequate control of factors other than the variable under investigation and followed by analysis according to acceptable statistical procedures.[10]

The reader must realize that good research can be reported without statistical analyses ever being used and that good research can be performed without conforming to the guidelines presented herein. The above definition provides a baseline on which to begin and to establish the operational elements of research.

Students often are overheard saying that they must go to the library to do research. Although a review of the literature is a pertinent activity or phase in performing research, the process of reviewing literature is hardly synonymous with most definitions presented. Research is sometimes referred to by colleagues as being synonymous with problem solving. A differentiation must be made between research and problem solving because their purposes and processes are different. Research is a search for new knowledge or verification of beliefs and has a definite objective through the controlled process of scientific inquiry. Problem solving is a systematic approach to the solution of a problem or objective through action or thought. Problem solving does not require exact and precise elements of scientific inquiry nor does it require quantitative data analyzed by statistical procedures. Problem solving deals with "everyday" decisions. The differences between research and problem solving then are contrasted by the degree of precision, control, or demand placed on their processes. Research is a more rigorous process than problem solving, and, although both methods are important in physical therapy, they should not be used synonymously. Wandell[11] has stated that the purpose of research is to uncover new information, whereas the purpose of problem solving is to solve an immediate problem in a distinct setting.

TYPES OF RESEARCH

Research is often divided into two types, basic and applied. Basic research is referred to as pure research. The research undertaken is usually selected because it will reveal knowledge about a wide area[12] or knowledge common to all professions.[13] Basic research is implicitly or explicitly intended to increase understanding of the causes or function of whatever is being studied.[8] Pure research may be associated with experimentation on animals.[14] It tends to be abstract and general and, although basic research may lead to practical application, it is not begun with specific use.[15] Applied research is often called clinical research or clinical trials, and sometimes is called action research, particularly in educational circles. Applied research is concerned with applying or gaining knowledge in the practice of physical therapy. This latter research very often attempts to determine the efficacy of therapeutic procedures and is implicitly or explicitly intended to increase understanding of methods of therapeutic and educational delivery.[7] Ritchie[16] has pointed out, however, that it is no longer possible or wise to make a distinction between pure and applied research, since the two are often combined in modern approaches to improving human welfare.

I would like to introduce the idea of micro- and macroresearch. Microresearch is when researchers investigate at the cellular, tissue, or organic levels to uncover causes of an event or condition. Macroresearch, on the other hand, is when researchers determine associations between events or conditions, using statistics to show strengths or bonds between the associations. Both micro- and macroresearch are applied in a sense because they strive to show why or how the events or conditions are linked together; the difference is only at the level of investigation.

WHY RESEARCH?

According to the definition of a profession, members have the responsibility to develop and add to its body of knowledge through research.

Research is imperative for the survival of a profession[6,17] and is the cornerstone of a profession although excluded from being an art or technology. Only through research can a profession open its theory, principles, and procedures to inspection by the scientific community.

Watkins[18] referred to the 1944 report of the Baruch Committee on Physical Medicine when stating that more basic and clinical research was needed for the proper development of rehabilitative medicine. Physical therapy in North America has grown out of a need for better health service for patients and has developed sound educational techniques for teaching that body of knowledge which has evolved through the years. The history of the development of the health professions and sciences shows that the organization of teaching and professional service preceded formalized research.[19] Research evolves from curiosity or a need to test the existing knowledge and procedures; in a developing profession, old information is often converted into a new frame of reference.[20] The rate of growth of a profession will be proportional to the rate at which its body of knowledge grows and the amount of energy given to reearch.[4]

The members of a profession cannot wait for things to happen or for bits and pieces of fact and information to filter down from the research of other disciplines.[6] A profession must incorporate the idea and identify the need for research in its curricula for the initial preparation of its members. Research instruction must not be supported only from an educational point of view; the educational institution must also support research through its line item budget.[17] The quality of the end product of research instruction during the educational preparation of members of a profession will be demonstrated by professional growth and application to the profession's service.

Because physical therapy was established out of an identified need and has subsequently developed its educational system and treatment procedures, research is needed to support and add to the present body of knowledge. The time has come to augment the art with the science so that physical therapy can emerge as a science with clinical relevance.[21]

To be minimally effective in clinical practice, a physical therapist must be able to determine a patient's condition (within or outside of normal limits), to determine what rehabilitative approach to take, and to modify the approach whenever the patient's condition warrants change. Research provides answers to the therapist's questions, the reliable techniques for assessment, and the best approaches to patient management. Research is essential for developing a scientific approach to clinical practice, that is, establishing objectives clearly, establishing efficacy of new approaches to patient management, and being systematic in making observations of the patient's condition and reaction to treatment.[8] It permits judicious selection of treatment once the therapist has assessed the patient. Research, in addition to demonstrating the effectiveness of treatment, must also realize its goals relative to time and cost.[21]

Research is essential for developing inquiring attitudes among physical therapists. The therapist must constantly be able to recognize and challenge authoritative thinking and insist on evidence (observations, tests, valid and reliable inferences) for such thinking and beliefs. Physical therapists must challenge techniques passed on from therapist to therapist (ecclesiastical succession).[3] Instruction in research can assist the student in how to effectively question and apply the methods of scientific inquiry.

Today, accountability is preeminent because of rising health costs. Clinical misjudgment arises as a potential ethical issue. Should physical therapists, or any health worker, deliver treatment which has not been substantiated for effectiveness? Physical therapists sometimes manage patients by using new treatments learned at workshops. These treatments may not have been subjected to controlled study to establish their effectiveness for a particular physical condition. These newly learned treatments or procedures may not work, or may at best be only placebos. Is the physical therapist unethical if he or she elects to use treatments that may not be effective in combating the problem that the procedures are intended to erase? Research is needed prior to clinical application of new methods and procedures. We cannot defend ourselves against skepticism and accusations of inefficiency or lack of integrity unless our treatments are effective.[22]

Research is essential for establishing positive habits of thinking, controlling, confirming, and acting; it does not just initiate action through the richness of clinical experiences with thought and control. Physical therapists must not accept what others say or everything that is written, but must ask—is this really so? After asking, solutions (research) must be pursued to answer the question.[16] Movement has been vigorous to establish the efficacy of intervention, theory, and the status of physical therapy.

WHO SHOULD RESEARCH?

Members of the profession are likely to be the best researchers for building the body of knowledge of that profession. The members are likely to have a better idea of the needs for research and can best design strategies to meet those needs.

The researcher must possess certain qualities to perform successfully. Interest in a particular area or problem of the profession is important because an uninterested researcher is unlikely to advance new ideas.[12] The researcher must be motivated to endure tedious work and be willing to devote much effort and time to the research endeavor. The researcher must possess considerable knowledge of the area being investigated, must be curious, and ever asking, "why?" Creative thinking and perceptive and critical observational abilities are also essential characteristics for the researcher. Of course, training in the procedures of conducting research and in the methods of analyzing the results generated by the research process is essential. The development of positive attitudes toward research among members of a profession is generally the responsibility of the programs offering the initial preparation for the professionals, whereas the molding and production of researchers is the responsibility of programs of graduate studies. Opportunities to perform research during pursuit of graduate studies is conducive to learning because the student is no longer preoccupied with mastery of accepted knowledge, but rather, can direct attention to solving the unknown.[23] Many physical therapists also learn research methods at their place of employment.[24] Fitness for the enterprise of research is best expressed in Table 1.1 by the world renowned scientist, Walter Cannon.[25]

Although advanced study (master or doctoral levels) is helpful in research preparation, research must not be limited to just these levels of study. Research is a rational and reality–oriented process and belongs to those persons who can meet and handle the process appropriately (that is, the elements [qualifications] of scientific inquiry). The clinical researcher is the physical therapist who functions as a clinical practitioner and as an investigator. As a clinician, the therapist can best identify the needs for research, the kinds of questions that need to be asked. As a researcher, the therapist can influence directions of therapeutic approaches. These roles can and should be performed simultaneously. The roles of teaching and research should likewise function together.

The clinical therapist might ask, "What are the benefits derived from adding research to practice?" The question can be answered in several ways. Clinical research makes the practice of physical therapy more stimulating and less routine than it otherwise would be. Clinical research is a source of positive reinforcement to the therapist because it provides a feeling of accomplishment derived from formulating a research question; observing or collecting and analyzing data; and reporting results to colleagues at meetings or in professional journals.[8] Research provides a more effective clinical practice because it provides answers for determining the

Table 1.1
Qualifications of a Researcher

Curiosity	Knowledge of mathematics
Imagination	Observational ability
Critical judgment	Good memory
Honesty	Patience
Variety of experiences	Ability to write clearly
Technical skill	Critical (tactful) judgments of peers
Ingenuity	Humility

most effective approach to patient care. Research provides a body of knowledge for improved quality of patient care.

Research provides the satisfaction of discovery, forms extensive friendships among colleagues or former students, provides practical and reliable approaches to direct patient care, and uncovers truth. Rewards of research are also gained through the recognition accorded by peers and seeing the spreading influence from research results.[25] Research may also provide the freedom to develop one's own ideas or a degree of concentration and interest in a certain question.[16] The ultimate goal of most researchers is simply to advance knowledge.

WHERE RESEARCH?

The School

Universities serve a valuable function by providing resources for research. Schools with graduate programs are obligated to create research and development products through student theses and dissertations. When disseminated to members of the profession information from these products enhances theory, supports clinical techniques, and demonstrates accountability. Universities with good research programs have strong commitments from faculty, students, and clinicians. Each benefits through productivity, available equipment, objectivity, and intellectual environment.

Responsibilities for research in physical therapy must not be granted solely to the student. Faculty of physical therapy programs must also engage in research. Treatment, education, and research are recognized basic functions of a comprehensive center of health activity,[26] and the faculty are functional components of the center. The attitudes of students and the quality of research emerging from the center are dependent on the knowledge, astuteness, interest, motivation, and direction of the faculty. Faculty serve as role models for students and, if students do not observe or participate in ongoing research in their own discipline, they might conclude that research is not a priority of the profession and can be eliminated from busy work schedules.

The Clinical Setting

The practitioner must play a vital role in the profession by performing research where the application of research is essential. The practitioner's purpose is the same as that of the students and faculty of physical therapy programs, that is building a body of knowledge for improved quality of patient care.

Practitioners working in clinics located near physical therapy schools benefit by contributing patients to research projects, overseeing student projects, and affiliating themselves with other researchers. Coordinated efforts among the different institutions helps build strong research programs.

Today's student of research methods may eventually become the director of a clinical department. If positive attitudes toward research are developed by the student, then physical therapy research activity in the clinic may someday be a commonplace function of the practitioner. The director of a department engaging in research should be trained in research and management.[26] Leadership in clinical physical therapy calls for certain criteria. Management must not only accept and approve of research activity in physical therapy, but must also schedule work to allow for conduction and analysis of research and to arrange for adequate space, equipment, and money. In other words, the leader must establish and support a climate of "vigorous intellectual ferment."[27] Proper management also calls for careful selection of staff. Staff present ideas that facilitate creativity and develop the new, the daring, and the different. Staff consists of persons trained in research and motivated to perform research, yet willing to function in the regular capacity of clinical therapists. A collection of selected staff can stimulate and inspire each other; research enhances their job satisfaction and self–respect.[27] Clinical research will improve quality physical therapy.

The Association

The professional organization can provide impetus for research activity through direction, monetary support, and recognition. The Research Committee, the Section on Research, the Foundation for Physical Therapy and the journal, PHYSICAL THERAPY, are arms of the American Physical Therapy Association. The Research Committee has developed long–range plans for fostering research in the profession, whereas the Foundation for Physical Therapy has been established to endow research activity. The establishment of research centers supported by Foundation funds will help the profession in directed research. Other physical therapy associations have similar mechanisms. The Chartered Society of Physiotherapy has a Research Advisory Board;[28] in 1975, however, the Specific Interest Group of the Association of Chartered Physiotherapists in Research was formed. This latter group promotes research activity among physiotherapists in the British Isles and has made considerable progress.[29] The Canadian Physiotherapy Association's counterpart is the Clinical Studies Division.[30]

Bohannon and LeVeau stated that research is perceived separately from practice and that practitioners believe their approaches to patient care are effective although research findings may differ. They suggested that students and practitioners be prepared to be consumers of research and increase the availability of research information to enhance the professional's use of research findings reported in the literature.[31]

DIFFICULTIES ENCOUNTERED IN PHYSICAL THERAPY RESEARCH

Problems confronting schools, students, and physical therapy clinicians are presented separately only to call attention to specific difficulties or situations. The difficulties in research are not universal and are being alleviated in many areas.

The Clinic

Practitioners often hesitate to attend presentations of original research or read research reported in their professional journals because they do not understand what is being presented. The formal education of practitioners prior to 1965 did not regularly include instruction in research methods.[24] The lack of instruction in research has produced an understanding gap between authors of research reports and physical therapy practitioners who often do not understand research reports.[32] Some suggestions for correcting the problem are: (1) that practitioners return to academic institutions periodically to refreshen their academic knowledge and to learn about research; and (2) that researchers conduct workshops for orientation in research methods and interpretation.[33] An insufficient understanding of research is not necessarily unique to practitioners; it may also be a shortcoming among students and faculty. The lack of understanding may have previously been a deficiency of the philosophy of the profession, but that is now being corrected.[24]

Difficulties encountered by clinical therapists conducting research are different from those encountered by faculty members. Physical therapists are employed to treat patients and, therefore, most of their time is expected to be directed in patient–oriented activities. Physical therapists have not educated the public, physicians, and administrators to the idea that they are researchers and that research is an integral part of their duties. Since the process of research is not measured easily for its immediate results or productivity (for example, number of patients treated per day), the employer may be reluctant to allocate the therapist's time for research activity. Of greater significance is the failure of research to contribute immediately to the financial success of a facility. Research does, however, increase costs of operation.

The responsibility of overcoming obstacles for clinical research is not only that of the department's leadership, but also that of every department member. Physical therapists must organize educational and public information programs to dispel any misunderstanding about the therapist's role in research. The best approach to alleviating any adverse concepts by critics is to demonstrate the ability and effectiveness to perform research in the clinic. All clinicians should not conduct research, but large clinics having several or more therapists should have one or two researchers who are permitted sufficient time and support to investigate clinical questions. Large physical therapy departments may consider establishing a "research arm" with a few therapists devoting a percentage of their time to research.

The School

Most schools in the United States and Canada with entry levels of physical therapy education offer some degree of research instruction.[24,34,35] This commitment to research instruction at the initial level of education will eventually dispel the image of not doing enough research.[17,36] Some schools do not place emphasis on laboratory experiences where an atmosphere of research–like activities prevails. Perhaps a more common and dangerous problem is the lack of research monies in line item budgets of physical therapy schools. Some directors of schools have not established research as a high priority among faculty, and these faculty, in turn, have not received financial support for research activity. Funds, when received for research, may enrich instruction through state–of–the–art equipment and new experiences. Support monies encourage student and faculty research. Faculty who have not been trained in or have not engaged in research often are appointed, or they are not sufficiently interested in or committed to research. Faculty frequently have excessive teaching commitments that prevent time for research. Some faculty believe their major responsibility is teaching, and they ignore the fact that educational information is derived from scientific inquiry. Research provides new ideas or knowledge and improved technology while dispelling or confirming previously accepted knowledge. If no research is performed by faculty, then the same information is passed on from year to year. What new information is passed on is borrowed from other professions and applied to physical therapy without being validated for physical therapy. As a result, therapists apply the information to treatments before the information is tested under rigidly controlled conditions. Groups who continuously borrow information and adapt it without the scrutiny of controlled experimentation are not professionals and do not command recognition of the scientific community.

Students will perform research when research is demonstrated to be an integral part of their education. Research cannot be demonstrated only through curriculum, but must be supported by a departmental atmosphere of intellectual curiosity and scientific inquiry through action. Students gain experience and insight from scientific inquiry through required projects at the initial level of education and through required thesis work at the graduate levels. Enthusiasm for and participation in research by faculty are contagious, and the condition soon becomes an indigenous characteristic of the educational program. The intent of exposure to or training in research is not to make all physical therapists into researchers. An acceptable blend of theory, research, and techniques needs to be developed among physical therapists. The present need for research is greater, however, than the current supply of researchers. If the advancement of knowledge is dependent on research and intelligence and if participation in research is a requirement of physical therapy, then intelligence must be a principal criterion for admission into physical therapy education.[4] The entry level curriculum must continue to produce graduates who will critically evaluate and compare clinical procedures. The universities must be successful in producing such students if physical therapy is to continue its growth and take its place among respected health disciplines.[3] Since the majority of physical therapists do not go on to higher levels of education, they must learn the research process at the entry level or through continuing education. The efforts of the universities may be reaping dividends, because the submission of research papers to annual conferences has reached a point where many good papers are rejected on the basis of volume and competition.[37]

Perhaps the response of an anonymous student, when asked about the problems of performing research in physical therapy, epitomizes the situation:

> The greatest area of concern in productive research for physical therapy is the lack of therapists involved in or qualified to perform research. Our educational system does not always provide the necessary background for the student to have a precise understanding of research. As students, we are more concerned with learning treatment techniques that are already established. We concentrate in these areas because our grades are dependent on learning concepts. Even though we might have a problem which needs research, we push it aside to get the grades to obtain a degree. Once we are out working, we again push it aside because our employer is more concerned with services and economics. Our educational system needs to provide the background emphasis for research and make known the opportunities available for students interested in performing research or becoming researchers.
>
> Anonymous Student

STIMULATION TO ENGAGE IN CLINICAL RESEARCH

During the initial education of physical therapy students, frequent laboratory sessions in most courses tend to stimulate students. Students learn to measure, test, assess, and make conclusions as a result of laboratory exposure. Assignment for interning in facilities having therapists who engage in research is another approach to stimulating interested students.[36]

Administrators of the clinical facility and the faculty of the physical therapy school must be convinced that therapists have a role in clinical research. Only when encouragement and support by clinical administrators and faculty are given will the research atomsphere flourish.

NEEDED AREAS OF RESEARCH

Physical therapists function traditionally as clinicians for direct patient care, as educators, administrators, and consultants. All areas germane to physical therapy are areas requiring research. Since physical therapists are predominantly providers of health services, substantial energies should be directed toward the scientific aspects of the profession and the delivery of physical therapy services.

Some specific areas identified for research are:

1. The efficacy and value of therapeutic procedures and physical agents.[36,38–40] Facilitation and mobilization techniques, electrical stimulation, lasers, biofeedback, therapeutic exercises and aids to enhance muscular strength, and comparison of physical agents and their combinations for treatment of specific conditions are all examples.
2. Tests and measurements in the assessment of physical conditions and in the analysis of motion.[36,38,40] Development of improved clinical techniques for measuring muscular strength, gait, edema, and treatment effectiveness are needed along with demonstrated validity and reliability of the techniques and instruments of measurement.
3. Rehabilitation engineering of devices for assisting the physically handicapped[38] and for achieving optimum design of the therapist's equipment.
4. Growth and development defects and ways of improving physical function.[40]
5. Practices of accreditation, registration, licensure,[4] and standards for physical therapy services.[41]
6. Curriculum construction, legislative planning, cost studies,[42] competencies of practice, and effectiveness and impact of specialization.

The April 1979 issue of PROGRESS REPORT of the American Physical Therapy Association invited ideas on priorities in physical therapy clinical research. The report of the mail–in survey listed the priorities as: (1) treatment outcomes, (2) physiological effects of treatment, (3) methods of patient assessment, (4) pathological mechanisms, (5) delivery of services, and (6) psycho–social aspects. Later, in June 1979, the Research Committee held a clinical research hearing in which individuals presented testimony on research priorities. These results indicated that treatment outcomes were suggested as needing research. Even today these identified areas of physical therapy need to be researched.

ESTABLISHING RESEARCH

The establishment of research in a facility (clinic, school, program) requires thorough and deliberate planning,[26,43] administrative support,[8,26] and employment of therapists prepared to practice, research, and teach.

The development and implementation of any new activity within a facility must necessarily derive administrative support. Research requires trained personnel, ideas, money, space, and "a climate of vigorous intellectual ferment."[27] Each criterion is administratively related. Above all, the administrators must be convinced of the necessity and value of physical therapy research. The administrator can be identified as the director of a department or program or as the director of a hospital or school.

Administrative Support

When establishing research in the clinic, some attention must be given to the administrative aspects. Without the support and encouragement of the clinical administration, the aspiring researcher has a harder than usual task.

The therapist's working conditions can encourage or discourage research. The researcher needs job security with guarantees that an approved research project can be completed.[25] Many researchers were hurt financially (unemployment) when federal funds were reduced or withdrawn in the late 1960s because their salaries and projects were funded solely by research grants ("soft monies"). Freedom to perform without undue interference from administrators is helpful to the researcher, as is the absence of administrative pressure and reduced numbers of written reports. Uncompromising deadlines or measurable end-products can destroy pilot or burgeoning research. Access to pertinent literature is very important. Professional in–service programs are beneficial to the researcher because they provide a forum for ideas and communication. Sympathetic official attitudes are encouraging because they condone the objectives and activity of the researcher, provide an "aire" of endorsement, and negate prejudices.[25]

"I do not have enough time to do research because I am expected to treat patients," is often voiced as a deterrent to clinical investigations. Since when has intellectual curiosity been confined to certain periods of the day? Do ideas or questions of a clinical nature occur only when certain periods of the day are designated for research? The answers to these questions should be obvious, but time is essential to perform literature reviews, write proposals, analyze data, and report results. Efficient therapists find time during the work day for activities other than direct patient care. Research can and should be integrated into the regular patient care program. Physical therapists must measure treatment outcomes and, if treatments are delivered under controlled conditions, the therapists can evaluate the effectiveness of his or her interventions. This is a form of research and invites reporting and scrutiny. Research really is a part of direct patient care because it answers questions and improves quality of care. Finding time to do research is the responsibility of the individual rather than of the administrator. Silvermann[8] has provided suggestions for selling the research idea to administrators. Results obtained and published from research provide a means of accountability. Published reports can be counted and the findings can be used in the administrator's talks to community groups or to the board of directors. Ongoing research is likely to convey local, state, and national recognition to the facility and therapists. This type of recognition is looked on favorably by administrators because it brings notoriety and possibly attracts money.[8]

Research is an excellent way of evaluating clinical programs and revealing objective information. Practitioners assess, observe, and measure, so that a systematic approach with controls built in could deliver important findings for supporting objectives. The systematic approach would probably not interfere with ongoing activity because it is really what physical therapy is about. Data gathering is part of any effective treatment program.[8]

Research Funding

Research studies require instruments that invariably require financial support for construction, operation, or maintenance. Large amounts of money are needed in some studies for equipment and salaries of research assistants. Monies are either obtained internally, from sources within the institution or facility, or externally, from sources outside the institution. Internal funding is usually made in small amounts to assist pilot studies; external funding is obtained from sources such as government, organizations, and foundations. The latter award large amounts of money but are very competitive and require special applications and time. A researcher can usually expect one year to elapse between submission of a grant application and initiation of the project, if successful in obtaining external funds. The researcher is advised to plan projects well in advance of anticipated target dates when hoping to use external funding; he or she also should be prepared for possible rejection of financial support. The interested researcher can find assistance in grant writing by asking those having prior experience, by reading books, and by attending workshops.

Funds for physical therapy research should improve with increased numbers of persons conducting investigations and when institutional administrators, government officials, members of the medical community, and the consuming public recognize the role of research in the profession.

HOW RESEARCH?

Many different methods are described for use in research; some are identical in purpose and technique but are given different names by different disciplines. Different methods are devised for studying different areas, because one method may not be adequate or flexible enough to fulfill the needs of all areas. All methods of research however, have commonalities. All methods require the collection of information relevant to the subject; the collected data must be verified, analyzed, and interpreted, and the findings must be presented in some orderly fashion. Some hows or methods of the research process are presented in the following chapters.

SUMMARY

This chapter has provided an introduction to the scientific method of research by discussing the what, why, who, and where of research, and discussing the types of research. Attention was called to areas of needed research in physcial therapy and to problems encountered in establishing or conducting research. Table 1.2 provides an overview of the research process discussed in this book.

Table 1.2
Cumulative Summary of the Research Processes Presented

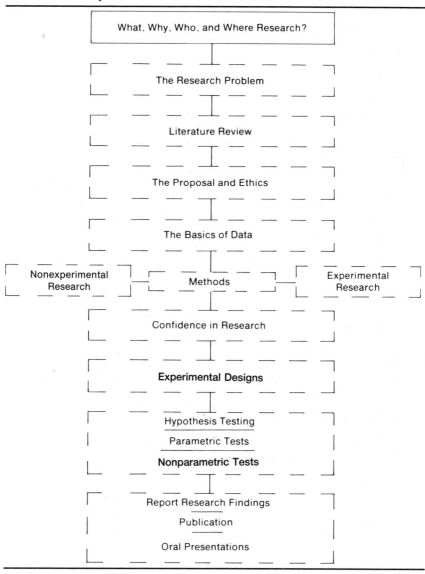

REFERENCES

1. Fowler HW: A Dictionary of Modern English Usage, E. Gowers (ed), ed 2. New York, Oxford University Press, 1965
2. Random House Dictionary of the English Language, Unabridged ed. New York, Random House, 1983
3. Peat M: Physiotherapy: art or science? Physiother Canada 33: 170–176, 1980
4. Worthingham C: The development of physical therapy as a profession through research and publication. Phys Ther Rev 40: 573–577, 1960
5. Greenwood E: The elements of professionalization. In Vollmer HM, Mills DL (eds): Professionalization. Inglewood Cliffs, NJ, Prentice–Hall, Inc, 1966
6. Hislop HJ: The not–so–impossible dream. Phys Ther 55: 1069–1080, 1975
7. Kerlinger FN: Foundations of Behavioral Research, ed 2. New York, Holt, Rinehart and Winston, Inc, 1973
8. Silverman FH: Research Design in Speech Pathology and Audiology: Asking and Answering Questions. Englewood Cliffs, NJ, Prentice–Hall, Inc, 1977
9. The national commission for the protection of human subjects of biomedical and behavioral research: the Belmont Report: ethical principles and guidelines for the protection of human subjects of research. Washington, DHEW Public Health Service, 78-0013, 1978
10. Report of the American Public Health Association Task Force. Am. J Public Health 47: 218–234, 1957
11. Wandelt M: Guide for the Beginning Researcher. New York, Appleton–Century–Crofts, 1970
12. Wilson EB Jr: An Introduction to Scientific Method. New York, McGraw–Hill Book Co, 1952
13. Steinhaus AH: Why This Research? In Hubbard AW (ed): Research Methods in Health, Physical Education, and Recreation. Washington, Am Assoc Health Phys Educ Rec, 1973
14. Campbell EWR: Introduction: The purpose of research. Physiotherapy 56: 480–481, 1970
15. Cox RC, Best WL: Fundamentals of Research for Health Professionals. Laurel, MD, RAMSCO Pub. Co., 1982
16. Ritchie AE: Considering research. Physiotherapy 56: 110–112, 1966
17. Basmajian JV: Professional survival: the research role in physical therapy. Phys Ther 57: 283–285, 1977
18. Watkins AL: Some research problems in physical therapy. Phys Ther 29: 443–447, 1949
19. Hines HM: What research means to a profession—its growth and continuation. Phys Ther 31: 450–451, 1951
20. Houtz SJ: Challenge of the scientific method. Phys Ther 31: 465–467, 1951
21. Gowland C, Clarke B: Research: Why Bother! Physiother Canada 32: 270–274, 1980
22. Ottenbacker KJ: Evaluating Clinical Change: Strategies for Occupational and Physical Therapists. Baltimore, Williams & Wilkins, 1986
23. Hellebrandt FA: Graduate study—a key to research and writing. Phys Ther 40: 257–260, 1960
24. Currier DP: Research in Physical Therapy Schools. (Unpublished survey.)
25. Cannon WB: The Way of an Investigator: A Scientist's Experiences in Medical Research. New York, Hafner and Co, 1965
26. Moffroid MT, Hofkosh JM: Development of a research section. Phys Ther 49: 1208–1214, 1969
27. Greenblatt M: Conducting a research department. Hosp Community Psychiatry 13: 580–581, 1962
28. The Research Advisory Board. Physiotherapy 52: 126–127, 1966

29. Partridge CJ: Progress in research. Physiother 68: 353, 1982
30. Clinical Study Council. Physiother Canada 23: 184, 1971
31. Bohannon RW, LeVeau BF: Clinicians' use of research findings: a review of literature with implications for physical therapists. Phys Ther 66: 45–50, 1986
32. Lehmkuhl D: Let's reduce the communication gap: Part I, the question what and why? Phys Ther 50: 61–63, 1970
33. Ruffer WA: Who should make research applicable? J Health Phys Educ 40: 41–42, 1969
34. Currier DP: Research in programs of initial physical therapy education. Physiother Canada 29: 211–213, 1977
35. Report of the Royal College of Physicians of Edinburgh on co–operation between medical and other health professions. Physiotherapy 63: 228, 1977
36. Griffin JE: What's the answer. Phys Ther 50: 259, 1970
37. Michels E: Paper submissions hit all–time high. Progress Rpt 10: 5, 1981
38. Basmajian JV: Research or retrench: the rehabilitation professions challenged. Phys Ther 55: 607–610, 1975
39. Fowler WM: Physical therapy and research. Phys Ther 49: 977–982, 1969
40. Hislop HJ: The doctorate in physical therapy. Phys Ther 48: 1325–1326, 1968
41. Chase HC: Some current research in the allied health professions. Phys Ther 51: 771–776, 1971
42. Magistro CM: The 1976 presidential address. Phys Ther 56: 1227–1239, 1976
43. Schrenk R: Research: Stepchild of medicine. Am J Clin Pathol 34: 268–269, 1960

2

The Research Problem

The human mind is our fundamental resource.
John F. Kennedy

If research is a process used to find facts or add to a body of knowledge (theory), then the process must have a beginning. Accumulating facts without any preconceived idea of which facts to gather or which are relevant would be disastrous. An organized plan is essential for gathering the facts. The first step in the plan for beginning research is to formulate the research problem.

WHAT AND WHY A RESEARCH PROBLEM?

Definition (What?)

The simplest way to define a research problem is to state a question. The question must be answerable, that is, a solution to the question must be possible. A problem can be an "irritation" which stimulates a person into doing research to answer the question or to eliminate the irritation.[1] The problem can be something that needs solving, an unresolved situation. The problem can be an idea which a person has for developing an approach to treatment or a new product.

We all have had questions to which we have sought answers. Often we asked another person, perhaps a teacher or a peer, and received a satisfactory reply. Sometimes we did not get a satisfactory answer to our question and had to seek a solution through library or textbook search. Our questions in these illustrated situations were answered by simple methods; however, not all of our questions or problems may have simple answers or solutions.

Too often people do not seek answers to their questions unless the answer is quickly and easily available. These persons are not curious and are not potential researchers. The persons who search for an answer, establish a formal organized plan to acquire an answer, and use methods of scientific inquiry to get the answer are researchers. The researcher is motivated to eliminate the irritation by obtaining a satisfactory answer to his question. Thus, research begins when answers to the question cannot be found.

The Value of the Research Problem (Why?)

The unanswered question is important because it directs or stimulates the curious and motivated person to seek an answer and can be responsible for starting research or scientific investigation. The stated problem can help direct the researcher and lead to an investigation through which a scientific approach is used for its solution. The specific information resulting from the research enables the researcher to make generalized statements based on the empirical observations from the research process. The reasoning process is deduction. The results of the research can serve as a basis for prediction and control of the phenomena studied.[2] The basic value of the research problem is to stimulate research that will lead to new scientific knowledge through the solutions to the problem. Research findings often lead to other interesting and significant problems to be studied.

IDENTIFYING A PROBLEM

How does one go about identifying or locating a research problem? For some persons, identifying a research problem or asking a research question may be more difficult than solving it. Since various circumstances serve as starting points for identifying an answerable question, certain attributes or activities can assist the student in identifying or locating a research problem. Suggestions on how to locate or identify research problems are valuable for the conduct of research necessary to complete a course in clinical investigations, a thesis, or a dissertation.

Necessary Attributes for a Researcher

In Chapter 1 the desirable qualities of a researcher were discussed and listed. Some of these qualities are repeated for the purpose of emphasizing their importance in research.

One of the first considerations is the student's or researcher's attitude toward the scientific method or the advancement of the profession. A positive attitude consists of interest, curiosity, and motivation. Perhaps interest is the key characteristic that aids in identifying the problem and seeking a solution. The student must be enthusiastic or interested in a particular area or the research process will be a distasteful experience. Having an interest in a particular problem can help direct the student in the pursuit of a solution and help the student to enjoy the experience. A student who finds routine dissection distasteful might develop an interest in dissection when it can be used to solve a defined problem of considerable personal interest. Students with enthusiasm and interest in what they are doing usually will find the research experience enjoyable. Some students may even continue in research as a result of this initial experience or exposure. The disinterested researcher does not usually contribute new ideas to a body of knowledge.[3]

Technical knowledge in the area of planned research is important.[4-9] The student must know a body of knowledge well to identify situations or areas which require additional facts or information before improvement can be achieved. The experienced researcher has little difficulty in identifying problems in a particular body of knowledge; his trouble is that he usually cannot find enough time to conduct the experiments necessary to answer all of his questions or solve the identified problems in his field of interest. The experienced researcher identifies new problems every time a research project or study is in progress.

The person who recognizes the deficiencies in a particular area will have an easier time formulating the problem to be solved through research. The student must be able to identify problems requiring research and he must know how to design an experiment to answer the question being asked. He must know how to select and operate the instrumentation used to measure or collect data. He must know how to record data and interpret the findings in light of the evidence collected. He must be able to describe adequately the problems, methods, and design used to collect data, and to present the results through oral and written presentations.

By far the most important attribute is thinking. Ritchie[4] has stated: "Don't accept what people say or write; ask yourself, or others, or the literature—is this really so, what is the evidence, how good is it, could I verify or disprove that point, how would I go about it and what would I need?" The selection of a research problem requires study, thought, and planning guided by imagination and critical judgment.[2] Thinking requires time and its process sometimes gives the impression of idleness. Administrators often frown on this aspect of research because some do not consider this process productive; thinking is difficult to measure in terms of productivity. Thinking is essential because it is the process which puts pieces of the puzzle together for organizing and starting the research. In addition, the identification of a problem requires that the researcher have imagination, originality, and critical judgment.

Acquired Essentials of the Researcher

Training in methods of research is essential for the student undertaking a project of scientific inquiry. Academic programs of physical therapy are structured to help students in research.

The programs offering initial preparation in physical therapy help the student to develop positive attitudes toward research and teach the student how to interpret the research literature. Programs of graduate studies prepare physical therapists in how to conduct research and encourage research through course work, independent studies, and theses. If proper training is provided in research then clinical physical therapists will further their interest in it by establishing research in their clinical programs. Students of physical therapy at all levels would then be exposed to research during clinical affiliations. Physical therapy's body of knowledge would grow, methods of health delivery would improve, and development of new and improved approaches to quality care would flourish. Training in research methods is essential for the survival of a profession because trained personnel will continue the required efforts to build the profession's body of knowledge. This book attempts to provide introductory training in research by covering elements of physical therapy research.

Although research is a tool of science, the skills of research must be learned just as the physical therapist learns anatomy and physiology. Research contains a body of knowledge composed of designs, methods of analysis (statistics), instrumentation, and writing. Each area of research requires degrees of competency which, in turn, command time for acquisition. Competency in research is acquired over a long period of time and not by successfully completing a single course or thesis. Whatever extent the exposure is to research, each experience contributes toward the necessary competency in research. On–the–job training and apprenticeships have proved to be excellent approaches for acquiring research skills.

Acquisition of knowledge in a particular field builds competence. Several approaches to gaining knowledge can be taken by the potential researcher. The formal approach is to pursue course work in the area of interest by matriculation, workshops, or continuing education. The informal approach to learning is to pursue organized and continuous reading on a subject. This approach is very effective for acquiring knowledge in a specific area and has the advantage of flexibility, for example, reading predominantly research literature at the convenience of the researcher. Reading numerous research reports provides a variety of styles and inputs, which enhances understanding. Enormous amounts of reading on a special subject will produce one area of competency essential for performing research.

Activities Leading to Problem Identification

An idea or problem may be born from a casual observation in the clinic. Therapists or student therapists encounter situations with equipment, assessments, procedures and techniques, curriculum, and peers or administrators, which may present difficulties.[6] These difficulties may be identified as research problems if immediate solutions are not available or if the identified questions cannot be answered by problem–solving methods. If physical therapists record ideas and problems encountered during their daily experiences, then research becomes their primary activity. Many everyday difficulties do not have immediate solutions or answers because solutions or answers are unknown.

A problem might be the result of a gap in a body of knowledge. An example of such a problem might be expressed by the question: Are proprioceptive neuromuscular facilitation techniques effective in restoring muscular function in a patient when there has been brain damage? Filling gaps that exist in current knowledge can link theories with techniques. Because of these gaps, techniques used in the clinic often are not based on theory and facts.

A theory is a guess, conjecture, or a group of postulations. Many theories exist in physical therapy, and practitioners often conjecture about the best therapeutic approach to a particular patient problem. Theories are not facts and contain generalizations which can and must be tested by rigorous scientific study. Researchable problems can be derived from theories, generalizations, and conjectures because they enable the researcher to make predictions about a wide range of circumstances. The results of investigating a postulation contribute to the theory by confirming or contradicting all or parts of the theory.[10]

Reading and analyzing the literature in a particular area of interest is perhaps the most satisfactory approach to identifying research problems.[1,4,6,7] As the student or researcher continues to read on a subject, a sizeable fund of knowledge will be built. As the reading program continues, not only is a stronger base of knowledge built, but the student becomes an authority on the subject because chances are, he possesses more information than the "average" colleague. Constant reading and analysis of the literature enables the student to identify deficiencies and strengths in knowledge, inconsistencies, and trends; most important, it may stimulate ideas for research. Research reports often suggest or indicate further studies which need to be conducted. Accumulating a list of promising research problems in the form of index cards is very helpful. The list can serve as a repository of reference and recall and can be reviewed periodically by the researcher for selection of the most promising problems.

The student should confine literature reviews to the particular area that holds his interest. The literature is voluminous, so limiting reading to one or two areas of professional interest is a practical approach.

Controversial issues should be examined. Different points of view on issues or contradictory research findings may provide new ideas for solution or resolution of the controversy. The literature contains research reports in which controversies are frequently discussed in the introductory phase of the report. Controversies of note have been associated with research on isometric exercise, the role of the vastus medialis, the effects of proprioceptive neuromuscular facilitation procedures, and the effect of faradic current in eliciting contraction of a denervated muscle. Professional exposure to intellectual discourse in courses, workshops, meetings, and informal discussions may assist the student in identifying areas of controversy within the profession.[7] Research can be designed to help solve a particular controversy that interests the researcher.

Observation in other settings can be helpful in providing ideas or a fresh approach to a research problem.[1,4] Seeing research in progress or consulting with others who are engaged in research can be stimulating as well as helpful to the inexperienced researcher. Researchers usually enjoy discussing their work because of their enthusiasm to advance knowledge and their willingness to gain or exchange knowledge with others. Exposure to other investigators or settings may also prevent duplication of efforts and costly equipment or convince the student of the vastness and complexity of a particular problem. Visitation and observations of research in departments outside of his or her own may enable the student to modify plans, abandon an idea, or provide the creation of a challenging problem to solve.

A final activity or source leading to a researchable problem is replication of previous studies. Many of the studies reported in the literature are "one shot" investigations that have not been replicated to show consistency of findings. The entry-level or masters student can often make a valuable contribution by repeating a study conducted by someone else to confirm results. Replication of findings of previous work strengthens theory and principles or occasionally uncovers doubtful or questionable conclusions. Borg and Gall[11] suggest that replication of a good study can be a better experience for some students than conducting an original study of poor quality, but warn that replication should be done only if it can make a significant contribution or clear up questionable areas in the original study, or when doubt is cast about the accuracy of a previous work.

CONSIDERATIONS IN SELECTING A PROBLEM

Once a problem has been identified, the researcher must examine it thoroughly for certain considerations before reaching a decision for proceeding.[7] Some departments (clinic, program) or facilities (hospitals, universities) may have established criteria to be followed before beginning research. In the event no formal direction is required when selecting a research problem, a few considerations are suggested to assist the beginning researcher. Most of the considerations are interrelated.

Interest, Training, and Knowledge

These criteria have already been noted, but once the problem has been identified, the student or researcher must ask whether the problem is sufficiently interesting to pursue and devote the time required to seek the solution.[7] The researcher must be curious, motivated, and interested in the specific problem identified. Although a basic aim of research is to advance knowledge, most research is initiated because of the personal interest the investigator has in the specific problem. Interest may be more difficult for students in the academic setting than for physical therapists in the professional setting. The student is strongly advised to have considerable interest in the problem before undertaking the required project.

The researcher's technical knowledge and skill must be considered when doing research. In the case of a student, the question of whether the student possesses sufficient competency and training to handle the process of problem solving arises. Projects are pursued usually near the end of a course of study, for example, the fourth year of an undergraduate program or the last year or term of a graduate program. Researchers often begin their research experience by collaborating with others, such as an experienced researcher or faculty member. Some neophytes serve apprenticeships before conducting research independently. The researcher's knowledge of a particular area is usually evident during the review process of a planned study. Inadequacy in any one of these criteria would be disastrous to the researcher and to the research, particularly in terms of energy and time lost.

Sophisticated approaches to the solution of a problem should not be considered if the approaches require special training and knowledge not readily available to the student, or if long periods of training would be required. Of course, qualifications may be the reason the student enrolled in the program to begin with; for example, the student may have had the problem in mind and then selected a graduate program because of the faculty and facilities of the graduate program. The situation would be ironic if the student wanted to do research which required electromyographic equipment but the program did not have faculty competent to teach or to direct research in electromyography.

Solvability of Problem

The student may select an interesting problem, but the problem may not be answerable for various reasons. Perhaps the problem is concerned with a condition or trait that cannot be defined sufficiently to plan an approach to its solution. The problem may be too broad or too complex for a solution within the capability of the available personnel or facilities. It is therefore necessary to select a problem for which a solution is possible within the framework of the facility and time and background available to the student.

Professional Contribution

The value or gains of the research must be considered by the researcher before commencing a study or even before seeking approval for the study.[3,4,8] At some point the researcher must defend and justify the selected problem. The results obtained from the research process must be worthy of the energy, time, and costs incurred. The expected contribution does not have to be dramatic or world shaking; however, it should make some contribution to the profession by adding to the body of knowledge; improving the conditions or operation of techniques; improving instrumentation or quality of care; or in some way providing answers to questions that will decide an issue, stimulate further research, or be relevant to physical therapy.

The researcher must ask whether the problem is too small (trivial) to be of any value or whether the problem is too large (complex) to be answered in a single study. Administrators of research funding or committees granting approval for research are demanding accountability of the researcher and research more than ever. Pursuing knowledge for its own sake is given scrutiny by those in authority to approve research; potential application of the research findings to improve human welfare is often given priority in approving research projects. The feasibility of all planned projects is challenged before proceeding with the research.

Availability of Technology, Equipment, and Facility

If the technical background of the researcher is inadequate in a specific area, consultation with experts must be arranged. For example, a statistician, electrical technician, or photographic technician might need to be consulted on experimental design and analysis, hardware instrumentation, or illustrations, respectively.

The problem may be selected which can be solved, but its solution may depend on expensive sophisticated equipment not available to the student. Sometimes arrangements can be made for the research to be conducted away from the student's department or through collaboration and direction of another adviser. Some research requires the purchase of equipment and supplies or the rental of space or costs for travel. The researcher must arrange for these necessities prior to commencing the project. The approving authority may be in a position to support the project financially or to advise the researcher where monies can be obtained. Requests for grants to support the research may have to be made by the researcher. Equipment may have to be borrowed.

The availability of the sample or population of subjects, events, or attributes to be studied must be considered. A problem may be identified but if the sample processing characteristics to be studied are not available or if the numbers are insufficient to answer the question, the research cannot proceed.

The researcher must also arrange his schedule so that sufficient time is available to complete the research process, from problem through publi-

cation (Table 1.2). The idea in this section is to give the utmost consideration to the available technology and facility when selecting a problem for
research.[7,8,12]

DELIMITING PROBLEMS

Once the problem has been identified for its research possibility, the
problem must be delimited. One of the difficulties students have in selecting a problem for investigation is that their problem is too global. The
student does not realize that the selected problem is too complex or broad
and that it cannot be solved through a single investigation. The problem
must be narrowed so that the question can be answered. A general problem should be subdivided into many questions which should be solved
separately; then, information gathered can be pieced together.

The student might be interested in knowing how the knee extensors
should be exercised for greatest enhancement, a complex, or global, problem. Subproblems of muscular force must be considered, such as type of
exercise (static, dynamic–concentric, eccentric, isokinetic) and influ-

Table 2.1
Global and Delimited Research Problems

Global problem
  How can the muscular force of the quadriceps be enhanced?
Delimited problem (subproblems)
  Types of Exercise
    Which type of exercise is best for increasing strength of the quadriceps? (static, dynamic-
      concentric, eccentric, isokinetic?)
    Do different exercises have specificity?
  Influencing factors in exercise
    What is best rate for performing dynamic exercises?
    What number of repetitions is best for increasing strength? (4, 6, 8, 10, 12, or 14 repeti-
      tions?)
    What number of repetitions is best for increasing muscular endurance?
    What is best load for achieving optimal strength gains? (40, 50, 60, 70, 80, 90, or maximum
      percentage of strength?)
    What is the ideal frequency of performing exercises? (1, 2, 3, 4, or 5 times/week?)
    What are the retention periods of strength gains? (weeks, months, or year?)
    What joint angles are optimal for performing static exercises?
  Stabilization Effects
    Do arm positions affect force generated?
    What effect do various hip positions have on the force generated?
    Does the backrest increase the ability of the quadriceps to generate force?
    How do design factors of equipment influence the force a muscle can generate?
  Facilitating Aids
    Does activation of reflexes during exercises influence strength gains?
    Does a wedge affect strength gains or force generated by the muscle?
    Does electrical stimulation of muscle during exercise affect strength gains?
    Do facilitating patterns of movement increase strength more than conventional positions?

encing factors (rate, repetitions, loads, frequency, and sets). Positioning (joint angles, hand grasping, support, inclination of seat), effects of facilitation, and assessment of strength also must be considered. If body positioning is selected as the problem, then the placement of the hands, angle of the hip joint, support or nonsupport for the back, the position of the knee (angle, static, or dynamic type of exercise), and inclination of the thigh by inclining the seat angle or by use of a knee wedge must be given serious consideration. Each of the subproblems might be used for a single investigation, but only the composite of all subproblems will answer the question: How should the quadriceps be exercised for greatest enhancement of force? Table 2.1 shows an example of global and delimited problems.

The delimitations guide the research by establishing limits or boundaries, by narrowing the selected problem, and by defining the scope of the investigation.[9] Sweet and Moir[13] have suggested that the problem be defined by listing independent variables in four categories: (1) treatment variables (type, duration, intensity, consistency); (2) subject variables (age, sex, physical status); (3) therapist variables (age, sex, experience, employer, professional attitudes); and (4) condition variables (type, severity, location, concurrent problems, intervening time between events). These authors listed independent variables to isolate variables to keep their effects constant (control), to determine effects of variables, and to achieve quantitative evaluation.[13] Assistance is usually required in delimiting the problem before the plan can be designed. Lloyd[14] has made some suggestions which may be of some assistance for breaking down the research problem. He suggested an orderly arrangement of information about the problem as:

1. Identifying the field of science in which the problem is located.[14] The question of how to enhance quadriceps force during exercise can again be used as the problem. The problem may interest physical therapists, physical educators, and sports medicine personnel.
2. Listing known major variables.[14] Variables (things that can be manipulated or measured) might include: types of exercise; rate, repetitions and frequency of exercise; stabilization measures of hand grasping, hip angle, back support, inclination of seat; and force-generated exercises.
3. Listing the type of data required. This list requires thought on the specific variable or variables to be measured.[14] The data in our example of a global research problem are measurements of force, tension, or torque.
4. Locating methods of gathering the data.[14] The kinds of instruments and procedures which have been used for obtaining data of force, tension, or torque must be considered and identified. The process of delimiting the problem involves assembling facts about the problem, verifying that

the problem is real and answerable, and knowing how to go about resolving it. Once a problem has been identified, we are ready to proceed with the process of verifying and organizing its solution.

LIMITATION

Limitations to a research project are not the same as delimitations. Limitations are conditions or variables not under the control of the researcher. The limiting conditions can influence the outcome of the investigation. Individual variations of the subjects in the study may cause limitations. The type of measuring device, the type of subject who volunteers for the study, or the method of selecting the subjects also may be limitations to the study and may influence the outcome. The economics of undertaking a solution to the problem and the moral issues concerning risk must be considered and could lead to certain limitations. The researcher, however, is obligated to control as many variables as possible.[7,9]

The delimiting of a researchable problem is the beginning of a process to converge on a specific issue within a general or broader subject area. Although a researchable problem requires a solution, it cannot be tested in question form. A question demands a response or reply which may still contain several ideas or concepts not subjected to the trial or scrutiny of controlled experimentation. A delimited problem must be narrowed further, that is, reduced to its component parts. In practice, the problem is identified for readers of the research plan (Chapter 4) or the published report (Chapter 12) as the gap in a theory, controversy of issues, or even the ineffectiveness of a treatment procedure. The component parts of the problem, hypotheses, and objectives filter out surplus or unrelated information contained in the problem.[15] The formulation of hypotheses reduces the problem to conditional relations which can be tested by the research process.

A hypothesis is a proposition that can be tested; it is a subdivision of a problem used in experimental research that involves causes and comparisons. A working hypothesis is a well-written statement of the problem indicating the variables (measurements subject to change) of interest to the investigator. It may point out the particular relation between the variables to be studied. For example, the problem to be investigated may be the effect of 50 pulses per second (pps) frequency electrical stimulation on the arterial blood flow to muscle. The variables to be studied are "50 pps frequency electrical stimulation" and "arterial blood flow to muscle." A scientific hypothesis is a conjecture or assumption about the science associated with the delimited problem. The delimited problem may also be converted into a statistical hypothesis that can be tested precisely. An example of the latter may be that no relation exists between the variables studied and could be stated as: "No significant difference exists between measures of blood flow when using 50 pps frequency electrical stimulation and when not using 50 pps frequency electrical stimulation.'' Statistical hypotheses and statistical hypothesis-testing will be discussed in detail in Chapter 10. The objectives or purposes define the boundaries under which the investigation will be conducted and describe the end-product which is expected to emerge from the research process.

Table 2.2
Cumulative Summary of the Research Processes Presented

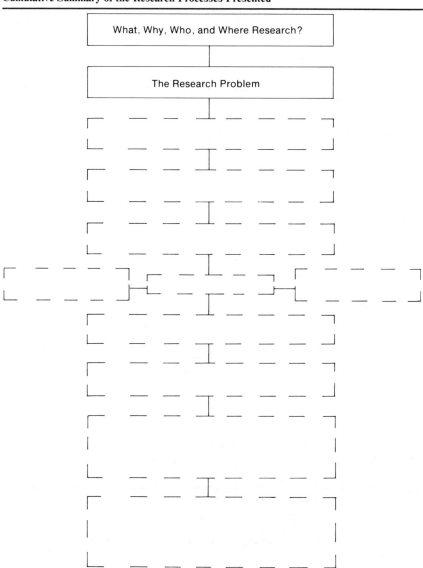

SUMMARY

The research problem is a question that must be answered by some organized process. The problem may be identified by recognizing everyday difficulties and experiences: gaps in a body of knowledge and controversial issues in a profession. Once identified, the problem or question must be delimited to a form that can be solved or answered. Before engaging in further steps of the research process, the investigator must take into consideration: his interest, training, and knowledge of the problem area; the solvability of the problem; the solution's contribution to the profession; and the availability of technology, equipment, and facilities.

Research is a process of thought and action, it requires direction from an identified problem. Remember the statement:

"For everyone who does something, ten others had the same idea but they only thought about it."[14]

Table 2.2 summarizes the research processes presented thus far.

REFERENCES

1. Wandelt M: Guide for the Beginning Researcher. New York, Appleton–Century–Crofts, 1970
2. Trelease SF: How to Write Scientific and Technical Papers. Cambridge, MA, The M.I.T. Press, 1969
3. Wilson EG, Jr: An Introduction to Scientific Research. New York, McGraw–Hill Book Co, 1952
4. Ritchie AE: Considering research. Physiotherapy 56: 110–112, 1966
5. Bernard C: An Introduction to the Study of Experimental Medicine. New York, Dover Publications, Inc, 1957
6. Van Dalen DB: Understanding Educational Research, ed 4. New York, McGraw–Hill Book Co, 1978
7. Clarke DH, Clarke HH: Research Processes in Physical Education, Recreation, and Health. Englewood Cliffs, NJ, Prentice–Hall, Inc, 1970
8. McLaren HM: So you want to conduct a clinical study. Physiother Canada 25: 219–224, 1973
9. Broer MR, Mohr DR: Selecting and Defining a Research Problem. In Hubbard AW (ed): Research Methods in Health, Physical Education, and Recreation, ed 3. Washington, Am Assoc Health Phys Educ Re, 1973
10. Gay LR: Educational Research: Competencies for Analysis and Application, ed 2. Columbus, OH, Charles E. Merrill Pub Co, 1981
11. Borg WR, Gall MD: Educational Research: An Introduction, ed 3. New York, Longman, 1979
12. Silverman FH: Research Design in Speen Pathology and Audiology: Asking and Answering Questions. Englewood Cliffs, NJ, Prentice–Hall, Inc, 1977
13. Sweet RL, Moir SB: Some elementary guides for performing research into the effects of physiotherapy treatments. Aust J Physiother 44: 85–90, 1973
14. Lloyd LE: Techniques for Efficient Research. New York, Clinical Publishing Co, Inc, 1966

15. Andrew CO, Hildebrand PE: Planning and Conducting Applied Research. New York, MSS Information Corp, 1976

3

Literature Review

> There is a dead medical literature, and there
> is a live one. The dead is not all ancient, the live
> is not all modern. There is none, modern or ancient,
> which, if it has no living value for the student, will
> not teach him something by its autopsy.
> *Oliver Wendell Holmes*
> *Medical Essays, "Medical Libraries"*

The literature review is a fundamental ingredient of the scientific method and ranks high in its potential for contribution to the research effort. The importance of the literature review has been mentioned as valuable for locating a research problem. The literature review may even be the first step in some research because a command of a body of knowledge may be gained through reading, or the inspiration of the research problem may begin as a result of a literature review. The library is the vehicle of the literature review and exists for the purpose of information retrieval; it should be a part of the researcher's paradise.

Although students taking a first course in college English are usually introduced to the library, its contents, and its system of operation, the research tools may not be exposed as such. This chapter offers suggestions to assist the beginning researcher with the literature review. The literature review is a process of acquiring depth and understanding of the published information in a particular area. The literature review may assist the student in locating and identifying a research problem; it certainly is essential for a logical or chronological approach to the basis of the research.

WHY THE LITERATURE REVIEW?

Before proceeding with the writing of the formal research proposal (plan of research), a survey of literature relating to the problem must be undertaken. The reasons for this often laborious task are:

1. To ascertain originality of research. Although all research does not have to be original, the literature review can be used to determine

whether comparable research has been published. The library is often used when pursuing an answer to a question which has been unanswered by associates or readily accessible reference sources. After reasonable or exhaustive but futile review of literature pertinent to the question, the researcher can reasonably be sure that the problem is original or, at least, that the answer has not been reported in the literature. For example, in reviewing literature on how to increase the capacity for tension development in the quadriceps femoris muscle through resistive exercises, the researcher may have noticed that no research study had answered why a wedge is placed underneath the knee when a subject is performing strengthening exercises for the quadriceps femoris muscle. The scientific approach to answering the question could have been considered original by the investigator since a thorough review of the literature did not provide any evidence or reason for a knee wedge used in strengthening exercises. Justifying originality is not the most valid reason for the literature review. The researcher must know what has or has not been published about the particular problem. If the solutions or answers to the problem had been reported to the extent that the question really had been answered, then the researcher might have been remiss in the selection and conduction of another study on the same problem. The review assists the researcher in determining the feasibility of conducting a study on a particular problem.[1]

2. To provide ideas for solving the problem. The investigator can formulate methods for answering the question by reading reports of studies which answered questions similar to the question under review. Approaches in technique or instrumentation used in measuring or collecting data similar to that required by the investigator can be found in published research reports. Inadequacies of previous studies can be identified and avoided with a thorough review of literature pertinent to the researcher's selected problem. Interpretations and discussions of other authors are important to the researcher in formulating a problem or in seeking approaches to interpreting the outcome in the planned research. The theoretical information is valuable when the completed research is being written for publication. Information contained in the literature review helps to form background information for the examiner and to assist in the interpretation of the results. Information gained from the review of literature provides the researcher with insight into understanding the importance of the answers to the question and the importance of these answers to the area investigated. One of the contributions of any research report is the stimulus which a certain aspect of the study provides to another researcher. The findings of a study are like links in a chain because one researcher reviews literature to identify and formulate a research idea, and his completed report provides

similar impetus to another researcher who, in turn, builds on to the body of knowledge.[1] Almost nothing is new in research, but reported findings of studies are extensions of what has already been done.

Literature reviews will often uncover controversies between reported findings of research or controversies in accepted concepts because of the lack of research replications. Continuous reading in a particular area of interest will increase the reader's knowledge of the subject.

3. To avoid repetitious findings. Occasionally a review of the literature uncovers several studies similar in scope and design that reveal insignificant findings. Replication of studies to confirm findings was mentioned earlier; however, when such repetitions occur several times in a specific area of the literature, they have outlived their purpose. Further replication of these studies serves no usefulness in research, and the student is discouraged against spending additional time with the particular problem. A strong possibility exists that additional studies using similar approaches in the particular area will yield insignificant findings.

PLANNING THE LITERATURE REVIEW

Primary Literature

Certain published materials are more appropriate than others for providing information about the particular problem or area of interest. These primary materials (periodicals, books) are written by members of the profession and, therefore, contain topics similar in nature and content to yours. For example, if the researcher is planning to study the effects of muscular length on force, the literature primarily concerned with the problem would be studies central to the stated problem; studies of joint position on performance, studies of types of exercise, or studies of the velocity of motion. Primary sources are, therefore, materials central to the particular problem being investigated.

Secondary Literature

Materials allied or related to the problem or area of interest but more peripheral than central are secondary sources.[1] Materials containing studies which investigated muscles other than those under consideration, or studies which investigated other influencing factors on muscular force would be secondary to the example given above. Secondary sources for one problem may be primary for another. The nature of the problem determines which sources are most central and of greatest value to the researcher and which sources are helpful but only background information. Secondary sources are those in which abstracted information is sufficient as a reference, whereas primary sources are those cited in detail in the written portion of the study or considered most pertinent to interpretation or discussion of results. Primary sources might also be the reprints or reproductions in your files. The secondary sources might be those materials skimmed over but containing some usable information.

REVIEWING PROCESS

Because of the voluminous amounts of literature, the task of reviewing can become overwhelming unless the researcher has a plan to guide in the review. Procedures used to conduct the review may vary with the person, familiarity with the library, the demands of the subject or area being reviewed, and the detail desired.

Medical Subject Headings (MeSH), appearing as the second part in each January issue of the **INDEX MEDICUS,** is a useful source for identifying key words used in a health science library. The MeSH enables the researcher to choose and categorize key words used in locating topics in **INDEX MEDICUS.** These key words are useful later when preparing the research findings for publication. MeSH contains an alphabetized list of subject headings, cross-referenced for locating closely related words ("see," "see related," and "see under"), and a categorized list that provides general headings relating to the trends of the medical literature.

Listing any relevant words associated with the statement of the selected problem is helpful. In seeking literature related to strength variations of the quadriceps femoris muscle with and without the use of a knee wedge during exercise, one could list such key words as: wedge, isometric exercise, strength, force, muscular tension, leg position, joint angles, joint motion, and knee. These key words are guides to indexes, card catalogues, books, and other primary sources containing pertinent information. Additional key words can be found following the titles in the January issues of the **INDEX MEDICUS.** This particular index is one of the most useful in the library and to the researcher.

Bibliographies accompanying the pertinent research reports of other researchers are valuable to the investigator. References are cited at the end of the relevant articles and can be used to locate more detailed information. Using the bibliographical information provided with each article of interest is an excellent means of obtaining additional information and references.

The examiner is often confronted with the decision of whether unpublished studies warrant review. The published report is usually given greater credit by editorial committees than is the unpublished report. Some editorial committees are reluctant to accept an unpublished report or personal communication as a reference in published articles. Theses and dissertations are examples of studies often cited in the literature as unpublished reports. If a study is good enough to conduct and be cited as a reference, it should be good enough to publish no matter whether the hypothesis was supported or not by the outcome of the study. Unpublished reports that have been cited by an author are often difficult to obtain or may require excessive periods of time to acquire. Research is never completed until published, therefore unpublished studies may be viewed as incompleted research. This point of view may be narrow because theses and dissertations can contain valuable literature reviews, but because of their inaccessibility to many readers, theses and dissertations are not readily accepted by many researchers.

The review should encompass major sources of literature published on the particular topic; major sources include periodicals, but not exclusively. Pamphlets, published proceedings of seminars, and up–to–date books are also good sources for the literature review, but must be valued for their excellence of pertinent information. The review provides the researcher with other researchers' thoughts and actions on similar problems. The literature review therefore, is an essential resource for apprising the researcher of all pertinent writings of a particular time and on a particular subject. If you have any difficulties in the review process, for instance in locating sources or a particular topic, consult a librarian.

A decision about when to terminate a literature review must be made by every researcher. The nature of the subject often dictates the termination of the review; for example, only a few references may be available on a specific topic and this may lead to an early termination. The usual approach is to begin with current references and work backward in time. Each published report reviewed will contain cited references of earlier work, and the researcher can judge their value and decide whether further review of the literature is necessary. Some journals may not accept references which go past 10 to 20 years from the current date. References reported years earlier than the current year may be valuable resources to the researcher and are acceptable in publications if given pertinence by the researcher. The researcher should terminate the literature review when enough support is available for providing sufficient background for pointing out the specific problem and its need for research. The literature review is flexible and may include few or many references which are current or go back more than 20 years. The point is that each reference used by the researcher must be of value to the planned study. In the published report, the researcher cites the pertinent reference sources.

PERSONAL ABSTRACT FILE

Each potential reference reviewed should be indexed and filed in a personal reference file. Isolation of each reference on a single index card or attached cards is important because, as review of the literature continues, considerable information is collected. The researcher should choose the size of the card (7.6 × 12.7, 12.7 × 20.3 cm) on which to record bibliographical and abstract information and notes. Since different journals have distinct formats for listing literature cited, authors should follow the journal style for presentation of references. The bibliography usually includes the authors' and coauthors' names as listed, title of article or book, periodical name or abbreviation (abbreviation according to **INDEX MEDICUS** or **LIST OF JOURNALS INDEXED IN INDEX MEDICUS** for the current year), volume number, pages, month, and year; or, for a book, city of publisher, publisher of book, and year of publication.

Many research reports contain an abstract preceding the introduction of the report, and this abstract is really a summary of the report. The abstract provides sufficient information to determine whether the report is pertinent to the research problem. If additional information is required of any particular report, then the method, results, and discussion can be summarized and recorded on the card. Also, key words relating to the content of the report are good to list at the top of the card (right–hand corner). Because background information leading to the purpose of the research and to the problem is often written in chronological fashion, the cards can be arranged chronologically in the files. The cards can be used for instant retrieval of information. Extraction of all important information from each research report is essential during the initial review so that efficiency can be maintained. Computers make this task convenient and greatly improve storage capacity. Cross-indexing by using key words makes the file serviceable.

INFORMATION RESOURCES

Abstracts

A number of journals provide readers with an abstracting service, which can save time in locating the original reports. Of course, abstracts are limited in the information provided, so caution must be exercised when using these resources. Abstracts should be considered as secondary sources of literature review. Abstracts of literature are generally located near the end of each journal issue. Chapter 12 discusses the content and format of published abstracts. Book reviews are also given space in many journals. The reviews usually call attention to the subject material contained in the book but do not provide detailed information about a subject, as do abstracts of literature. Such journals as **PHYSICAL THERAPY, ARCHIVES OF PHYSICAL MEDICINE AND REHABILITATION,** the **AMERICAN JOURNAL OF PHYSICAL MEDICINE, PHYSIOTHERAPY CANADA,** and **PHYSIOTHERAPY** provide abstracting services in most issues.

Biological Abstracts

This is a semi–monthly publication; each entry includes bibliographic citations and abstracts. Each issue contains an Author Index for retrieval of references based on author or corporate names, a Biosystematic Index with references according to gross taxonomic categories, a Generic Index of the names of genus–species, a Concept Index of broad concepts, and a Subject Index for retrieval of references based on specific subject words. About 250000 reports are covered yearly in **BIOLOGICAL ABSTRACTS** and **BIORESEARCH INDEX.** The latter is a monthly publication that indexes biology–related material not covered in **BIOLOGICAL AB-STRACTS.**

Excerpta Medica

This is a monthly international publication that monitors, abstracts, translates, classifies, and indexes biomedical literature. More than 5000 journals are routinely indexed; in addition, books, reported literature, and conference papers are also included. The index is divided into 42 sections covering the entire medical field and seven index sections which cover special areas. Sections may be subscribed to separately (for example, Rehabilitation and Physical Medicine). Usual arrangements are by subject but semi–annual and annual subject and author indexes are available.

Muscular Dystrophy Abstracts

This booklet is presented by the Muscular Dystrophy Association and **EXCERPTA MEDICA** and is a service of abstracts from current world literature covering muscular dystrophy and related disorders and areas of basic science pertinent to their conditions. Twenty two to twenty four issues are published yearly along with an annual **INDEX** by Subject and Author.

JOURNALS

Listing all journals of interest to physical therapists would be futile because of the diversity of interests and the numbers of available journals. Libraries have a master file of all journals contained in a particular library and this file is accessible to patrons. Since research is usually first reported in journal articles, journals are primary sources for seeking information for investigative work on a particular topic. Selection of the journals appropriate to the investigator's topic depends on the subject being pursued. Individual issues of a journal preceding the current year are bound together in a cloth volume, usually for each calendar year. The index for a particular year is located near the end of each bound volume. Issues for the current year are separate from the bound volumes of a particular journal and are usually placed on special racks or shelves. Because current issues of journals for the present year are separate, the contents of each journal issue must be consulted individually. The current copies of a particular journal do not circulate or have restricted circulation. Special indexes for journals are available and are valuable sources for locating special articles.

INDEXES

Some journals have periodic indexes in addition to the volume index, which is usually part of the December issue of the particular volume. The **RESEARCH QUARTERLY,** research journal of the American Alliance for Health, Physical Education, and Recreation, had 10–year indexes beginning with 1930 and a 30–year-index from 1930 through 1959. These indexes are filed by author and subject.

Sixty–Five–Year Index of Physical Therapy

The **SIXTY–FIVE–YEAR INDEX OF PHYSICAL THERAPY,** Journal of the American Physical Therapy Association, contains a table of contents, subject index, and an author index. This issue includes categories different from previous issues, cross-referencing of subjects, editorials, and Letters to the Editor in categories for the years 1921 through 1985.

Fifty–year Cumulative Index: Archives of Physical Medicine and Rehabilitation

This index spans the years from 1929 to 1969. The index includes a 50-year history of the journal, cumulative indexes of authors and subjects, page index by volume and month, and a list of medical abbreviations.

Fifty–year Index of Physical Therapy

The **FIFTY–YEAR INDEX OF PHYSICAL THERAPY,** Journal of the American Physical Therapy Association contains a table of contents in addition to subject and author indexes. A pagination index lists the pages by volume and month and covers the years from 1921 to 1970.

Five–year Index of Physical Therapy

Five–year indexes have been published by **PHYSICAL THERAPY** since 1970. In each index a Table of Contents is used to list subject headings; an author index at the end of each publication cites the work of authors by a numbering system.

Physical Fitness/Sports Medicine

PHYSICAL FITNESS/SPORTS MEDICINE is a quarterly index published by the President's Council on Physical Fitness and Sports. This bibliography includes citations from more than 3000 periodicals. It began in 1978 and all citations are in English.

Current Contents: CLINICAL MEDICINE

This is a weekly booklet that reproduces tables of contents of more than 850 of the world's journals. This booklet saves time in locating medical information. About 136000 journals and book titles in medical and allied health sciences are published yearly. Each issue lists about 175 contents and features current book contents, title world index, author index and address directory, and a publishers' address directory.

Index Medicus

This is a comprehensive index to the world's medical literature and is published monthly. Several thousand journals are indexed completely or selectively. Each issue contains a subject and author index. The Subject Index is alphabetized according to key subject headings with each subject heading containing the title of English language or translated articles; author; journal by special abbreviation; volume; pages; and date article was published. The Author Index contains the author's name and bibliographic information. The January volume lists the key words and all journals included in the indexing process.

CUMULATED INDEX MEDICUS is the annual INDEX MEDICUS, which is a cumulation of monthly publications into author volumes and subject volumes of citations. Subject headings, JOURNALS INDEXED, and BIBLIOGRAPHY OF MEDICAL REVIEWS are included in the annual editions.

Science Citation Index (SCI)

This publication contains volumes arranged as Citation Index and Source Index. The Citation Index is a listing of references found in footnotes and bibliographies of journals covered by the SCI. The first authors of the cited references are listed alphabetically. Previously published works by the cited authors are listed for the time period covered by the SCI edition. Each entry in the volume shows cited author, citing author, year cited article was published, name of publication, year article was cited, volume number, and pages. Separate sections of the Citation Index include a Patent Citation Index listing the patent number, name of inventor, reference year, and other items.

The Source Index contains the listing of the articles of the cited authors. The descriptions are first listed by primary author, second by co-authors, and then by cross-reference.

Some suggestions for the use of indexes may help in locating research articles in journals:

1. Explore various subject headings by listing key words contained in the topic or related topics.
2. Begin with a specific subject heading before using general headings.
3. Start the literature search with the latest index volumes and then proceed to older volumes.
4. Explore each index volume systematically before proceeding to another volume.[2]

REPRINTS

If a published report is particularly useful, then a reproduction or reprint should be obtained. A reprint of an article is valuable for convenience and efficiency in retrieving the information. A reprint can be placed in your personal file and is available as needed. Reprints make maximum use of library time, contain complete references, and reduce errors caused by abstracting. Reprints of recent references (within the past 2 years) can be obtained by writing directly to the author and requesting a reprint of the article. Authors generally have reprints of their articles and are usually willing to send a copy on request. The address of the author often accompanies the article at its beginning or ending. Figure 3.1 is an example of a postcard which can be printed or typed in advance, is economical, and is applicable to most requests for reprints. Pertinent information required for the postcard is illustrated. The label or printed address can be removed and used by the sender to address the envelope containing the requested reprint. This approach eases the mailing process for the sender.

BOOKS

Books on most areas of health care are available in medical libraries or through a medical library. Books give basic material in varying degrees of depth according to the book's purpose, but are not the most up–to–date sources of information. Books require more time to write and publish than journals, thus losing some immediacy. Their bibliographies offer important sources on a topic.[3] Consult the card catalogue of your medical library for their book holdings. The card catalogue uses either the Dewey decimal or the Library of Congress system for classifying and locating books. Card

Mr. John Doe
Department of Physical Therapy
Podunk Hospital
Podunk, CA 94126

Dear _____ :

I would appreciate receiving _____ reprint(s) of your article entitled _____

_____

which appeared in _____

_____

Thank You,

                 (your name)
                 _____
                 Program in Physical Therapy
                 University of Null
                 Blackbird, PA 17261

Fig. 3.1.   Postalcard for requesting reprints.

catalogues are arranged according to a cross–reference system consisting of subject, author, and title cards. Each card pertaining to a particular book contains identical information, but the order of information is peculiar to the function of the card. The card catalogue contains only those documents owned by that particular library, and cards provide little information about the content of the books.

LIBRARY REFERENCE RESOURCE PUBLICATIONS

Books in Print

This is an annual index to general books currently available from about 20000 American publications and lists about 719000 titles. Authors Index and Titles Index, Publishers Index, and Subject Guide are arranged in separate volumes. The Author Index includes author, title, price, publisher, series, whether the book is illustrated, edition, year the book was published, and the type of binding. The Titles Index lists titles, author, price, and publisher. The Author Index is more inclusive than the Titles Index, but the Titles Index provides an alphabetical listing of American publishers.

Subject Guide to Books in Print

Listings in this volume give author, title, publisher, current price, and year of publication. The listings represent books from more than 1900 American publishers with some 646268 books appearing about 813098 times under 65096 headings and 54564 cross-references. Books in preparation are also listed.[4]

British Books in Print

This book is an annual index to general books offered currently by British publishers.

Bowker's Medical Books in Print

Medical books currently available from American publishers are indexed. This resource is published annually but is also a subset of BOOKS IN PRINT.

INTERLIBRARY LOAN

The purpose of this service is to make available for research, materials not owned by or missing from the local library. The Interlibrary Loan service will usually provide photocopies of requested articles rather than make the journal available, but the service will not provide photocopies of entire publications (books). Books can be obtained by the local library from other libraries in the system with relatively short waiting periods (2 to 3 weeks). Usually there are no charges to users for loans or photocopies if the requests do not exceed a certain number, usually less than 10 articles per request. The library personnel will advise you if charges will be made.

Theses, dissertations, and microfilmed copies of sources are also available through interlibrary services.

Special forms for requesting materials are available at your library. Information usually needed on the special forms is your name and associated facility or department; status (student or faculty member); work phone number; complete bibliographical information of the requested book or article (Chapter 12 discusses bibliographical material); source of reference where book or article is indexed; and date when the library is to discontinue its search if attempts to locate the requested material are unsuccessful.

The Interlibrary Loan system is a valuable service to physical therapists working in small hospitals and towns where medical libraries are not available. The researcher should check the services of the local or secondary

Table 3.1
Regional Medical Libraries

Regions	States			Libraries
1	CT	NH	RI	New York Academy of Medicine
	DE	NJ	VT	2 East 103 Street
	ME	NY	Puerto Rico	New York, NY 10029
	MA	PA		(212) 876-8763
2	AL	MS	VA	University of Maryland Health Sciences Library
	FL	NC	WV	111 S. Greene Street
	GA	SC	District of	Baltimore, MD 21201
	MD	TN	Columbia	(301) 328-2855
3	IA	MI	SD	University of Illinois at Chicago
	IL	MN	WI	Library of the Health Sciences
	IN	ND		P.O. Box 7509
	KY	OH		Chicago, IL 60680
				(312) 966-2464
4	CO	NE		University of Nebraska
	KS	UT		Leon S. McGoogan Library of Medicine
	MO	WY		42nd. and Dewey Avenue
				Omaha, NE 68105
				(402) 559-4326
5	AR	OK		University of Texas
	LA	TX		Health Science Center at Dallas
	NM			5323 Harry Hines Boulevard
				Dallas, TX 75235-9049
				(214) 688-2085
6	AK	OR		University of Washington
	ID	WA		Health Sciences Library
	MT			Seattle, WA 98195
				(206) 543-8262
7	AZ	HI		Louise Darling Biomedical Library
	CA	NV		University of California
				Los Angeles, CA 90024-1798
				(213) 825-1200

school library regarding interlibrary loans. Libraries make books and journals available to those researchers who cannot obtain materials at their own facilities. If interlibrary services are not available locally, contact the Regional Medical Library serving your state (Table 3.1).

OTHER MANUAL RESOURCES

Libraries contain many other resources for information not included in this book. Some defy the classifications given but are useful to the researcher. Two such resources are: Medical Device Register—US & Canada. This directory of medical suppliers began in 1988. It contains a keyword index of 6000 names of medical products, a directory of products with over 50000 supplier listings, a trade name index covering more than 3000 products, supplier profiles listing every supplier in the directory, and a supplier geographical index ordered by state and zip code. A medical specialty panel name is assigned by the Federal Drug Administration (FDA) whenever a standard product name is used in the directory. Physical medicine is the name assigned to the products that most physical therapists use.

Scientific Meetings

This is a listing of forthcoming national and international meetings of technical, scientific, medical, engineering, and management organizations. The listing is published four times each year.

AUTOMATED REFERENCE SERVICES

Literature review can be time consuming if exhaustive reviews are required. Even if reference materials are available in a large medical library, considerable time is spent in cross-referencing and checking the many sources to prevent exclusion of particular report which may be of great value. An overwhelming volume of literature exists on most topics. Automated systems have developed through the sponsorships of the Federal Governments of the United States and Canada to help the scientist retrieve information from computerized storage systems. In cooperation with The National Library of Medicine in Bethesda, Maryland, and The National Science Library in Ottawa, Ontario, the libraries of government departments, agencies, and other research and specialty libraries in North America provide resources and services of great value to the researcher. The national libraries provide resources and services not always available locally. If the local library has access to the appropriate electronic equipment, publications or bibliographies can be transmitted immediately. Costs incurred for these services may be based on the number of years surveyed, whether the survey is "on–line" or "off–line," or simply on a flat-fee basis. Arrangements for paying these costs vary widely. In some cases the library budget has provision for these costs; in others, the department to which the requester belongs pays. Or the individual requester may have to pay in advance, from five to twenty five dollars. The requester is advised to determine each institution's policy regarding payment before making use of automated service.

Key words from **INDEX MEDICUS** (see Reviewing Process) are used in automated literature searches. Libraries offering these services will have a form to be completed. This form will require listing key words that describe or categorize the topic you wish searched for references. Library personnel are available to assist in selecting search words and planning search strategy in the event that you are unfamiliar with the procedure.

Many universities have on–line computer terminals linking them to an information retrieval system such as Lockheed **DIALOG, SDC/ORBIT, ERIC,** and **DATRIX II** systems. Such systems increase the availability of multiple data bases, broadening the researcher's ability to retrieve citations, dissertations, and abstracts. Some data bases can be searched by the author's name, key words in the article, date of publication, and titles. Charges vary from system to system based on computer time and printout entries. The user is advised to seek the librarian's advice on selecting pertinent data bases, additional automated services, and costs.

Medlars

MEDLARS (Medical Literature Analysis and Retrieval System) is a computerized search service of journal articles listed in the **INDEX MEDICUS.** The service became operational in 1964 for indexing international biomedical literature and preparing bibliographies of scientific articles on request. The bibliographies searched do not include articles published prior to 1964. Citations are given to the person requesting the service and contain the title, author(s), journal, volume, pages, date, and whether the article is written in a language other than English.

Articles indexed are from **INDEX MEDICUS, INDEX TO DENTAL LITERATURE,** and the **INTERNATIONAL NURSING INDEX,** and contain citations to medical and health–related journals.

Regional Medical Library

The Regional Medical Library (RML) system has been established by the federal government and serves as the major medical library resource in each of the seven regions in the United States. The RMLs provide library and ancillary services to libraries and health professionals through interlibrary loans, reference service, and training. The RML system provides backup support to researchers and hospitals not having computers. Within the seven regions, more than 300 medical libraries have terminals for **MEDLARS**. The locations of the RML libraries by region are given in Table 3.1.

Medline

MEDLINE (**MEDLARS** on Line) is a newer and speedier version of **MEDLARS**. Because of its initiation in 1974, **MEDLINE** has a smaller data base than **MEDLARS**. The system is computerized and bibliographical information on a specific subject is available immediately from a computer readout. The citations span journals listed in the **INDEX MEDICUS**.

Microfilm

Microfilm provides the researcher with the original article. The reader can read any page of the article on a large viewing screen; the film can be advanced, dropped, or regressed at a rate controlled by the researcher. The film permits easy storage of material, in lieu of the original copy, which would require larger storage facilities. Consultation with the personnel at the information or circulation desk of your library will determine whether the service is available and to what extent.

Special Indexes

KWIC (Key–Word–In–Context) and **KWOC** (Key–Word–Out–of–Context) are computer–based systems for printing bibliographical titles according to a preselected series of key words. The key words of a title are sorted out and printed in alphabetical order and called a "permuted" index, because every time a key word in a title is located the desired article will appear. The system was designed to be an efficient method of reducing time required for scanning long titles or subjects; and, therefore, a long title will not be cited in its entirety. **KWOC** differs from **KWIC** by providing the complete citation in a single–entry listing (author, title, and source).[4,5] The student should consult with local library personnel for additional information about these systems and their availability.

SUMMARY

Without familiarity with the resources of a library or an organized approach to the library search, the process of literature review is difficult and time consuming. The researcher must be familiar with the valuable sources in the library, such as the card and periodical files, indexes, reference resource publications, automated reference services, and interlibrary loan services. An organized plan that outlines the topics to be

QUEEN MARGARET COLLEGE LIBRARY

covered and various possible services providing information about the topics is necessary before beginning the library search. This section has provided a few guides for the literature review in preparation of an investigation. Used properly, the library can become a paradise for you in the research process. Table 3.2 provides a summary of the research processes presented thus far.

Table 3.2
Cumulative Summary of the Research Processes Presented

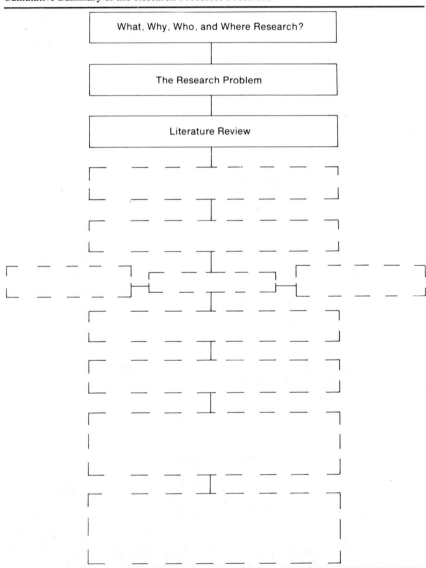

REFERENCES

1. Clarke DH, Clarke HH: Research Processes in Physical Education, Recreation and Health. Englewood Cliffs, NJ, Prentice–Hall, 1970
2. Treece EW, Treece JW, Jr: Elements of Research in Nursing, ed 3. St. Louis, C.V. Mosby Co, 1982
3. Prince B, Makrides L, Richman J: Research Methodology and Applied Statistics, Part 2: The Literature Search. Physiother Canada 32: 201–206, 1980
4. Herner S: A Brief Guide to Sources of Scientific and Technical Information, ed 2. Washington, Information Resources Press, 1980
5. Seefeldt V: Searching the Literature. In Hubbard AW (ed): Research Methods in Health, Physical Education, and Recreation. Washington, Am Assoc of Health Phys Ed Rec, 1973

SUGGESTED READINGS

Leiper C, Richardson M: Aids to conducting a literature search. Physiother Canada 25: 225, 1973
Morton LT: Research and the library. Physiotherapy 56: 119–120, 1966

4

The Proposal and Ethics

What a man's work comes to! So he plans it . . .
Robert Browning
Bells and Pomegranates

The proposal is an important component of the research process and serves as a foundation from which an investigator can begin to conduct a study. Although students should logically complete a course in research methods prior to work on a proposal, the proposal is presented early so that, for those courses requiring a written research proposal from students, sufficient time can be provided for its completion. Succeeding chapters discuss necessary details that explain the research process and provide the essentials for completing the proposal. This section deals with the salient features of the formal research proposal, of the review process, and of its preparation. Some ethical considerations and guidelines for research on humans are discussed also.

WHAT IS A RESEARCH PROPOSAL?

A research proposal is a document that outlines a planned project or investigation. The proposal is sometimes called a protocol. The proposal is a design of a research study outlining the problem, a procedure for data collection and analyses, and a presentation of the resources for the investigation. It is an organized plan of the proposed research and serves the same function as a blueprint.[1]

WHY A PROPOSAL?

No research involving human subjects should be attempted unless some authoritative source representing the institution in which the research will be conducted reviews and approves the proposed study. One of the main purposes of a research proposal is the production of a document for review prior to the initiation of the study; the document outlines the manner in which the investigation will be conducted. Because of legal aspects, a review of proposed research is necessary to determine that the rights and welfare of the subjects involved are adequately protected and that the risks to a subject are outweighed by the potential benefits or value of the information gained.[2]

The general purposes of a written proposal are: (1) to place in writing the investigator's organized plan for conducting the project, (2) to provide a guide for the investigator to follow during the conduct of the project, (3) to provide a vehicle for review and a document which can be judged for its scholarly merits, (4) to establish limits and criteria to be followed and adhered to throughout the conduct of the project, and (5) to provide a measure of accountability for those involved in the project.

Placing the proposal in written form compels the researcher to organize ideas and think. Setting ideas down on paper reduces error and prevents important aspects of the study from being overlooked. The written proposal becomes a reference establishing controls and modes to be followed during the conduct of the study. The written proposal facilitates evaluation by others. The proposal should be reviewed by peers for their assistance prior to being submitted for formal review. Peer review can correct flaws and assist in making improvements. Occasionally a great idea is not valuable in the eyes of others, thus an informal critique of the proposal by others can save time, effort, and cost.

Research usually requires financial support, which makes the proposal extremely important for acquiring funds. Funding sources require a proposal in which the procedures to be used are effectively described.[3]

The proposal may, in turn, be judged on: (1) its value or contribution to a body of knowledge; (2) the competency of the principal investigator; (3) the availability of facilities (time, space, equipment, funds, and personnel) to conduct the project; and (4) conformity to ethical or moral principles for human or animal investigations.

PROPOSAL REVIEW

Any undertaking in which a physical therapist, university faculty member, staff member, or student investigates or collects data on human subjects for research must be reviewed by an institutional review board in accordance with federal regulations. Most health–related facilities (hospitals, universities, organizations, and clinics) support the concept of, or a program of, scientific investigation, including applied and basic research. If such a program exists in a particular facility, a research committee or another body is usually established (Institutional Review Board–IRB).

The review committee may be a permanent committee, such as a utilization committee, ethical review committee, research committee, or a human assurance committee; or it may be established specifically for review of a research proposal. The committee might be composed of senior or recognized clinicians and investigators employed by or associated with the particular facility. The composition of the committee must command the respect of those submitting reviews as well as personnel of higher authority by its maturity, experience, and wisdom. A member of the committee cannot be involved in review of proposals in which he has a professional responsibility except to provide information on request by the review committee.[2] The structure, tenure, and composition of the committee is established from need and is controlled locally.

The committee has the responsibility of reviewing research proposals and ensuring that all investigations in the facility are conducted under the highest ethical, moral, and legal standards. The committee ensures that the welfare and safety of all subjects undergoing study are adequately protected by the investigator and his or her co–workers. The committee guarantees that the risks to a particular subject are less than the potential benefits, or the importance of the research findings. The committee also determines the acceptability of the proposed research in terms of feasibility, as well as standards and regulations of the facility and government. Where monies are available to support approved research proposals, the committee may have the added responsibility of establishing priorities of support.

The committee is usually responsible to a governing board or some group of higher authority. Minutes and actions of all committee meetings are recorded and maintained for review or audit whenever the need is presented.

Under federal regulations, three ways exist for processing a researcher's proposal to conduct a project: (1) by exemption certification, (2) by expedited review, and (3) by full review. Research activities eligible for exemption certification are: (1) commonly accepted educational activities, such as instructional strategies and their effectiveness on curricula and classroom management; (2) educational tests if confidentiality of subjects is observed; (3) surveys and interviews with subjects not identified; (4) observation of public behavior; and (5) investigation of records, existing data, documents, and pathological specimens. Exceptions to these activities may include: (1) studies using prisoners, the mentally disabled, and patients in federal hospitals; (2) situations when subjects studied can be identified; (3) use of minors; (4) observation of the public behavior of minors; (5) techniques exposing subjects to discomfort and harassment beyond that commonly encountered in daily living; and (6) situations involving the deception of subjects. Exemption certification is granted through the IRB.

Federal regulations permit an expedited review. The expedited review involves a few members of the IRB, but approval is granted by committee action on recommendations of these few members without the researcher's appearance before the group. A proposal is eligible for expedited review if the research activities involve only minimum risk and involve one or more of several specified categories. The specified categories considered for expedited review are: (1) collection of excreta and external secretions (for example, sweat and saliva); (2) recordings of data using noninvasive procedures conventionally used in clinical practice (for example, temperatures and electromyography-EMG); (3) collection of blood samples by venipuncture, of limited quantities over a specific period of time; (4) voice recordings; (5) moderate exercises; (6) group behavior and characteristics; (7) approved drugs; and (8) study of existing data, records, documents, and specimens (for example, pathological, nail clippings, hair).

A full review by the IRB constitutes all proposals not falling under one of the previously cited categories or activities. Invasion of the body other than for blood samples by venipuncture requires a full review (for example, needle or wire electrodes in EMG, new devices, and drugs). A full review requires the researcher to appear in person before the committee as well as providing each committee member with a copy of his or her proposal prior to committee disposition of the proposed study.

Persons planning to submit a proposal for IRB review and approval are advised to obtain local or institutional regulations and procedures prior to preparation of the proposal. Regulations vary by institution, are subject to change, and follow federal rules and guidelines.

The student will probably be faced with a different organizational structure for research activity at the university. Universities may have specific review mechanisms for research; a particular procedure for faculty to follow and a separate procedure for students. The university may decentralize the authority to its colleges for review. Universities, however, usually establish central committees with the final authority for approving research studies. The decentralized reviews, in this structure, constitute peer reviews serving to improve proposals before reaching the central review committee for disposition. Student research projects, including theses and dissertations involving human subjects and animals, can often receive an expedited review by delegated members of the central review committee if the study does not invade the body of the subjects. The review process may take 2 to 4 weeks before approval is given by the central review committee. Whatever the local situation may be, some form of review and approval is necessary to perform research studies where animal and human subjects are involved.

FORMAT OF THE PROPOSAL

Local facilities supporting research conceptually and monetarily often have a specific or suggested format to be followed when submitting a research proposal. The format of the proposal presented here is a guide for those potential investigators who do not have a specific format to follow at their facility or who want to supplement an available format. The contents of any format should, however, provide pertinent information to answer anticipated questions of the reviewers. Table 4.1 outlines the essential questions to be addressed in a research proposal. A sample proposal can be found in Appendix, Table A.

The entire proposal must be worded precisely so that the reviewer's time is not wasted by redundant or superfluous writings. Good writing is concise and a good proposal is worded to convince the reviewer that the proposed research merits approval. Avoid jargon or verbal gestures which merely add space or confuse the reviewer. Writing, like research, is basically a logical flow of reasoning and must flow smoothly and logically from step to step. Sufficient detail must be presented to answer the reviewer's anticipated questions and to avoid raising concerns about the problem or the investigator's scholarly ability. A research proposal should not exceed five typewritten pages.

The following subject headings are major divisions of the proposal, but are discussed only briefly here to clarify the headings. Detailed discussion of the contents or information essential to the writing of the proposals are provided throughout this book.

Title of Research Study

The words in the title should be concise yet sufficient to give the reviewer a good idea of what the project is about or what is being proposed for study. The title may reflect the nature of the major problem or be a statement of a subproblem. Although the title must be free of excessive or redundant wording, brevity should not reduce clarity.

Name and Title of Investigators and Participating Facilities

The principal investigator's name and title are listed first and then names of other investigators follow in order of contribution to the study. An investigator's title may be the highest earned degree or position that provides some indication of scholarly ability or competence.

The participating facility is usually the place of employment of the investigator(s) or place where the research is to be conducted. This information is important to the reviewer who must judge the competency of the investigators and the adequacy and availability of the facility(ies).

Objective of the Study

A brief statement of the problem is helpful. If the statement is that of a major problem, then the subproblem to which the proposal is addressed must also be stated. Not all studies have subproblems, but many do, and a

Table 4.1
Essential Components of the Research Description (Proposal)

1. Objectives.
2. Past pertinent experimental/clinical findings.
3. Characteristics of sample; criteria for inclusion/exclusion.
4. Method of subject recruitment; who will seek it; method of consent.
5. Study design.
6. Research procedures.
7. Potential risks.
8. Procedures protecting against risks, confidentiality.
9. Benefits versus risks.
10. Incentives offered.
11. Sources of data collection.
12. Consent document.

proposal is submitted for approval each time a subproblem is studied. Sometimes subproblems must be studied (pilot project) before major problems can be solved or major questions can be answered. An example of a major problem is "How can the force of contracting muscles be increased?" A subproblem may be "What is the effect of various hip angles on the quadriceps femoris muscle force during dynamic resistive exercise?" The example of a subproblem is related to the major problem and is one step in answering "How can the force of contracting muscles be increased." Perhaps the researcher is only interested in the effect of various hip angles on the force generated by the quadriceps femoris; then the problem statement concerns the effect of hip angles and not other methods of increasing muscular force.

Perhaps the researcher does not wish to pursue further research in the area of enhancing muscular force during resistive exercise and is only interested in seeking an answer to "What is the effect of various hip angles on the quadriceps femoris muscle force during dynamic resistive exercise?" In this situation the only problem stated is "What is the effect of various hip angles on the quadriceps femoris muscle force during dynamic resistive exercises?"

After reading the problem statement, the reviewer has an idea of what is to be studied, but the reviewer does not know the aim or purpose for studying this particular problem. Purpose (goal, objective, aim) and problem statements are not the same.[4] A problem is defined as an answerable question and an objective is the purpose or aim for answering the questions. Objectives grow out of the problem statement or from previously researched questions and pave the way for gathering new information. Objectives can provide direction to the study.

If a single objective is to be achieved by the research, a succinct statement of purpose of the the study should be stated. If more than one objective is to be achieved, the objectives should be listed in outline form to reduce wording and to catch the reviewer's attention. The objectives must be specific and listing them in order is helpful to the researcher and reviewer for establishing priorities of effort and emphasis.

The problem and objective must be delineated so that the plan of the study will enable data to be collected and analyzed in such fashion that answers to questions or tested hypotheses are possible.

A stated hypothesis or question in this section takes the place of a problem statement. The remainder of the proposal is built from the foundation provided by the stated problem and the study objective.

Significance of the Study

The investigator must explain why time and effort should be spent on the study. This section is a justification of why the research should be conducted or a defense of the stated objectives. An argument must be presented on what the study is expected to contribute to the problem or to a body of knowledge. The investigator's familiarity with the problem should be displayed during the discussion. The discussion must be in keeping with the objectives and the problem and must not be too broad or overstated.

The investigator should provide supporting statements for the practical or theoretical importance of the research and state whether the proposed study is a replication of former research, a step in advancing knowledge (area of little or much research), or whether the answers to the problem will open up new areas of research.

Related Research

By this time the researcher has read many studies related to the problem or is familiar with what research has been done in the area of interest. Only the most pertinent studies supporting the investigator's argument should be cited in this section, and then only the highlights of the cited studies are discussed. The investigator must present the information in a logical sequence, sometimes chronologically, to demonstrate his knowledge of previous research (his or others). The story must convince the reviewer that previous research has not answered the question or tested the hypothesis stated by the investigator.

If any current studies overlap the problem of the proposal, the investigator should show how his proposal differs from those studies or how it will complement them.

Technical flaws of previous research should be pointed out in the discussion. In the event that little or no previous work has been reported in the area of the proposed study, the investigator should cite studies most closely related to the proposed study.

Most of the discussion has implied importance only to original work. The student who is doing classroom projects or a master's thesis need not be so concerned about originality. Original studies require confirmation, especially if no other studies have been reported that refute or confirm the conclusion or inference. Replication of a study should be possible by reading the Methods sections of a report. A replication of another study is treated similar to an original approach when writing the proposal. The reviewer must devote as much time to the review and render a judgment of the significance of the replication as for an original approach, so do not pass up a good opportunity to confirm or refute another person's work. Read **PHYSICAL THERAPY** and many reported studies which need replication will emerge.

Procedure of the Study

This section is the principal part of the proposal and is, therefore, the part given the most detail; it should be organized, well written, and concise. Information included in this section will be given close scrutiny by the reviewer. The section should provide the operational aspects of the problem and objectives, including method of selecting samples and gathering data, controls, measurements, statistical design, safeguards, and how the findings will be presented. Sometimes an outline form is preferred and reduces the length of the section for the convenience of the reader. Subheadings of various contents are desirable and assist in reading and identifying aspects of particular interest to the reviewer.

1. Sample. A brief description of the subjects (sex, age, physical or mental status) and welfare of subjects (safeguards, consent form) are to be included. If humans are not used, descriptions of the sample characteristics and condition(s) are provided. The protection of the rights and welfare of subjects participating in an investigation is extremely important and a detailed discussion will follow at the end of this chapter.

Although the size of the sample is important, an accurate number of subjects required cannot be given at this point because needs change or attrition of subjects occurs during the process of the study. The size of the sample affects the outcome of the experiment and should be sufficiently large; however, the size of the sample effects is dependent on the type of experiment conducted. For example, few subjects may volunteer for projects involving noxious conditions, but many may volunteer for projects where conditions are pleasant and require minimal consumption of the subject's time. The investigator must be the judge about the size of the sample needed to meet the objectives of the study. Usually larger sized samples are needed for relation studies than for comparative studies. When using analysis of variance, a repeated measures design will conserve more on numbers required than a randomized design. Chapter 5 discusses sampling methods and Chapter 9 discusses design.

The rule is to provide sufficient information about the sample or the subjects' characteristics, how the subjects will be obtained, the approximate number of subjects needed, and how the subjects' welfare will be safeguarded (hazards to be encountered or ill effects). The nature of the consent form must be included with the proposal; a sample of a consent form is in Appendix, Table B.

2. Method. A description of how the study will be conducted should include controls to be used, units of measurement, tools or equipment, and techniques and conditions. These details should indicate how data are to be gathered. If you merely state that a plethysmograph is used to measure the arterial blood, you are not supplying enough information. Blood volume is measured by a venous occlusion plethysmograph. The instrument is air–filled, water–filled, or electronic, and is manufactured by several companies. The manufacturer's name and address is footnoted in the published report, because providing information now, although not essential, is helpful to the researcher for later use in writing the report for publication.

In the case of a descriptive study, the measuring instrument could be the oral interview, mail questionnaire, or attitude scale. In thesis work, the student is usually required to describe the type of instrument used, rationale for its selection, and its validity and reliability data. Submission of the paper instrument is a good idea so that the reviewers can formulate judgments about the adequacy of the instrument for meeting the objective and problem of the study.

3. Design. The design of the study should be described (see Chapter 9 for details). The character of the hypothesis, the variables involved, the method of selecting subjects, and the restrictions placed on the study should be considered in the design. The design must permit the testing of hypotheses. For example, if the hypothesis involved comparing the effectiveness of training with isometric contractions versus contractions caused by electrical stimulation and combinations of these contractions with respect to increased muscular strength, the study might involve comparing the strength over time (final or posttest strength) of four groups. One group serves as a control (no exercise), while the other three groups (isometric, electrical stimulation, and isometric plus electrical stimulation) serve as experimental groups. A design involving four groups would be required in the study. The availability of subjects and the residual effects of the training modes determine whether the groups are to be selected randomly or whether the modes could be repeated over one group of subjects (see Chapter 5 for methods of selection). A brief description of the controls of the independent variables (Chapter 5) is recommended so that provisions for minimizing variability of data during the data gathering are taken. Some variables are identified for the study by asking, "What effect does training by electrical stimulation of specific current characteristics have on the force developed by the quadriceps femoris muscle?''

Since the dependent variable (strength or force) involves subject variation (motivation, size, sex, and age), administration of pretest strength should determine whether groups of subjects are similarly matched prior to beginning the various modes of training. The design should indicate the number of groups included in the investigation, how the groups are selected, and whether there will be pretests and posttests.

In experimental research, the investigator has a number of designs from which to choose. The complexity of designs depends on the number of independent (modes of exercise) and dependent variables (strength measures) involved in the study.

4. Analysis. The procedures for analyzing and synthesizing data are given. Although statistical designs are not mandatory in research, statistical methods are valuable to the researcher who deals with data containing variation. Often conclusions about data are based on a degree of uncertainty, and statistics enable the researcher to make a logical decision based on the most probable outcome, which may not have been obvious to him without the assitance of statistical measures. The statistical design used in analyzing the data should be stated in name; for example, a two-tailed paired t-test at the 5% level of significance. Enough cannot be said for selecting the appropriate statistical design before the study begins. Many studies have been published in which the statistics were determined in retrospect to the collected data. Data should never be collected and then some statistical design found to fit the data; fit the data to the design. The full information contained in the data will not be obtained unless the researcher plans in advance the kinds of information he or she wishes to gather through selection of the types of tests, the test routines, and the appropriate methods of analyses. Once data are collected the researcher is limited to the choice of appropriate analyses because statistical designs are only appropriate to specific data–gathering designs. The planning and selecting of techniques for analyses of data are procedural and ethical issues which must follow rules of scientific inquiry.

Time, Space, and Availability of Equipment

1. Time. Researchers need a time frame for perspective and to keep the study on schedule. The existence of deadlines and other commitments requires careful budgeting of time for research studies. A time frame or schedule consists of a listing of the study's major phases (e.g., proposal preparation, reviews, subject selection, gathering data, analyzing data, and report preparation) and the expected completion time associated with each phase. Allow time for the process of obtaining funds, purchasing, and delivery of equipment. Allow for delays so that you can meet your completion date. The Gantt method is a chart listing major phases to be completed on the left–hand side and the time allowed for their completion across the top.[5,6]

Researchers frequently work on a 3–year schedule. While collecting data for a study in the present year, researchers are also preparing the report of the prior year's study and writing the proposal for next year's study. The time schedule is valuable when placed in the proposal because it permits the researcher to display his schedule for the conduction of the investigation, and it allows the reviewers to assess the appropriateness of the allotted times.

2. Space. Special rooms may be required for the study; appropriate negotiation for the use of the rooms may be necessary; if so, this should be indicated. Acquiring space may require special improvement funds for which approval must be given. If space is available, then so indicate in the proposal.

3. Availability of Equipment. The types of equipment to be used have been identified and described earlier, but what if the equipment must be purchased, borrowed, shared, or repaired? The reviewer must know whether the costs to be incurred are justified and whether equipment is immediately available or its use must be negotiated.

Cost Analysis

Every administrator is interested in the costs of performing research. Costs may be incurred indirectly in the salary of the physical therapist, who spends time conducting the research rather than treating patients. Costs may also be incurred in equipment and supplies, additional personnel, computer time for data analyses or costs for a statistician to analyze the data, art work for illustrations and slides of the findings, literature searches with computers, renovation or special improvement of work areas, and construction of equipment not commercially available. There also may be hidden costs that occur after the study has been approved and funded.

Reviewers must make decisions about the proposal regarding contributions and the costs of obtaining information. The proposal is a form of advertisement to sell the merits of the researcher's efforts, time, and costs in doing the study. The manner in which the proposal is written is very important; you must convince others of your scholarly abilities in a single document. Sometimes you may be invited to defend the proposal verbally or to answer committee questions. Many times these advantages are not available to the investigator. Granting agencies often require lengthy proposals written on special forms which they make available on request. In the student's situation, the proposal must convince readers or a committee that the student is adequately prepared to perform the study in question. It would be ironic for a student majoring in sociology to request approval for a study in the biochemical effects of 10 minutes of ultrasound on ligamentous structures of rats. The researcher must also be aware of meeting review deadlines for submission of the proposal. Do not hesitate to seek assistance in writing the proposal or in performing the study.

THE PILOT STUDY

After identifying a researchable problem, the student or researcher may have some questions about its feasibility. Concerns may center on the data-gathering methods, such as the adequacy of the measuring instruments and controls, scoring techniques, unanticipated flaws, and desire to try alternative procedures. Expenditure of time and costs in completing the study may also be of concern. The pilot study may be the solution to these problems.

The pilot study is a preliminary research trial. It requires most of the research process to be implemented but on a smaller scale than that of a major study. Pilot studies use fewer subjects than major research projects, but each and every procedure is followed, including analysis of the gathered data. The pilot study serves as an evaluation of the researchable problem and is often used to assess the quality of student theses and dissertations.

The pilot study provides valuable information not only to the novice, but also to the experienced researcher, who can use the study for improving hypotheses and data-gathering procedures, for determining time needed to complete a major study, for reducing flaws previously overlooked, and for obtaining feedback from subjects. The original research proposal almost always will be modified as a result of a pilot study. Information gained from the pilot study will improve the subsequent research. Many of the studies reported in the literature are results of pilot work but are not often reported as such. These "one shot" studies frequently need confirmation and larger numbers of subjects, and therefore, further research.

STUDENT RESEARCH PROJECTS

Student research projects are a part of the curricula of many programs offering initial preparation in physical therapy. The purpose of student projects is to acquaint students with the principles of the scientific method, which involves identifying a research problem, developing a design for investigation of the problem, undertaking an investigation, and writing a report that describes the outcome of the project. Projects include the methods and instruments discussed in later chapters. The learning that takes place during the project provides the foundation for appreciating the elements of physical therapy research and serves to increase the understanding of research above that which is presented in a didactic course.

The procedures for developing and conducting the project follow the systems approach shown in Table 1.2 and elsewhere in the book. At this point you should be able to develop a research problem and be giving some thought to its organization and how to write a proposal. Although the proposal cannot be completed without understanding the material presented in subsequent chapters, much of the proposal can be written at this point. In the event that assistance is needed in identifying a research problem, the following section lists some titles of past student projects. No attempt has been made to select only quality project titles; the listing merely identifies areas of interest to former students. The appropriate method for solving the identified problem follows each title.

Topics Selected by Students

Initial Preparatory Level.

From a Physical Therapy Affiliate Program[7]:

Effect of massage in reducing edema of the hand. Sellers BJ, Haefner B (comparative)

Effects of stroking massage in reducing edema of the foot. Stearns L, Price S (comparative)

Effect of local massage on the skin temperature of the hand. Beattie DP, Christopher HR (comparative)

Thermal effects of massage to the hand using a power medium. Canfield J, Kluthe M (comparative)

From the Medical College of Georgia, Augusta, Georgia:

Determination of normal values for radial nerve conduction velocity. Humphries R, Currier DP[8] (comparative)

Physiological effects of passive exercise on cardiopulmonary function. Smith K[9] (comparative)

Physical therapy recipients in nursing homes: the criteria for selection. Adams P (survey)

Use of a backrest in strengthening knee extensor muscles. Richard G, Currier DP[10] (comparative)

Interrator reliability in manual muscle testing. Gunnels CA (correlational)

Validity of the orthokinetic cuff in reducing spasticity in the wrist. Freeman B (comparative)

Use of isometric maximum to predict one repetition maximum for progressive resistance exercise. Calzada A (correlational)

Connective tissue laxity in subject having Barlow syndrome. Evans P (correlational)

Effect of adhesive strapping in the prophylactic care of the ankle joint. Rammel M (comparative)

Effect of the inverted position on the heart rate, blood pressure, and respiratory rate in the normal adult. Gilbert R (comparative)

Motor conduction of the anterior interosseous nerve. Craft S, Currier DP, Nelson R[11] (comparative)

Conditions of employment of the 1975 physical therapy graduating class in a four-state area. Price S (survey)

From the University of Alberta, Edmonton, Canada:

Combined effectiveness of standardized physical therapy and biofeedback–induced foot warming exercise. Ogiwara S (comparative)

Short–wave diathermy combined with manual mobilization as a method of increasing range of motion in the treatment of "frozen shoulder." Strong M (comparative)

Comparison of two methods of postoperative management following geometric knee replacement. Woytiuk M (comparative)

Comparative effects of passive positioning and exercise on arterial insufficiency disorders. Anderson M (comparative)

Capsular lesions of the glenohumeral joint: a comparative study of active and passive treatment programmes. Millar B (comparative)

Comparison of the treatment of "tennis elbow" using ultrasound with hydrocortisone and ultrasound without hydrocortisone. Morgan F (comparative)

Assessment of the mobilization techniques of Maitland to increase the range of movement on the chronic "frozen shoulder." Crocker M (comparative)

From Lincoln Institute, Melbourne, Australia[12]:

Influence of motivation on the performance of an exercise (comparative)

Effects of three different exercise regimens on endurance (comparative)

Strength gain comparison between progressive resisted exercise and regressive resisted exercise (comparative)

Dosage time required for lengthening hamstring muscles (comparative)

From the University of Kentucky, Lexington, Kentucky:

Effect of increased abdominal muscle strength on forced vital capacity and forced expiratory volume. Simpson L[13] (comparative)

EMG activity in shoulder muscles during exercise in sagittal planes and diagonal patterns. Smiley C (comparative)

Do good physical therapy students make good physical therapists? Scott MJ (survey)

Normal values for two–point discrimination and reliability of a two-point discrimination instrument. Walder J, Bathke J (normative)

High voltage electrical stimulation and blood flow. Carlson D (comparative)

Energy cost during gait of a hemipelvectomy amputee. Kennedy PJ, Glasgow SC (case report)

Graduate Studies Level.

Theses[14]:

Comparative study of selected aspects of today's basic professional education for physical therapy in India and the United States of America. Mapleton AJ

Electromyographic and cinematographic findings in a novel motor skill development by walking with a simulated below–knee pylon. Ho SBL

Comparison of the isometric strength of the extensors at the metacarpophalangeal joint. Barnes WJ

Circling behavior on the rate produced by direct drug stimulation of the globus pallidus and caudate/putamen. Springer AP

Effects of vibration on the Achilles tendon reflex. Coogler CE

Attitudes of physical therapists toward patients and health professionals. Sorensen AM

Evaluation of the back abdominal strength ratio with the cable tensiometer. Bendinsky A

Conservative management of low back pain in the chronic state: a comparative study of two different techniques of treatment. Fernando CK

Dissertations.

From the University of Kentucky:

The effect of one session of delayed onset muscle soreness inducing resistive exercise on serum creatine kinase, white cell blood count, edema, and plasma volume, Franklin ME

Effects of short-term, medium-frequency electrical stimulation on normal, partially denervated, and denervated rat skeletal muscle, Greathouse DG

Effect of variation in the burst mode and carrier frequency of high amplitude electrical stimulation on muscle fatigue and pain perception of healthy subjects, Rooney JG

SOME ETHICAL CONSIDERATIONS

Widespread concern about the ethics of medical research has evolved ever since the Nuremburg trials. Ethical questions associated with the use of human and animal subjects are being raised more today than ever. The welfare and rights of humans have been violated in medical research. Because of these violations, a formulation of declarations has been developed to outline proper ethical principles involved in the acceptable use of human and animal subjects in research.[15] In 1964, the World Medical Association established some guidelines for persons engaged in research on humans (Table 4.2). This declaration has served as the basis for the regulations for testing new drugs under United States law and also as the basis for the guidelines of the Medical Research Councils of Great Britain,[16] the United States,[17] and Canada,[18] and for a large number of universities and hospitals. These approving bodies attach great importance to the ethical acceptability of experiments involving human subjects.

Laws have been written in response to political pressures caused by public emotional reactions to violations of ethical principles. The laws represent efforts to protect the rights and welfare of every human. Ethical considerations arise because of uses to which research has been put, misdeeds of persons conducting research, and appropriations of public funds to support research.[19]

Risk and Responsibility

Research often involves uncertainties which may, in turn, involve risks. Physical, psychological, and social injuries are considered potential risks when a subject participates in activity involving uncertainties.[19] Infringement of privacy and psychological damage, such as emotional upset, public embarrassment and humiliation, loss of self respect, or loss of dignity are considered potential risks, as well as physical discomfort, exposure to pain, or other physical harm. Because people are protected from unjustifiable assault, research involving humans must be justified for its contribution to scientific knowledge.[20]

The term research applies to those procedures carried out on humans for the purpose of contributing to knowledge. Behavioral research and questionnaires are included under guidelines for research involving human subjects. The researcher is asked to show how subjects (normal or patients) will benefit from the experimental intervention, what controls will be exercised to ensure the safety, welfare and rights of the subjects, and how subjects will be informed about potential risks. Potential risks must be balanced against potential benefits. A new approach to treating a condition is not a guarantee it will be effective or will replace the old approach. Controlled trials are essential to determine the efficacy of new

Table 4.2
Declaration of Helsinki

I. Basic Principles

1. Clinical research must conform to the moral and scientific principles that justify medical research and should be based on laboratory and animal experiments or other scientifically established facts.

2. Clinical research should be conducted only by scientifically qualified persons and under the supervision of a qualified medical man.

3. Clinical research cannot legitimately be carried out unless the importance of the objective is in proportion to the inherent risk to the subject.

4. Every clinical research project should be preceded by careful assessment of inherent risks in comparison to foreseeable benefits to the subject or to others.

5. Special caution should be exercised by the doctor in performing clinical research in which the personality of the subject is liable to be altered by drugs or experimental procedure.

II. Clinical Research Combined with Professional Care

1. In the treatment of the sick person, the doctor must be free to use a new therapeutic measure, if, in his judgment, it offers hope of saving life, reestablishing health, or alleviating suffering.

If at all possible, consistent with patient psychology, the doctor should obtain the patient's freely given consent after the patient has been given a full explanation. In case of legal incapacity, consent should also be procured from the legal guardian; in case of physical incapacity the permission of the legal guardian replaces that of the patient.

2. The doctor can combine clinical research with professional care, the objective being the acquisition of new medical knowledge, only to the extent that clinical research is justified by its therapeutic value for the patient.

III. Nontherapeutic Clinical Research

1. In the purely scientific application of clinical research carried out on a human being, it is the duty of the doctor to remain the protector of the life and health of that person on whom clinical research is being carried out.

2. The nature, the purpose, and the risk of clinical research must be explained to the subject by the doctor.

3a. Clinical research on a human being cannot be undertaken without his free consent after he has been informed; if he is legally incompetent, the consent of the legal guardian should be procured.

3b. The subject of clinical research should be in such a mental, physical, and legal state as to be able to exercise fully his power of choice.

3c. Consent should, as a rule, be obtained in writing. However, the responsibility for clinical research always remains with the research worker; it never falls on the subject even after consent is obtained.

4a. The investigator must respect the right of each individual to safeguard his personal integrity, especially if the subject is in a dependent relationship to the investigator.

4b. At any time during the course of clinical research the subject or his guardian should be free to withdraw permission for research to be continued.

The investigator or the investigating team should discontinue the research if in his or their judgment, it may, if continued, be harmful to the individual.

approaches. The researcher must have some justification for studying the new approach and a reasonable explanation of its potential benefits.

In general, the clinical therapist uses different and new therapeutic measures if, in his judgment, they are within the aims of the treatment requested by the referring physician. The therapeutic measures used must be consistent with "accepted" forms of therapy stated in licensure acts. The therapist obtains the patient's approval informally when rendering a full explanation of what the treatment is and what can be expected from the treatment. This situation does not require a formal written consent. The physical therapist can combine clinical research with professional care to the extent that the research is justified by its therapeutic value for the patients. In all incidences the therapist must obtain prior approval for controlled clinical trials (review committee, referring physicians, and patient by written consent). The objective of all new therapeutic approaches should be acquisition of fresh physical therapy knowledge to improve the quality of therapy.

Practitioners find the concept of withholding treatment from patients perplexing. If the treatment to be investigated is known to be effective, it is unethical to withhold it from the patient. If the effectiveness of the treatment is unknown or equivocal, it is unethical to continue its use or use it without appropriate controlled evaluation.[21]

When risks are unknown, a controlled trial using animals may be required. Ethics also cover the use of animals in research. Principles of ethics safeguarding the comfort and humane treatment of experimental animals have been developed by the American Psychological Association, and a statement of how animals will be treated in experiments is required in all proposals involving them.[22]

The conduct of experimental studies is controlled directly by persons and approving bodies at respective work facilities, and indirectly through meetings and journal articles. Opinions and discussion among professional groups generally precede the acceptance of resolutions and principles or passage of rules.

Informed Consent

Explaining the nature and purpose of a treatment procedure to a patient is generally left to the judgment of the physical therapist, and the patient usually accepts this explanation without question. This approach does not fulfill the ethical codes of research protocols. When the treatment is novel, the physical therapist is wisely advised to make extra efforts for the patient's comprehension. Since the conduct of clinical research raises moral and ethical questions, informed consent is essential.[23] Today, facilities of employment require the therapist in experimental research to obtain written consent from the subject prior to the research study. In general, the researcher is obligated to give full details about risks and benefits involved in the research to those participating and those responsible for minors who will participate.

The information required in each informed consent is given in Table 4.3.[2] Forms will vary from facility to facility but the information required will be similar. An example of a consent form is found in Appendix, Table B.

Guidelines for Research

Experimental and descriptive research involving human subjects is necessary to further scientific knowledge and to improve physical therapy. Some general rules of conduct are presented to assist the therapist interested in conducting research on humans; these rules serve only as guides. Specific rules are mandatory when applying for government research grants and when working for institutions. The researcher must obtain the specific information concerning ethics and consent for particular applications.

Table 4.3
Elements Required in the Informed Consent Form

1. Title of proposed study.
2. The first paragraph is a statement of agreement to participate which includes the subject's name and the names of the investigators.
3. Explanation of expected duration of the subject's participation, as well as the location of the research project.
4. Principal investigator's name.
5. Description of study in narrative layman's language (200 words or less). Explain purpose, procedure, experimental effect.
6. Describe risks, benefits, and any discomfort that subjects can expect.
7. Indication of antidotes or alternative treatments available, that no form of compensation or medical treatment is available from researcher but is provided at expense of subject's health care insurer.
8. Offer to answer subject's questions about the study.
9. Inform subject of choice to withdraw from participation in the study at any time without prejudice.
10. Indication that participation is voluntary and assure subject of anonymity of data.
11. Disclaimer for medical care and compensation.
12. Indicate whom to contact for answers about the research, whom to contact in event of injury, and that a copy of the consent form will be given.
13. Signatures:
    Subject
    Witness
    Date
14. Statement that procedure was explained in detail, followed by the signature of the researcher.

Principles for Human Research.

1. Any research must be justifiable for its scientific value.
2. Even if the inquiry has scientific value, it must not be pursued if benefit is outweighed by risk to the subject.
3. The research must be conducted by scientifically competent people.
4. The research must be conducted under a sound design or proposal and be carried out according to the design, although the design may be modified on approval of the review committee that had originally approved it.
5. Care must be taken throughout the study to see that the subject is not harassed, and the research must be terminated if there is risk of harm, either physical or emotional.
6. The subject should be entitled to withdraw at any time.
7. No subject should be used in research unless he or she has given free consent after being fully informed. In the case of a child or mentally incompetent person, the consent of the legal guardian should be obtained and risks must remain minimal for these subjects. A child is usually defined as a person under 18 years of age.[2,20,24]

Principles for Behavioral Research. Sometimes a complete explanation in advance of the purpose of behavioral research can invalidate the results. These guidelines follow the ethical standards of the American Psychological Association.

1. When a person is involved as a subject in a research project, his or her permission must be obtained.
2. Whenever possible the nature, purpose, and results of the research should be described to those persons directly or indirectly involved.
3. Subjects should not be coerced to participate in a research program; they should be free to withdraw whenever they desire.
4. Only when a problem is significant and can be investigated in no other way is the investigator justified in giving misinformation to research subjects or exposing research subjects to physical or emotional stress.
5. When the possibility of serious aftereffects exists, research is conducted only when the subjects or their responsible agents are fully informed of this possibility and nevertheless volunteer.
6. The investigator seriously considers the possible harmful aftereffects and removes them as soon as permitted by the design of the experiment.[25]

Principles for the Use of Data Gathering Instruments. The gathering of data, such as answers to questionnaires, inventories, interviews, and other data–gathering instruments are considered descriptive research and are concerned with the matter of privacy.

1. Any research which includes the use of questionnaires should have scientific or other meaningful purpose and value.
2. Questionnaires should be designed and administered by competent persons.
3. Care should be taken insofar as is consistent with the purpose of the study, that information acquired be absolutely essential to the study and be as free as possible from embarrassing questions.
4. Participation in such studies should be voluntary, and care should be exercised to ensure that subtle pressures are not used to obtain participation.
5. Answers to questionnaires should be kept confidential, and, when possible, anonymity should be afforded. Codes and ciphers must be kept in secure places; transfer of data between places (shipment and delivery) should have careful controls; and provision for the destruction of all edited and obsolete data on punched cards, printouts, tapes, and other records must be made. Computer transmission of data may be restricted in certain studies.
6. Subjects should be free to withdraw at any time prior to or during the administration of a questionnaire; they should be informed in advance of this right.
7. Subjects must be given a clear and understandable explanation of the purpose of a questionnaire prior to its administration.[2,24]

The objective of laws, principles, and guidelines on research ethics is to ensure protection of the rights and welfare of the subject. Comparative and descriptive research represent a delicate balance between the health professions and public opinion and legal limitation. The researcher must accept responsibility for his or her actions by carefully weighing the way the research is conducted. The law, principle, or guideline encompasses every potential situation encountered in research.[22]

POLAR QUESTIONS ON ETHICS

Students pursuing instruction in research have been asked about their positions on two questions dealing with ethics in research. The questions address problems at opposite extremes (polar) and represent situations which students may face some day. These are the student responses:

1. A professor performs and publishes research based on your proposal submitted in partial fulfillment of a course in research. What is your reaction?

A professor's performance of research based on a student's proposal is perfectly ethical as long as the student is informed of the professor's intention and use of the proposal and has the expressed consent from the student for its use. If feasible and out of courtesy the professor should invite the student to participate in the experimental solution of the problem. The student will be somewhat limited in ability to complete the experiment, thus, the collaboration would serve as a valuable learning experience to the student. When the report is published, the person having greatest responsibility for the completion of the study should be the author listed first. Mutual agreement or a contract to this effect should be made before the study is begun.

Anonymous Student

2. A student performs research in partial fulfillment of a course or thesis requirement and uses a professor's expressed research problem, laboratory, and equipment. What is your reaction?

A professor should not be reluctant to allow a student to conduct research using the professor's idea, laboratory, and equipment. This arrangement permits a faculty member with research and teaching responsibilities to generate and oversee many more research studies than he would otherise have time to complete on his own. This arrangement provides guidance to the student, while the student gains valuable experience. The professor usually has facilities and equipment at his disposal which may not be available to the student. Each contributor to the research should receive due credit. A mutual understanding of each person's role is necessary before the onset of the study. The interaction of student and professor in research allows for initiative, enthusiasm, and expertise, which is necessary in the performance of research.

SUMMARY

The research proposal is a document outlining a planned project or investigation. The proposal serves as a guide for the investigator to follow during the project; provides a vehicle for review and a document judged on its own merit, while establishing limits and criteria to be followed throughout the project. The proposal also provides a measure of accountability of those engaged in the project.

The proposal must be written concisely and convincingly. It should include the following information:

1. Title of the research study
2. Name and title of the researchers and participating facilities
3. Objectives of the study
4. Significance of the study
5. Related research

6. Plan of the study
7. Time, space, and availability of equipment
8. Cost analysis

Because the researcher asks questions, pries into the mind, and samples the physiological characteristics of a subject, the issue of ethics is raised

Table 4.4
Cumulative Summary of the Research Processes Presented

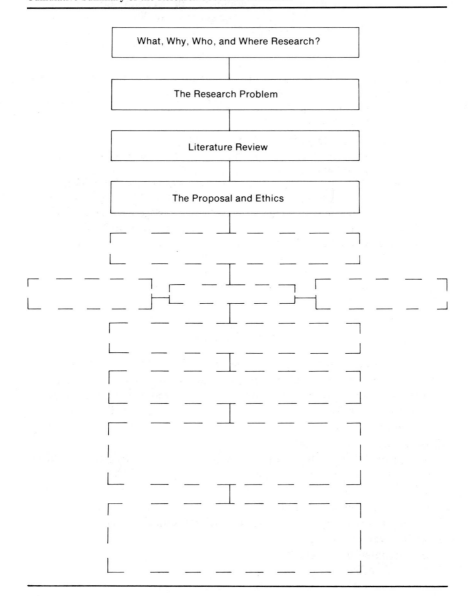

by the public, legislators, and those responsible for approving studies. When writing the proposal and conducting the research, the investigator must consider the moral and ethical issues and state in the proposal how the rights and welfare of subjects will be protected. The researcher must obtain the consent of the volunteers.

Some titles of previous research projects have been listed to assist readers in formulating a research problem and proposing a title for a project. Table 4.4 provides a summary of the research processes presented thus far.

REFERENCES

1. Treece EW, Treece JW Jr: Elements of Research in Nursing, ed 3. St. Louis, CV Mosby Co, 1982.
2. Code of Federal Regulations 45CFR46: Protection of Human Subjects (HHS). Washington, U.S. Government Printing Office, 1983
3. Makrides L, Richman J: Research methodology and applied statistics, Part 7: Writing the research proposal. Physiother Canada 33: 163–168, 1981
4. Wandelt M: Guide for the Beginning Researcher. New York, Appleton–Century–Crofts, 1970
5. Archibald RD, Villoria RL: Network–Based Management Systems (PERT/CPM). New York, John Wiley, 1967
6. Gay, LR: Educational Research: Competencies for Analysis and Application, ed 2. Columbus, OH, Charles E. Merrill, 1981
7. Schneiderwind W, Burke J: Physical Therapy Affiliate Program: An Introduction to Research. Carville, LA, US Department Health, Education, Welfare, 1970
8. Humphries R, Currier DP: Variables in recording motor conduction of the radial nerve. Phys Ther 56: 809–814, 1976
9. Smith K: Physiological effects of passive exercise on cardiorespiratory function. Phys Ther 56: 295–297, 1976
10. Richard G, Currier DP: Back stabilization during knee strengthening exercise. Phys Ther 57: 1013–1015, 1977
11. Craft S, Currier DP, Nelson R: Motor conduction of the anterior interosseous nerve. Phys Ther 57: 1143–1147, 1977
12. Wheeler JR: Student research projects: an innovative approach to learning. Physiother Canada 28: 99–101, 1976
13. Simpson L: Effect of increased abdominal muscle strength on forced vital capacity and forced expiratory volume. Phys Ther 63: 334–337, 1983
14. Theses and dissertations. Phys Ther 55: 58–60, 1975
15. Visscher MB: Ethical Constraints and Imperatives in Medical Research. Springfield, IL, Charles C Thomas Pub, 1975
16. Report of the Medical Research Council for 1962–1963 (Cmmd 2382). London, Medical Research Council, pp 21–25
17. American Medical Association Ethical Guidelines for Clinical Investigations. Chicago, Am Med Assoc, November 30, 1966
18. Medical Research Council; Extramural Programmes; 1966. Ottawa, Canada, Medical Research Council, 1966
19. Michels E: Research and human rights, 2. Phys Ther 56: 546–552, 1976
20. Cox KR: Planning Clinical Experiments. Springfield, IL, Charles C Thomas Pub, 1968
21. Makrides L, Richman J; Research methodology and applied statistics, Part 6: Ethics in human research. Physiother Canada 33: 89–94, 1981
22. Research Precautions of Ethical Standards. Washington, Am Psychol Assoc, 1963

23. Burdette WJ, Gehan EA: Planning and Analyses of Clinical Trials. Springfield, IL, Charles C Thomas Pub, 1970
24. Guidelines for Human Research: General Faculties Council. Edmonton, Canada, University of Alberta, 1972
25. Ethical standards of psychologists. Am Psychol 18: 56–60, 1963

SUGGESTED READINGS

Cox DR: Planning of Experiments. New York, John Wiley & Sons, 1958
Krathwohl DR: How to Prepare a Research Proposal. Syracuse, Syracuse University Bookstore, 1965
Slater SB: The design of clinical research. Phys Ther 46: 265-273, 1966
Wilson EB, Jr: An Introduction to Scientific Research. New York, McGraw–Hill Book Co., 1952
Michels E: Research and human rights. I. Phys Ther 56: 407–412, 1976

Part Two
ROOTS OF RESEARCH

5

Quantification in Research

I often say that when you can measure
what you are speaking about and express it in
numbers, you know something about it; but, when
you cannot measure it in numbers your knowledge
is of a meagre and unsatisfactory kind; it may
be the beginning of knowledge but have scarcely
in your thought advanced to the stage of science
whatever the matter may be.

Lord Kelvin

A vital part of the research process is the gathering of measurements or counts in a form appropriate for deducing reasonable conclusions. A scientific premise exists when a phenomenon can be measured, and if it can be measured, it can be understood. Research deals with existing phenomena and measured values of phenomena; therefore, it must deal with quantities, numbers, and facts.

The word "agree" means to correspond, conform, resemble, and concur[1] whereas the concepts "objective" and "subjective" can be considered as degrees of agreement. Objective means to exist independent of thought or outside of the mind, and subjective is the opposite, to exist in the mind or be dependent on thought.[1] The concepts of objective and subjective are considered in terms of amount or degrees of agreement. To be objective, an event, trait, or quantity must be agreed on unanimously; whereas to be subjective, the degree of agreement can vary with the event, trait, or quantity.[2] A group of physical therapists may "eyeball" the motion of a patient's glenohumeral joint and judge the range as 155, 160, or 165 degrees but after measuring the joint motion by an appropriate instrument, the motion is found to be 160 degrees. In the first approach the 160-degree motion could have been the value most but not all therapists agreed on, whereas every therapist observed the measuring instrument and agreed with the value indicated on the instrument. We say the first approach was subjective because the measurement was a guess or a product of thought or experience, whereas the second approach is considered objective because the measurement resulted in agreement, although a difference in the process of agreement could be distinguished. This represents degrees of agreement.

Instruments are used in education to measure the absorption of knowledge. Students are familiar with objective and subjective examinations. One examination is objective because a response is correct and all others incorrect to the question; another examination is subjective because the results are dependent on the judgment or mental belief of the professor (quality). The two examples are different degrees of agreement. Science is concerned with truth and reality; it is objective. Quantitativeness is objectivity.

Statistics is a branch of applied mathematics dealing with the organization, description, and interpretation of data obtained by observations and experiments. Examination and treatment of data with statistics enable the researcher to predict outcomes of related events or make generalities from the data with increased assurance of being correct.

Some comment about the use of statistics in a book or course on research methods is necessary. Most students who have conveniently avoided taking more than a single course of college mathematics are usually terrified by the word "mathematics." This book exposes the student to elementary statistics and scientific concepts because every physical therapist must know how to read and interpret the research literature to maintain professional competence. The therapist must think, act, converse, and write in scientific style. The way this book treats statistics should ease the apprehension of any student lacking mathematical background. Effort has been made to simplify the mathematical component. The student seeking a career in scientific research eventually must reckon with more sophisticated mathematical concepts than presented here. Statistics is a valuable tool to the researcher who constantly deals with animate objects with variations too complex and frequent to reason out through logic alone. Statistics is more often a friend to the researcher than not; the researcher works hard to build a body of scientific knowledge so that the student can understand some of the operations of the knowledge-building process.

The use of statistics in research does not prove that the findings are true or real. Statistics never did nor will ever prove anything. Statistics is a valuable tool for helping the researcher to make correct decisions, conclusions, and inferences, but statistics does not prove anything. Data are variable; people are variable; characteristics, traits, events, and measurements are variable in the type of research physical therapists perform. Because of the variability of some methods of assuring accuracy, we need to increase chances for making the correct decision or prediction, or instilling confidence in the research; statistics is the tool which helps determine the probability of making the right decision. The student must learn what probability means in research and how statistics will assist with decision-making.

Clinical therapists deal with patients who are different, yet have similarities. Twenty patients may be diagnosed as having rheumatoid arthritis, which is a similarity between the patients; on examination of these patients, however, you note dissimilarities. Treatment plans may be based on the dissimilarities. The function of statistics in physical therapy is to make optimal use of numerical data concerning the disease, patients, and the efficacy of the treatments while considering the similarities and dissimilarities.[3]

This chapter will establish the roots of scientific inquiry.

BASICS OF DATA

Variables

Research in physical therapy is concerned with animate and inanimate objects and numerical facts derived from data. A datum is a single observable or potentially observable phenomenon; a datum is a fact and can be a number (*data* are more than one datum).[4] A single datum can be a single observation, a single value, or a single measurement. A single isolated observation or value does not usually command attention in science because it does not provide sufficient descriptive evidence of traits, events, or phenomena. Science deals with quantities of information because of the variations in the universe; we therefore deal with data, not usually a datum. Data are collections of single observations of units, groups, or occurrences.

Data are a function of the problem or question and measuring instrument. Data vary from study to study but supply the researcher with the information needed to test the hypothesis or answer the question.[2] Data are quality or quantity representing elements or observations in an experiment.

A measurable characteristic, trait, or property is called a variable and a single measurement of a variable is a variate.[5] In a series of scores, effects, or characteristics, each unit may differ from another. A variable can change from one observation to another.[6] The differences between units of a variable are the quantities or qualities measured or assessed in research. Muscular force, heart rate, treatment time, latency, and methods of facilitation are a few variables that appear in physical therapy research reports. Most textbooks on statistics or research use the capital letters X and Y to denote variables.

Variables can be discrete or continuous. A discrete variable is a measurable characteristic that can assume only specific or limited values, exact numbers obtained by counting indivisible units. An integer (exact or whole number) is a discrete variable because it is a limited value. Real gaps exist between successive measures of discrete variables; the measures are not capable of infinite subdivisions. The number of patients sitting in the waiting room is an example of a discrete variable. Patients cannot be 5.5 or 10.3; they must number 5 or 10. If three transcutaneous electrical nerve stimulators are in use, and if an additional unit is put into service, the count goes from three to four without passing through any intermediate fractional values; at no time are stimulators slightly less than four or a little more than three. The measure of the variable is exact, and measurement proceeds by a series of gaps from unit to unit. The number of hospital admissions, the number of physical therapy clinics in London, heart rate, glands, or number of days in a month are other examples. Attribute is the term given and used for labeling variables that cannot be measured directly as numerical values. Physical therapists conducting descriptive research might be working with qualitative data which deals with male or female, fracture or no fracture, levels of membership, or colors of clinical uniforms. When numbers or units are assigned to attributes, like a frequency count, statistical analyses can be made. If attributes are countable characteristics, they are also discrete variables. The numbers of diathermy units currently used in different parts of the country are attributes which may interest physical therapists studying sociology or human ecology.

Continuous variables include muscular strength, distal latency of the median nerve, volume of water displaced by hands, and body weight. Measurable characteristics which can assume unlimited values are continuous variables;[7] they are approximate numbers obtained by measurement, capable of infinite subdivisions, without gaps existing between successive measures. If a therapist stimulates a nerve of a patient with 150 volts, the voltage is approximately 150 volts. The measured voltage may be more or less than 150 volts; to increase the stimuli to 160 volts, however, the force must pass through infinite gradations between 150 and 160 volts.

A continuous variable may be limited in practice to certain values by the measuring device (defined range), but theoretically could take on any value (unlimited). For example, latency of nerve is measured to the nearest tenth of a millisecond (3.6 msec), but if electromyography were refined to a more precise procedure, then the latency might read 3.589 mseconds. A group of young men is measured for their O_2 intake during a specified activity; the recorded quantities of O_2 per unit of time could conceivably fall into a series of numbers (0.75, 1.15, 0.92, 0.87, 1.26 liters/min), each having a different value. The series of different values constitutes a continuous variable, O_2 consumed per unit of time.

Variables can also be identified in research according to their function. Variables manipulated in the study are independent variables, whereas those measured as a result of the experiment are dependent variables. Examples of independent and dependent variables are shown in Table 5.1.

Table 5.1
Examples of Variables

Independent	Dependent
Cause	Effect
Treatment	Physiological response
Abscissa, X	Ordinate, Y
Controlled factors	Outcome
Manipulated variable	Measured variable
Material taught	Test score
Whirlpool bath	Increased joint range
Angle of hip	Quadriceps force

Derived Variables

Most variables in scientific inquiry consist of data which are direct measurements or counts[8] recorded as output of various instruments. Sometimes the values among two or more independently measured variables are best expressed as relations. Derived or computed variables are expressions of the relations between two or more quantitative variables; ratios, rates, or percentages.

A ratio can be a proportion or a relation between two similar variables. The ratio can be a single value, like a quotient (0.5) or a fraction ($^{50}\!/_{100}$). The quotient is preferred for computational purposes because of its ease in mathematical manipulation. In the classical study by Inman and coworkers,[9] the glenohumeral joint was found to move two degrees for every one degree at the scapulothoracic joint. The relation was expressed as a ratio of 2:1.[9]

A stated research question might be: Does the angle of the hip have any effect on the force generated by the quadriceps femoris muscle in strengthening exercises? The specific variables are identified from the question and shown in Table 5.2.

Table 5.2
Identification of Variables from a Research Question—Does the Angle of the Hip have any Effect on the Force Generated by the Knee Extensors?

			Independent	Dependent
Variable		A.	Angle of hip (degrees)	Muscular force (kg)
		B.	Type of exercise	
Variable factors		A.	Position of hands	Body size
			Support, no support to back	Cooperation
			Inclination of back support	Measuring instrument
				Researcher
		B.	Static	
			Dynamic	
			Concentric	
			Eccentric	
			Isokinetic	

A percentage is a form of a ratio expressed as a proportion. The percent ratio is a variable expressed as a proportion of a whole (100). The percent does not relate two variables.

Rates are also derived variables and are expressed as variables per unit of time. Rates are important in physical therapy. The distance a patient walks in a given unit of time or the time an impulse takes to travel over a segment of nerve are two examples of rates.

Population and Sample

A population is commonly considered to be the number of people living in a particular place or defined area. In research the meaning of population may or may not refer to the number of persons residing in a circumscribed area such as a city, county, state, or country. A population is all groups, collections, or aggregates of humans, animals, objects, materials, traits, measurements, events, or "things" in the world or universe. Population is the totality of observations of a defined variable, or all members of a particular species. This type of population in which every member is considered is an infinite population. In practice, a researcher cannot measure or observe every member in the world having the defined trait, so that the population often is defined to identify a specific group or size. If a physical therapist was interested in measuring the degrees of spasticity of the right biceps in every patient having a stroke, he could not complete the task in a lifetime even if people did not have strokes after the measurements began. Population is used in theory to include infinite variables; in practice, the population is often redefined to meet the needs of the researcher for study and for making inferences. The therapist could, however, define the population about which inferences are made from the data collected in the study. Population in this example could include all patients having strokes in Chicago, with the total observations confined to a circumscribed area already defined. The therapist could just as well have defined the population as all patients having strokes affecting their right–sided extremities and admitted to the therapist's hospital during the next two years. These types of redefined populations are called finite populations.

Not all individuals in a population can be measured because of economic, time, and physical constraints, so the therapist decides to measure only a proportion of the subjects representing the population. The specific part or proportion of the population selected for measuring the variable is called a sample. The physical therapist who defined his population as all patients having strokes of the right side and being admitted over a period of 2 years might measure only a proportion of the total number of patients appearing during the 2 years. The proportion of patients measured by the therapist constitutes a sample which will contain the numbers of patients established arbitrarily by the therapist. A sample is a subset of the population.[6]

Parameters and Statistics

If we were measuring a variable or variables among every person or trait in the world, we would be dealing with a value or measure called a parameter. A parameter is a value characteristic of a population and is the real or the true value. If heart rates of all physical therapy students could be measured during their first physiology examination, the average heart rate for all physical therapy students in the world would be a parameter. In statistics, parameters are usually assigned capital or Greek letters. On the other hand, if the heart rates of all physical therapy students attending the University of Kentucky were measured under the same circumstances as above, the average value recorded would be a statistic. A statistic is a value characteristic of a sample. Since only the students attending a particular university were measured from all physical therapy students throughout the world taking their first physiology examination, and since the students measured constituted a sample, the average heart rate now is a statistic. A statistic usually appears in small case or Roman letters.[6]

Using parameters in everyday verbal or written communication should be done with caution. Parameter is a mathematical term and defined as such[1] and should not be misused. Learn to communicate scientific terms appropriately, and do not use parameter unless discussing a value of a population in statistics.

Measurement

A substantial portion of research and clinical practice is spent assessing the subject and patient, respectively. Assessment requires measurement. Measurement is the assigning of numbers or quantities to behaviors, observations, functions, or objects according to rules.[10] Visual assessment and gross motor tests are common measurement systems used by physical therapists to evaluate motor functions.[11] The visual system does not include quantification of characteristics of the function; practitioners often support the soundness of the method, however, by anecdotal justification for objective measurement in clinical or research situations. Measurements in either situation must be measured, recorded, and studied appropriately to eliminate subjectivity.

Levels of Measurement

Measurement and quantification exist at several levels, depending on the mathematical and logical assumptions that are fulfilled. Measurements and analyses of numbers based on the higher level are considered more sophisticated than those of lower quality. The scale of measurement will determine the type of information obtained from data.

Caution must be exercised when using scales of measurement. Requiring specific levels of measurement in using statistics recently has been advocated in the physical therapy literature.[12] Stevens[13,14] developed the concept of scales of measurement and applied them to statistics. His concept has been refuted by statisticians. Lord argued that "the numbers do not know where they came from;"[15] Burke stated that the origin of numbers is irrelevant for statistical purposes;[16] Gaito wrote about inconsistencies in the use of scales of measurement,[17] that interval scale aspects were not important to the analysis of variance,[18] and that mathematical literature is not supportive of scale aspects as a requirement for use of statistics.[19] Although some researchers and textbooks advocate the concept of levels of measurement in selecting statistics, this book adheres to the mathematical belief that the rules of parametric and nonparametric statistics be followed rather than scales of measurement in using statistics.

Nominal Measurement. A nominal measurement is one in which numbers or labels have been assigned to differentiate, or represent, classes of objects, persons, or characteristics. The nominal scale is the weakest level of measurement because statements can be made only about presence or absence of equalities but not about quantitative differences between members of the category. The numbers identify, classify, differentiate, or label members of the category. They have no other function and cannot yield additional information about the events, effects, or traits. Classifying types of arthritis into categories such as osteoarthritis, rheumatoid arthritis, traumatic arthritis, and gouty arthritis are nominal types of variables or attributes. Attributes are countable characteristics when numerical values are assigned. Labeling academic courses by numbers, people by telephone or social security numbers, test subjects as numbers, addresses by postal code numbers, and athletes by their uniform numbers constitutes nominal types of values or discrete variables. Some scales of "activities of daily living" are assessed on the nominal level. A nominal measurement meets the minimal requirements of the definition of measurement, the assignment of numerals to objects or events according to defined rules.[13]

Ordinal Measurement. In ordinal measurement members of a category can be differentiated as having more of, the same, or less than a particular quality or trait than another member. A conditioned muscle contains less lactic acid than a nonconditioned muscle after a given amount of work. The exact amount of difference between muscles does not fall within the capability of the ordinal measurement. Because the ordinal measurement is higher on the hierarchical scale than the nominal measurement, it must also possess those qualities of the nominal measurement in addition to its own uniqueness of ordering or ranking members along some scale or dimension. The quantity cannot be measured in magnitude but can only reflect the relative position between members on the scale. Statements are not possible[7] about the quality of differences between members or the number of times one member is greater than or less than another. If the researcher chooses the ordinal level of measurement, he or she can only state that subjects having an above–knee amputation have shorter stride lengths than normal persons of similar height.

Interval Measurement. This level of measurement is more complex than the ordinal or nominal levels. Unlike the two levels of measurement already discussed, interval measurements use a scale of equal distances between points. The scale is given units of measurement, but the units of measurement are arbitrarily assigned. The interval scale is limited because the zero point is arbitrary. Temperature is the classical example cited. The distance between 10°C and 20°C is 10°C; similarly the distance between 20°C and 30°C is 10°C. One cannot state that 20°C is twice as warm as 10°C. The difference in magnitudes and zero points can be conceptualized if Celsius, Fahrenheit, and Kelvin scales of temperature are compared. Another example of interval measurement is calender time, because its zero point was assigned arbitrarily.[7]

Ratio Measurement. Ratio level measurement holds the highest position on the hierarchy and, therefore, possesses all the characteristics of the interval scale. The uniqueness of this measurement is its true or absolute zero point. This uniqueness enables the user to talk about the absence of something, for example, zero distance or zero time. Ratio judgments can be made about ratio data. It can be stated that something is two or three times as much as something else if it measures two or three times the number of units. The unit of measurement remains arbitrary, but the ratio scale allows us to multiply or divide each of the values by a specified number without changing the properties of the scale.[20] Many ratio level measurements are made in physical therapy research: nerve conduction velocity, length of a brace, treatment time, and volume of water displaced by an edematous hand are examples. Few ratio level measurements are used by social or behavioral scientists since zero intelligence or zero attitude cannot be measured.[21]

When a researcher discusses data or results of a study, his statements must fit the scale or level of the data collected in the study. The researcher must be aware of the measurement level and avoid making statements or judgments at ratio levels, for example, when data are ordinal. An awareness of these levels will help draw appropriate conclusions about data.

Rounding of Numbers

Before leaving basics of data, rounding of numbers in data should be mentioned. In published research reports, statistics are often reported to two figures to the right of the decimal point.

The rule in rounding decimal fractions to the nearest whole number is to drop the last place in the decimal fraction if it is less than 5. If the last place in the decimal fraction is greater than 5, the value to its left is raised by one. For example, the last figure to the right of the decimal is rounded up if the third figure is more than 5 (5.457 rounded up to 5.46) but is dropped if the third figure is less than 5 (25.342 dropped to 25.34).[22] This rule holds true for whatever degree of accuracy is desirable. Rounding may occur for any value whenever a decimal is used. If an integer (whole number) is used, then rounding is not necessary; 36 is not rounded to 40 but stands by its own value. The accuracy or precision of the unit is usually dependent on the measuring instrument. Stating a latency value of 2.9528 msec when using a clinical type electromyographic unit is pretentious because the instrument is not capable of yielding values of that precision. A value of 2.9 or 3.0 msec would be appropriate. The type of data, accuracy of the measuring instrument, or precision desired will determine the rounding-off procedure used in a research project.

ORGANIZATION OF DATA

Data obtained through surveys or experiments are often an unorganized collection of numbers which, on inspection, do not provide immediate information. For the collection of numbers to be meaningful to the researcher, the numbers must be arranged, summarized, or organized (arrays) so that pertinent information can be extracted.

Univariate Distributions

Univariate distributions are arrays that express a single variable. For example, suppose 10 people have the following strength values recorded from their left knee extensors; 50, 34, 26, 41, 37, 29, 45, 52, 30, and 46 kilograms (kg). These numbers, as a group, are not very meaningful to the reader, but if arranged in descending order of size, they become more meaningful:

52
50
46
45
41
37
34
30
29
26

An arrangement of this kind is called an order or rank distribution, but has only the advantage of providing the order of scores. The order of scores represents an array of a variable or univariate distribution.

Additional meaning or information may be obtained if the array (data) is classified or arranged into two groups: those having knee extensor strength over 35 kg and those having strength under 35 kg (Table 5.3). If we knew that strength of the knee extensors over 35 kg was high for 15-year old girls, we then could gain additional information from the grouping (Table 5.3). By examining the table further we can make other interpretations. We could say that 40% (4 of 10) of the subjects examined are under the cut–off point, or that 60% (6 of 10) were high for 15–year olds.

Frequency Distributions

Suppose we have recorded the latencies of the median nerve for 20 subjects as: 4.0, 3.5, 3.2, 4.0, 3.8, 4.2, 3.4, 3.5, 3.5, 4.0, 3.2, 2.8, 3.3, 3.8, 3.5, 3.4, 3.8, 3.4, 3.2, and 3.3 milliseconds. Now the values are arranged by order and frequency:

X	f
4.2	1
4.0	3
3.8	3
3.5	4
3.4	3
3.3	2
3.2	3
2.8	1
	$20 = n$

By ordering the latencies we see that several values appeared more often than once in the array. Grouping a series of numbers by frequencies is a convenient method of arranging data. A collection of scores arranged by order of magnitude and accompanied by frequencies is called a frequency distribution.[2] The latencies can be regrouped in still another fashion:

X	f
4.2–4.4	1
3.9–4.1	3
3.6–3.8	3
3.3–3.5	9
3.0–3.2	3
2.7–2.9	1
	$20 = n$

Table 5.3
Strength Data of Ten People

Strength (kg)	People
Over 35	6
Under 35	4

This arrangement is a grouped frequency distribution composed of data arranged within class limits (subgroups) to assist in the presentation of numbers.[23]

Research data can be presented by a group frequency distribution in still another fashion (see Table 5.4). The end points of the subgroups (classes) are class limits, class boundaries, or class intervals (e.g., 3.3–3.5). The midpoint between the upper and lower class limits of a class is called the class midpoint (e.g., 3.4).

Class limits are equal-sized divisions of the grouped frequency distribution; the lower (e.g., 3.3) and upper (e.g., 3.5) limits indicate the lowest and highest values recorded in a particular boundary or interval. The class limits are determined by subtracting the lowest value of a set from the highest value (e.g., 4.4 − 2.7 = 1.7). The remainder 1.7 becomes a quotient and is divided by the number of classes desired. In Table 5.4 the quotient 1.7 was divided by 6 (1.7 ÷ 6 = 0.28 rounded to 0.3) and 0.3 was established as the class size (the rule for rounding can be applied). The midpoint of a class is a value or measure halfway between the lower and upper limits of a class (e.g., 4.4 − 4.2 = 0.2 ÷ 2 = 0.1 + 4.2 = 4.3).

The group frequency distribution is a convenient arrangement when dealing with large sets of data as sometimes used in sociology, education, and psychology. Although no rule has been established, the usual practice is to group data into 10 to 15 classes.[24] The data ($n = 20$) of Table 5.4 were used for illustrative purposes only and do not correspond to recommended practices of using grouped frequency distributions with large sets of data (e.g., $n > 100$). This distribution, however, requires different statistical methods than for simple frequency distribution or raw scores and will not be discussed further in this book. The group frequency distribution is cumbersome when dealing with numbers having many digits (2537.485 and 3516.983). Another disadvantage is that the identity of the individual raw scores is lost in the grouping process. For example, the values of 116.8, 118.5, and 115.9 are lost in a class having limits of 115 to 119 and a midpoint of 117.

Table 5.4
Frequency Distribution of Twenty Scores with a Class Limit of 0.3

Limits	Midpoints	Frequency	Cumulative Frequency
4.2–4.4	4.3	1	20
3.9–4.1	4.0	3	19
3.6–3.8	3.7	3	16
3.3–3.5	3.4	9	13
3.0–3.2	3.1	3	4
2.7–2.9	2.8	1	1

Bivariate Distributions

Bivariate distributions are arrangements of paired values or observations of two variables. The bivariate distribution is used when interest centers on the relation of two variables. This will be used in discussing correlation in Chapters 7 and 10.

Frequency distributions are used to reduce a mass of data for increased understanding and ease of presentation. Frequency distributions are used routinely to describe observations grasped quickly and for presentation in tables. Remember that a series of numbers does not provide much information, but grouping the data into a meaningful distribution helps to extract additional information.

MEASURES OF CENTRAL TENDENCY

There are many other ways of describing data. Chapter 12 discusses tables and graphs for presenting data for group performance. A branch of statistics called descriptive statistics is used to describe data of a group. As mentioned earlier, a datum is of little value in applied research because a single observed score or value is likely to be unstable, unrepresentative of the true situation or condition, or unauthoritative. For example, if the physical work capacity of 100 children is measured and the range of scores varies from 500 to 1000 kg M/min, the child whose value is 1000 kg M/min may not be "typical" of the group if the majority of scores recorded were between 525 and 750 kg M/minute. For these reasons, large groups of numbers or scores best represent a characteristic or trait. Large groups of numbers or scores, however, become cumbersome; methods of descriptive statistics provide representation of a group of numbers with a single value, a statistic. Measures of central tendency are single values which supply information typifying the central performance of an entire group.[6] Any measure indicating the center of an array or series of numbers is a measure of central tendency.

Mean

The arithmetic mean is the sum of a set of measurements divided by the number of measurements in the set.[7] The mean is a measure that describes a typical, representative, or "average" value for a set of observations. The mean is the balancing point in a series of numbers. If you consider the force arm of a lever as a frequency distribution then the lever would be balanced if the fulcrum were at the arithmetic mean.[25] In other words, if the weight of the scores in the distribution is considered the force and the distance of the scores away from the fulcrum, the force arm of the level, then the force times the distance on one side of the arithmetic mean equals the force times the distance on the other side. The mean is considered a first-class lever, or teeter–totter.

We are familiar with batting average, average rainfall, grade-point averages, and average patient load. Since the term "average" is used for other measures of central tendency, the term "mean" is used in statistics and in scientific literature so readers do not confuse the measures of central tendency.

The formula for the mean is:

$$\bar{X} = \frac{\Sigma X}{n}$$

Computation of the mean can be illustrated in the following example consisting of the strength values recorded from the left-knee extensor muscles of 10 people. The sample contains 10 variates of the variable "strength".

X(kg)	
52	
50	$\bar{X} = \dfrac{\Sigma X}{n}$
46	
45	$= \dfrac{390}{10} = 39.0$ kg
41	
37	
34	
30	
29	
26	
$\Sigma X = 390$	

The Greek letter Sigma, Σ, is used to indicate the sum of these n observations. The symbol ΣX then directs you to sum all scores ($\Sigma X = 390$ kg). The formula for the mean directs you to divide the sum of scores by the total number of scores ($390 \div 10 = 39.0$ kg = mean). The symbol $\bar{X}$ (read X-bar) stands for the mean of the set of scores.

The mean has several important mathematical properties, but only two are discussed here. Any mean computed from a sample of size n is an estimate of a population mean, μ (pronounced mew). The sample mean is the most accurate and the most efficient estimate of the population's central tendency. The mean is affected by extreme scores in the distribution. The very small or the very large scores, which may not be typical of the majority of the scores in the distribution, influence the outcome. For example, if a distribution consisted of five scores, 1, 10, 12, 15, and 100, the mean would be 27.6, which is not typical of the scores 10, 12, and 15. Since the mean of a sample is the best estimate of the population mean, it is the most frequently reported measure of central tendency in the scientific literature.

Median

The median of n numbers of scores arranged in order of values is the middle number of the distribution if n is odd, and the mean of the two middle numbers if n is even. The median is also that point on a scale of measurements above and below which 50% of the scores fall. Examples of the median are:

Median of *odd* numbers of scores in a distribution (ranked): 4, 7, 9, 15, 20

The median is the middle number of the distribution. If n is *odd* as shown here with 5 scores, the number 9 is the median.
Median of *even* number of scores in a distribution: 2, 3, 8, 12, 14, 60
The median is the mean of the two middle numbers if n is even; therefore, the median is found by first locating the two middle scores of the distribution which are the numbers 8 and 12. Next find the mean of these scores by summing the values $(8 + 12 = 20)$ and dividing by 2, or $20 \div 2 = 10$. Ten is the median of the distribution.

The median is not distorted by extreme scores as is the arithmetic mean. For example, 1, 10, 12, 15, and 900 are scores of an odd-numbered distribution and 12 is the median, which is representative of the majority of scores of the distribution. The median is very easy to calculate and define and uses minimum mathematical computation. The median does not take into consideration the value of each score in the distribution. The median ranks the score occurring in the center of a set of data as the "middle" score. If scores are arranged in order, the score designated as the median has the same number of scores on either side of it.

Mode

The mode is the most frequently occurring value or score in a distribution. A distribution may have more than one mode. Examples of modes are 2, 4, 4, 4, 5, 6, 6, 6, and 6, where the number 6 is the most frequently occurring number and the mode; or 2, 10, 10, 13, 20, and 20, where the numbers 10 and 20 occur with equal frequency and more than any other score, so that the numbers 10 and 20 are modes. The mode is a nominal statistic and does not depend on the values of measures or their order. The mode is a count representing a particular trait.

CHARACTERISTICS OF MEASURES OF CENTRAL TENDENCY

Mean

The mean is used appropriately for measures which can be added and divided because of equal units of division on their scales. The calculation of the mean also involves adding and dividing; it is a statistic incorporating all scores of a variable in its calculation.[7] The mean can be used for subsequent arithmetical analysis of data.[6] The mean is the most stable or reliable measure of central tendency because it fluctuates less widely than the median and mode.[26] The mean is precisely defined and easy to calculate. It is the best estimate of its corresponding parameter of a population and is the only arithmetical measure that indicates size and position in a frequency distribution. The mean is good for describing data because it is the balancing point of a set of data. Although the mean is the preferred measure of central tendency in scientific research, it is one of the most abused statistics. When extreme measures are present, the mean is not the best representative of the measures and should not be used. Suppose a set of data contained scores of 1, 55, 60, 48, 62, 51, 52, 58, and 200. The mean of these scores is 65.2, a value larger than most scores, and is not representative of the data as the "average" or balancing point.

Median

The median is used when a measure of central tendency is needed to represent the middle value of a distribution. The median is not distorted by extreme scores; it is preferred to the mean when the scores of a frequency distribution are grossly asymmetrical.[7] This statistic varies less than the mode on repeated measurements of a variable. Although mathematical procedures are available for its calculation, they are limited and less satisfactory than procedures using interval and ratio data.[6] The median is a measure of position only and not a measure of relative status. It does not incorporate the magnitude of particular scores of the variable in its calculations.

Mode

The mode is used to indicate which score in a distribution has the greatest frequency. When plotting scores along a continuum, the mode is the highest point. It is a crude average that is not unique, because one or more modes may occur in a frequency distribution. The mode is a questionable measure of central tendency; its value may be a low or high score.[27] With repeated measurements of a variable, the mode varies more than the mean or median; therefore, it is less stable. The mode is nonexistent in continuous variables if the measuring instrument is precise enough to prevent two identical scores from being recorded.[24] The mode, when existent, is sensitive only to numerical counts.[6]

MEASURES OF VARIATION

Although the mean is the best measure for providing information about the central value of the distribution (centroid) and represents the entire distribution, the mean is only one point or measure of a distribution. Frequently the mean is not even a score contained among the scores of the sample. Other descriptive information about the distribution is, therefore, desirable. Perhaps you would like some information about how the scores in the distribution are spread or dispersed about the mean. The lowest and highest scores in the distribution, or the scatter of scores in one sample as compared to those scores of another sample, are interesting. The researcher is usually concerned with the reasons for causing or contributing to the variation in the data collected in the study.

The various ways scores scatter or spread within a distribution can be expressed by measures of variation or variability. Below are three distributions, each with the same size ($n = 5$) and each with identical means and medians. A cursory observation reveals that the distributions are different. How are the distributions different if their size, means, and medians are the same? The distributions differ in their degree of variability:

A	B	C	
1	6	2	
2	7	5	$\Sigma X = 40$
8	8	8	$\overline{X} = 8$
10	9	10	Mdn $= 8$
19	10	15	

Range

The range is the least complicated measure of variability because it is only a rough measure of scatter. The range is the difference between the largest and smallest scores in a distribution. The range for sample A is 18 ($19 - 1 = 18$), for B the range is 4 ($10 - 6 = 4$), and for C the range is 13 ($15 - 2 = 13$). By determining the ranges of the three samples we can easily determine which sample is more variable (sample A). The highest and lowest scores in a sample are customarily reported in research studies as the range. The range has several disadvantages:

1. The range uses only a part of the available information contained in a distribution because it involves only two scores.
2. The range does not provide any information about the numbers that are in a distribution or how the scores are distributed between the highest and lowest scores.
3. The range often becomes larger as the number of scores in the distribution is increased, which makes distributions of unequal sizes difficult to compare with each other.

Variance

A student of the life and behavioral sciences soon realizes that measurable characteristics vary. The weight, age, heart rates, nerve conduction velocities, joint ranges of motion, strength, and lung volumes of patients are different. Life would be boring if variability of measurable character-istics did not occur. Thus, the researcher needs some statistic to indicate the amount of variability in a set of data. The variance is a statistic that tells you how much the scores of a distribution deviate or scatter from the mean. A small variance indicates that most of the scores are relatively close to the mean, whereas a large variance indicates that most of the scores are some distance away from the mean.

Since the mean is the balancing point of a distribution of scores, basing the variations of the distribution on the mean as the starting point seems logical. The variance is formed from the squares of deviation scores from the mean. If you subtracted all scores from the mean, you would notice that some score differences from the mean (deviations) are positive because the scores are larger than the mean, and some scores are smaller than the mean, or even negatively labeled. If all absolute differences (de-viations) are added together, observing signs, the sum would be zero, but an old algebraic trick eliminates positive and negative signs by squaring the deviations. To illustrate:

X	Deviation $(X - \overline{X})$	$(X - \overline{X})^2$
2	-2	4
3	-1	1
$4 = \overline{X}$	0	0
5	$+1$	1
6	$+2$	4
$\Sigma = 20 \div 5 = \overline{X} = 4$	$\Sigma = 0$	$\Sigma = 10$

The formula which directs the above calculation is $\Sigma(X - \overline{X})^2$ and is the sum of deviations squared or sum of squares. If the above formula is used in the calculation of the variance of a large set of data, the work becomes tedious. Several formulas for calculating the sum of squares exist; these formulas use individual deviations from the mean when determining the variance, and they are all equally good.[26] The formula for variance sug-gested here can be used easily with electronic calculators:

$$\text{Formula for Variance: } s^2 = \frac{\Sigma X^2 - \frac{(\Sigma X)^2}{n}}{n - 1}$$

where s^2 is the symbol for the variance of the sample which is the best estimate of the variance of the population σ^2 (small sigma squared); ΣX^2 is the sum of all the squares (square each score and add up all the squares); $(\Sigma X)^2$ is the square of the sum (add up all the scores and square the sum; [e.g., $2 + 2 + 4 + 5 + 6]^2$); n is the size of the sample or number of scores (e.g., $n = 5$ in $2 + 3 + 4 + 5 + 6$); and $n - 1$ is a method, for certain algebraic reasons, of determining an unbiased estimate of σ^2. An unbiased statistic is one that shows no systematic tendency or trend to be greater or less than the parameter of the population.

Table 5.5 is an example of calculating the variance from a sample. The result of the example shows that the variance is a descriptive index of how each score differs from every other score; the variance is an average of the squared deviations from the mean.[28] The variance is a measure of deviation (dispersion, scatter, or spread) of scores about the mean. The variance is sometimes referred to as the second moment,[23] is a measure of variability not related to the size of the sample, and is independent of the mean. The variance reflects similarity or dissimilarity of the scores contained in the sample, and by examining the variance, we cannot determine the balancing point of the distribution of scores. The variance is not easily interpreted because its unit of measure is in squared terms of the variable. In the example, the variance of 4.89 is in centimeters squared (cm^2), but does not indicate area, because the original unit was measured as the diameter of the wound in units of centimeters. The researcher needs some statistic that will tell him or her about the size or magnitude of the variability throughout the distribution in the same unit as the variable. The variance is not reported in a research study as a descriptive statistic, but rather is used for further calculations and is often reported in the summary of analysis of variance.

Standard Deviation

Since the variation is in squared units, a measure of variability that is not in squared units but tells you something about the magnitude of the vari-

Table 5.5
Wound Size Before Physical Therapy (diameter in cm)

X (cm)	X^2		
5	25		
2	4	$\overline{X}$	= 6 cm
10	100	n	= 10
7	49	s^2	$= \dfrac{\Sigma X^2 - \dfrac{(\Sigma X)^2}{n}}{n-1}$
6	36		
5	25		
4	16		
8	64		$= \dfrac{404 - \dfrac{(60)^2}{10}}{10-1}$
7	49		
6	36		
$\Sigma X = 60$	$\Sigma X^2 = 404$		$= \dfrac{404 - 360}{9} = \dfrac{44}{9}$
			$= 4.88888^*\ cm^2$

* Note: 4.88888 rounded up to two decimal points = 4.89 cm^2 = Variance.

ation of the scores in the sample is desirable. The standard deviation is expressed in units of the raw data and is the square root of the variance. The standard deviation is also defined as the square root of the mean of the squared deviations from the mean.[6]

The formula for the standard deviation is:

$$s = \sqrt{\frac{\Sigma X^2 - \frac{(\Sigma X)^2}{n}}{n-1}}$$

where s is the symbol for standard deviation. The standard deviation is the measure of variability most frequently reported in the literature, although the variance is probably the most important measure of variability for statistical calculations. In the research literature the standard deviation is reported:

1. by spelling out the two words, standard deviation,
2. by abbreviating the two words, **SD**,
3. by reporting the value following the mean, 6.0 ± 2.21 cm,
4. or by using the symbol, s.

The standard deviation reflects the variability of scores within a sample and is based on how far the scores deviate from the mean. A large value for standard deviation indicates a large amount of variation within the sample, while a small value is indicative of little variation.

Coefficient of Variation

The researcher might wish to compare the magnitudes of standard deviations of similar populations; that is, he or she might want to know whether scores of a certain motor development test are more variable than scores by the same group of children on another motor development test. Making these comparisons by using the standard deviations would be very risky, because the scores of the different samples might also have different means or be derived from various study conditions. The standard deviation is based on the squared deviations about the mean of a specific group of scores and, when different standard deviations are compared with data having different means, the interpretations can be erroneous.

In order to compare the variability of different populations, a method of relative variation has been developed. The coefficient of variation is a ratio of the standard deviation and the mean in terms of a percentage; it has no units of measurement. The coefficient of variation is a very useful statistic for assessing variability among findings of different studies. The formula for the coefficient of variation is:

$$CV = \frac{s}{\bar{X}} \times 100$$

A high percentage indicates considerable variability in a set of data whereas a low percentage indicates a small amount of variability in the data.

Using the results of a group of children on two different motor development tests, the coefficient of variation might be:

Test A:
$$CV = \frac{0.25}{5.00} \times 100 = 0.05 \times 100 = 5\%$$
Test B:
$$CV = \frac{5.00}{50.00} \times 100 = 0.10 \times 100 = 10\%$$

Comparison of the coefficients indicates that the children's scores were more variable on Test B (10%) than on Test A (5%).

The coefficients of variation were used in the study on recording electrode placement in median and peroneal nerve conduction studies, in which latency and amplitude measurements were compared to ascertain the relative variability within the different measurements. Results of computing the coefficients showed that measurements of muscle action potentials were more variable than latency measurements, and, therefore, the physical therapist using these measurements can place more reliance on values of latency than amplitudes of muscle action potentials when assessing the functional integrity of motor nerves.[29]

Percentiles, Percentile Ranks, and Quartiles

Often the description of the relative position of a score in a distribution is needed, particularly in descriptive research (Chapter 6). The standard deviation is not always the best way to describe the spread of scores in a distribution. Percentiles, percentile ranks, and quartiles describe the spread of observations in a sample[28] and their relative positions.

A percentile is a score in the distribution which divides the frequency into hundredths (100 equal parts).[28,30] Suppose a certain percentage of subjects in a distribution have scores less than a specific value, and the value below which the certain percentage of subjects lies is the percentile. If 76% of subjects on a 50–item test score below 38, the value of 38 is the 76th percentile (P_{76}). The calculation of percentiles in Table 5.6 can be made from data presented earlier under Frequency Distributions.

Each score has limits (−0.05 and +0.05) taken as one–half a unit below and above the reported value. For example, a value of 3.3 msec will have limits of 3.25 and 3.35 milliseconds. In calculating the 30th percentile, the value below which 30% of the observations lie is six (0.30 × 20 = 6). Looking at Table 5.6, the sixth observation or subject has a value of 3.3 msec and the upper limit is 3.35 milliseconds. Thus, 3.35 msec is the value

Table 5.6
Latencies of Median Nerve (N = 20) in Rank Order

Subject	Latency (msec)	Subject	Latency (msec)
1	2.8	11	3.5
2	3.2	12	3.5
3	3.2	13	3.5
4	3.2	14	3.8
5	3.3	15	3.8
6	3.3	16	3.8
7	3.4	17	4.0
8	3.4	18	4.0
9	3.4	19	4.0
10	3.5	20	4.2

below which 30% of the observations lie, P_{30} = 3.35 milliseconds. Any percentile desired can be determined similarly.

Percentiles are calculated according to particular ranks. Percentile ranks are calculated according to specific values or the reverse process of calculating percentiles.[7] Look at Table 5.6 and select the 13th subject whose score is 3.5 milliseconds. The number of subjects having a latency below number 13 is 12, or 60% ($^{12}/_{20}$) × 100 = 60%). Number 13 occupies one-half of the value or distance between 3.5 and the next higher value of 3.8 msec (number 14), or 2.5% ($^{1}/_{20}$ × 100 = 5 ÷ 2 = 2.5%). The values between two observations must be considered for establishing percentile ranks corresponding to exact values. If the 2.5% is added to the 60% already obtained, the percentile rank of the value 3.5 msec is 62.5. Percentile ranks are used to express scores obtained in survey instruments (Chapter 6).

Quartile is a generic term for a score dividing the distribution into four parts or quarters. The first quartile corresponds to the 25th percentile, the second to the median, and the third to the 75th percentile. The quartile deviation is a measure of variability defined as half the difference between the 75th and the 25th percentiles. The formula for quartile deviation is:

$$Q = \frac{Q_3 - Q_1}{2}$$

where Q is the quartile deviation, Q_3 is the 75th percentile expressed as a quartile, Q_1 is the 25th quartile, and 2 divides the difference between the two quartiles in half. The 25th quartile of the data presented in Table 5.6 is 3.35 milliseconds. This value was obtained by multiplying N by 25% and adding the one–half unit above the value for the upper limit (20 × 0.25 = 5th subject, or 3.3 msec; 3.3 + 0.05 = 3.35 msec). The 75th percentile is

3.85 milliseconds. The quartile deviation is then found by placing the quartile values in the formula and solving for Q:

$$Q = \frac{3.85 - 3.35}{2} = \frac{0.50}{2} = 0.25 \text{ msec}$$

The quartile deviation is used for computing the Thurstone attitude scale (Chapter 6) and provides a quick and easy descriptive measure of the variability.

PROBABILITY

Students who have not taken a course in research methods or statistics are often overheard saying that something is true because "it" was proven by a research study reported in some journal. This faith in reported studies is encouraging to those who report research studies, but may be harmful. Researchers deal with probability rather than certainty when reporting their findings of a research study.

What is probability? Kerlinger has said, "Probability is an obvious and simple subject. It is a baffling and complex subject. It is a subject we know a great deal about, and a subject we know nothing about. Kindergartners can study probability, and philosophers do. It is dull; it is interesting. Such contradictions are the stuff of probability."[31] Probability is chance occurrence, likelihood, randomness.

Probability is a concept and method of estimating what might or should happen against what has happened. The researcher concludes or infers from what the collected data indicate; a risk is taken when making conclusions or inferences. Probability is not an absolute, but rather an estimate or a chance of something occurring. The findings of one research study do not make the situation absolute. Conclusions are based on a chance occurrence and, therefore, the decisions or inferences are not absolute. Sustained study or replication of research projects is really needed. The possibility exists that a single report is wrong or that a replicated study refutes the original study; on the other hand, the original study may be valid. Which study is then correct? Additional replication is essential to resolve the question. Researchers often ignore replication, thinking that only originality is meritorious. If the original report is never challenged then we continue to have faith in a concept that may be false. For years the vastus medialis was believed to be solely responsible for the last 15 degrees of full knee extension. This belief was challenged with the use of electromyography, and it is now believed that the vastus medialis functions in concert (phasically) with other components of the quadriceps femoris muscle to perform knee extension, and that all components of the quadriceps contribute to full extension of the knee. This is an example of one study for which no replication was performed for many years following the acceptance of a tenuous concept.

No intent is made here to discredit reports in any way. On the contrary, this book supports research and its processes. The point being made is that the researcher bases conclusions on the probability that the conclusions are true. The reader must understand probability theory and realize that there is always some possibility that the conclusions based on data of a "one-shot" study may be erroneous. Most of the time, reports are accurate and true and the authors of the report are truthful; conclusions are based on the collected data and the probability that the data are representative of the population or universe.

Historically, mathematicians developed the probability theory to win at gambling. Everyone has talked about his or her chances of winning something. Horse racing, card playing, batting in baseball, or staying alive while driving on a freeway are all problems in probability.[7]

THE NORMAL CURVE

The theory of errors states that chance events or occurrences in large numbers tend to arrange themselves in the form of a bell–shaped curve. This curve is called the normal curve, the bell curve, the normal probability curve, Gaussian curve, and the normal distribution (Fig. 5.1). The normal curve is a mathematical paradigm or standard which permits the researcher to compare collected data to the "ideal" and then to make

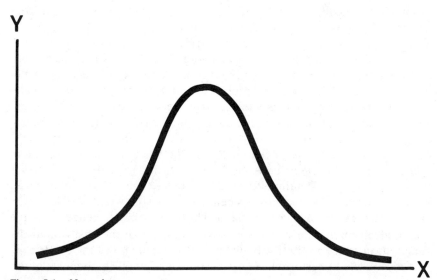

Figure 5.1.   Normal curve.

reliable conclusions, decisions, and predictions from the collected data. Few observable variables in research conform exactly to the normal curve when plotted, but frequently collected data approximate the normal curve. The normal curve offers convenience and practical application of mathematical theory through statistics.[31]

Figure 5.1 displays the normal curve, which is smooth, with the ends never touching the baseline (asymptotic). Asymptotic implies that the distribution contains an infinite number of data with no limits. The normal curve is representative of the population.

If you draw a broken line perpendicular from the midpoint of the peak to the abscissa (X), the point where the line bisects the abscissa represents the mean of the distribution (Fig. 5.2). Each proportion on either side of the mean (broken line) will be ½, or 50%, of the curve. If additional perpendicular lines (ordinates, Y line) are drawn from the inflexion points of the curve to the abscissa, the proportions can represent specific percentages or proportions of total area of the curve, or probability (Fig. 5.3). An inflexion point is a point along the curve where the curve changes in respect to the abscissa (X axis) from convexity (upward) to concavity (downward).[2] The proportions marked off along the abscissa correspond to standard deviation (SD) units because of the mathematical paradigm of the normal probability curve. In the normal curve, the mean is designated as zero and units to the right or above the mean are labeled positively as $+1$, $+2$, and $+3$ SDs. Units to the left or below the mean are labeled negatively as -1, -2, and -3 SD, respectively. The area between $+1$ and -1 SD represents about 68% (34.13 + 34.13%). The area between ± 2 SD

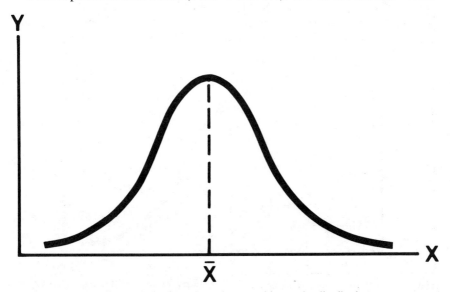

Figure 5.2. Normal curve showing where the mean bisects the distribution.

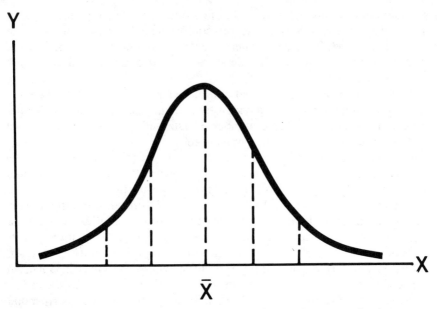

Figure 5.3. Broken lines are drawn from inflexion points to show proportional areas from the normal curve.

represents about 95% (47.72 + 47.72%) of the area, whereas ±3 SD is about 99% (49.46 + 49.46%) of the total area of the normal curve (Fig. 5.4). Additional units can be calculated since, in theory, the end lines of the curve are asymptotic (infinite) and never end; in practice, however, ±3 SD is usually representative of the total area. The curve is symmetrical and extends from plus infinity to minus infinity. The curve can now be used to

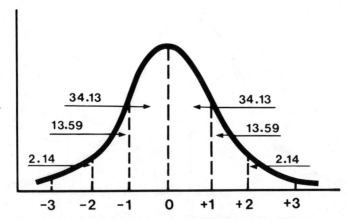

Figure 5.4. Normal curve showing areas (%) between ordinals at different standard deviations.

compare collected (obtained) research data to the ideal, normal, or standard paradigm.

If we measured 50 young women for maximum isometric force of the quadriceps femoris muscle with the knee positioned at 60 degrees from full extension and obtained a mean force of 60 kg and a standard deviation of 15 kg, we could interpret the data using the normal curve. We could say that about 68% of the scores fall between 45 and 75 kg (± 1 SD from mean; 60 ± 15). If we continued to measure the quadriceps femoris muscle strength of thousands of equal-sized samples of women under similarly controlled conditions, we could plot the mean values of the samples and find that overall (thousands), the mean values would follow a curve similar to the normal curve. Individual means will fluctuate by chance, but ultimately, the total group of means collected will cluster into the various proportions of the normal curve. Since testing infinite (population) numbers of subjects is not practical for time and money, small samples can be tested, the results can be compared with the normal curve, and reliable inferences can be made by the researcher about the population or quadriceps femoris muscle of all women in the world given rigidly controlled limitations of the selection criteria (age, mass, health, and physical activities).

GATHERING DATA

The purpose of research is to learn something about people, about events, or about specific "traits". To learn about these traits we gather information by taking several of them and studying the characteristics or variables of interest. After our study, we come to some conclusion—physical therapists are good people, hot packs are useless, or eccentric exercise is effective. To come to the conclusion, we must sample characteristics or data. We must take a portion of the defined population for study and, on the basis of the information contained in the portion selected, make a conclusion.

Making the correct choice of subjects or characteristics for the study will increase the likelihood of obtaining a representative population and, therefore, improving the generalization of the study results. If a physical therapist wants to study the effects of ultrasound on "frozen shoulder," the logical choice of subjects would be patients with frozen shoulder. Any patient having frozen shoulder may not be suitable. Frozen shoulder resulting from disuse (fractures or muscular paralyses) may not be the same as frozen shoulder from some acute inflammatory process. The point is that the study must be conducted on samples which are truly representative of a well-defined population. No perfect method exists for choosing a sample which assures an exact representation of the population. Successive samples taken from any population will differ among samples and from the population. The variation is called sampling variation and should be given consideration whenever conclusions are based on the data of a sample.[32]

An understanding of the concept of sampling is important to the researcher to avoid making incorrect conclusions from data. The method used to gather data can influence the outcome of the research and limit the statements made about the data of a sample (generalization). The method selected for gathering data will also help to determine statistical design of the study.

Advantages of sampling have been cited by Daniel and Coogler;[33]

1. Reduced cost. Measuring a particular trait on every member of a population is economically impossible if the population consists of everyone in the universe. If the population is defined as all staff members of a particular hospital, then there is no need for sampling because all staff members can be measured economically. Sampling, however, reduces costs of research by involving fewer items than contained in a large population.
2. Increased speed. Again, when dealing with a large population, you could not measure every member in a lifetime. Sampling enables the time commitment of the study to be within practical limits of the investigator's schedule.
3. Increased accuracy. By reducing the data in the study, all energy and time can be focused on the details of managing and interpreting the data.[33]

In research involving human subjects, a biased sample threatens the accuracy of the findings. Sample bias can be prevented by observing proper probability sampling formats.[34]

Models of Samples

The Random and Independent Sample. The random and independent sample is a method of selecting a portion of a population. Random implies that each member of the population has the same chance (probability) of being selected for the sample, whereas independent means that the selection of any one member in no way affects the selection of any other member.[2] Random sampling is used to generalize results to the population, to comply with the assumed premises of certain statistics, and to reduce biases likely to result from selection of other procedures.[35] This type of sampling is impossible in practice if the population is defined as the universe. Each member does not have an equal chance of being selected into the sample because of the infinite number of members. When defined populations are small, the random sampling method is used commonly. For example, if we sampled the physical therapists graduating in a particular year, the names and addresses could be obtained, labeled, and a sample of desired size drawn from the complete listing. This procedure would be random and independent if every new graduate had an equal chance of being selected into the sample, and if a selected graduate in no way affected the next selection into the sample. Tables of random numbers are available for the purpose of random sampling. The researcher places a finger over a spot on the table of random numbers without looking; the number underneath the finger is selected and the graduate's name having the corresponding number is selected into the sample. The procedure is continued until the sample quota is reached. Another procedure involves placing all numbers into a hat and selecting concealed numbers from the hat (lottery).

The Stratified Random Sample. This method is used commonly in public polls. The population is divided into subgroups or strata; each stratum contains a particular characteristic of interest, but only one characteristic is contained in any one stratum. Each stratum is sampled randomly and the various subsamples collected from the strata are combined into the desired sample.

An example will help clarify the procedure. Let us say that arbitrarily the Canadian Physiotherapy Association has 6000 members consisting of 1% (60) members having doctoral degrees; 10% (600) having master's degrees; 35% (2,100) having baccalaureate degrees; and the remaining 54% (3,240) having diplomas. Strata are represented by the numbers enclosed in parentheses. If the size of the sample was 10% (600) of the population (6000), then each stratum would contribute the percentage proportional to the population percentages. One percent (6) of 600 selected randomly from the doctorate stratum would constitute the partial sample representative of that portion of the population. Additional random samples would then consist of 60, 210, and 324, respectively, to compose the stratified random samples of members having various academic backgrounds. Stratified sampling works best when the variables of interest are closely related to the variables on which strata are based.[31]

Proportioning the strata is important if the researcher wishes to preserve the natural concentration of sections within the population. If 100 members of the Orthopaedics Section of the American Physical Therapy Association and 100 nonmembers of the Orthopaedics Section are surveyed, to determine whether the Section should be given special status by the Association, the outcome would be obvious. The survey should maintain the proportion of the two groups if stratified random sampling is the preferred method used. If there are 35000 members of the Association and 7000 are members of the Section, then the sample must include 20% from the Section and 80% nonmembers of the Section to maintain the proportion.

The Systematic Sample. This procedure is effective when a complete list of the members of the population is available for selecting the sample. If the researcher knows he or she has access to 100 children with cerebral palsy but wants a sample of only 25 for study, the systematic sampling method is appropriate. The population (100) is divided by the size of the sample (25) to obtain a quotient of 4 (100 ÷ 25 = 4). The researcher places the names of the first four children in a hat and selects the name of one randomly. Thereafter, every fourth name appearing on the list is selected until 25 children are in the sample. In practice, some researchers arbitrarily establish a systematic procedure other than the one discussed; for example, every other child with cerebral palsy appearing in the clinic where the researcher is employed is selected for study.

The Sample of Convenience. Researchers often accept volunteers or subjects into the study because the subjects are available to the researchers. In the hospital, the sample might consist of 20 patients having fractures of the humerus; in the university, it might consist of 30 volunteer students or the 50 rats purchased because these members of the sample are available or willing to participate. This method permits little choice of subjects chosen.[33]

Some statisticians have reservations about this technique despite its frequent use in research. The procedure is subject to biases.[30] If you wanted to determine whether a new approach to increasing muscular strength was effective, a hidden bias might be that all volunteers are highly conditioned athletes and strength gains normally would be slow in this group. The effects of the new approach to exercise might be overlooked or not be evident in this group because of the bias caused by conditioning. Limiting the population to only subjects conditioned similarly to those included in the samples has been suggested as an acceptable solution.[36]

The Cluster Sample. Another method of sampling that saves time and money and is convenient is cluster sampling. The population is defined and then nonoverlapping regions of subgroups (clusters) are formed. The cluster method seeks heterogeneity in the cluster. Clusters are composed of geographical or census units. Once the clusters are identified, several are selected randomly. When the randomly selected clusters are formed, samples from each are selected randomly and combined to form the desired sample size.

Suppose a researcher is interested in seeking information about a sample of patients having the Neer shoulder prosthesis over a particular period of time. Fifty hospitals where this type of shoulder surgery was performed during the designated period are identified. Ten hospitals are selected randomly from the 50 hospitals and then 2 cases are chosen randomly from each selected hospital to compose a sample of 20 patients.

CHARACTERISTICS OF THE SAMPLING METHODS

Random Sampling

The random sampling method is used when a population is defined by any subject being drawn independently for inclusion in the sample. Subjects are usually selected from intact groups. An intact group may include students of a particular school, all patients in a particular hospital on a given day, or all therapists assigned to a particular state chapter of the American Physical Therapy Association. It is a good technique for survey research. Random sampling has certain advantages: no prior knowledge of the traits or characteristics of the population are necessary; the larger the sample size the more representative the sample becomes because it approaches the population size; and most statistical analyses are appropriate.[37] Use of random sampling is difficult if the study requires patients with a particular condition because that type patient is not generally a member of an intact group. The intact group might, however, be feasible if time and money are available for studying patients over widely dispersed geographical areas. Random sampling requires that all subjects in the defined population be labeled or numbered; this may be costly and time-consuming. Other sampling methods which are available can gather the same information but much more economically than the random sampling method.

Stratified Sampling

This method of sampling is used when representativeness of a defined population is essential to the study. It identifies subgroup characteristics within the defined population and permits random sampling of subjects within the subgroups (strata). Stratified sampling increases in precision when the observed characteristic has some relation to the characteristic by which the subgroups are defined. Because the weight of subjects is related to their height, precision is gained for estimating height if the population is subdivided by weight. If the subjects in the strata are listed separately, the proportional samples are easily obtained. Although large numbers of subjects are required in the population, fewer numbers are needed than for random sampling. Stratified random sampling requires elaborate methods for estimating the population's parameters.

Systematic Sampling

The systematic sampling method is used to replace the random sample technique because of similarities or is used in conjunction with other methods (e.g., stratified). The method is generally inexpensive and rapid to complete. The procedures are easy to grasp. It differs from random sampling because each member of the population is not selected independently. Members of the sample are automatically selected once the first subject has been chosen. The procedure requires a list of subjects in the defined population, which can restrict its use because of the inability to list all members. Arrangement of subjects on the lists can cause trends or periodic variation, eliminating random selection. Systematic sampling is an acceptable replacement for random sampling if the list of subjects is in random order. Estimation of the population parameters is difficult.[37]

Cluster Sampling

Cluster sampling is used to reduce the large numbers of subjects needed for the random and stratified methods. It is well suited for studying intact groups; for example, students in classes of a school. It is used when it is impossible or impractical to obtain a list of all members of a defined population. Clusters are relatively representative of a population and save cost and time required by most other methods. The parts of a cluster are considerably more homogeneous than in random samples. Statistical analyses are difficult and the homogeneity of clusters results in some loss of precision. Subjects are not selected randomly but are drawn in bunches (clusters).

Convenience Sampling

This method is used when other procedures of sampling are not practical. Convenience sampling is frequently used in health related research because legal and ethical constraints require the researcher to obtain informed consent from human subjects prior to participation in the study. Although research has revealed that volunteers display distinguishing characteristics which may or may not require consideration when planning a study,[38] it is impossible to obtain informed consent from all subjects when selected randomly. Once volunteers have consented to participate in the research study, they can be assigned randomly to a control group or to different experimental modes. Considerable savings in time and costs result from using a sample of convenience. It affords little choice, however, about which subject will be chosen, and this may result in bias. Convenience sampling encourages selection of subjects in such a manner that random selection is not assured.[33] Although a sample of convenience does not meet the requirements of random sampling, it is acceptable provided that the researcher infers that the study results apply only to populations resembling the sample.[35] The population should be defined so that subjects drawn from samples compose a larger collection of subjects having similar characteristics.[33]

The student should be aware of the uses and shortcomings of the various sampling methods before engaging in research.

SUMMARY

Research involves the process of observing and measuring phenomena. When measured phenomena are quantified, mathematics can be applied to simplify interpretation. Quantitative measurements increase research efficiency; before an investigation begins, however, the researcher must have a clear understanding of the basics of data. Probability theory is an important concept in research and is the base of statistics enabling researchers to analyze data.

The mean, range, and standard deviation are the most frequently reported descriptive statistics in the research literature. The coefficient of variation is a good statistic for assessing variability among different studies reported in the literature.

Data gathering or sampling is important to the researcher to avoid making incorrect conclusions and predictions. Several methods of sampling have been presented.

This chapter has introduced the reader to the concept of quantitation in research. Table 5.7 provides a summary of which research processes have been presented thus far.

Table 5.7
Cumulative Summary of the Research Processes Presented

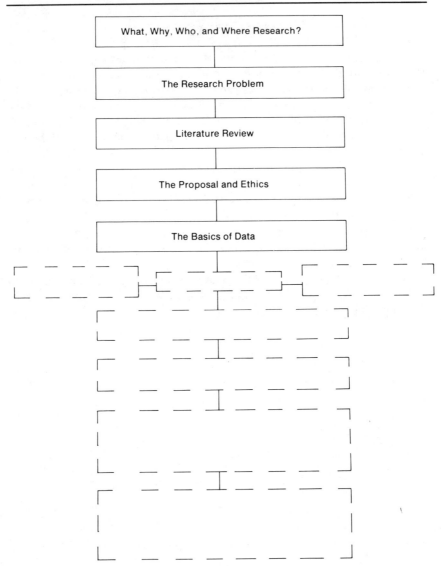

REFERENCES

1. Random House Dictionary of the English Language, unabridged ed. New York, Random House, 1967
2. Meyers LS, Grossen NE: Behavioral Research Theory, Procedure, and Design. ed 2. San Francisco, WH Freeman and Co, 1978
3. Curwen MP: Statistics in clinical research. Physiotherapy 56: 116–118, 1970
4. Wandelt M: Guide for the Beginning Researcher. New York, Appleton–Century–Crofts, 1970
5. Alder HL, Roessler EB: Introduction to Probability and Statistics, ed 6. San Francisco, WH Freeman and Co, 1977
6. Morehouse CA, Stull GA: Statistical Principles and Procedures with Applications for Physical Education. Philadelphia, Lea & Febiger, 1975
7. Ferguson GA: Statistical Analyses in Psychology and Education, ed 5. New York, McGraw–Hill Book Co, 1981
8. Sokal RR, Rohlf FJ: Introduction to Biostatistics. San Francisco, WH Freeman and Co, 1973
9. Inman VT, Ralston HJ, Saunders JB de CM, et al: Relation of human electromyogram to muscular tension. Electroencephalogr Clin Neurophysiol 4: 187–194, 1952
10. Michaels E: Measurement in physical therapy: on the rules for assigning numerals to observations. Phys Ther 63: 209–215, 1983
11. Peat M, Campbell G: Measurement in physical therapy. Physiother Canada 31: 132–136, 1979
12. Rothstein JM, Lamb RL, Mayhew TP: Clinical uses of isokinetic measurements: critical issues. Phys Ther 67: 1840–1844, 1987
13. Stevens SS: Mathematics, Measurement, and Psychophysics. In Stevens SS (ed): Handbook of Experimental Psychology. New York, John Wiley & Sons, Inc, 1951
14. Stevens SS: On the theory of scales in measurement. Science 103: 677–680, 1946
15. Lord FM: On the statistical treatment of football numbers. Am Psychol 8: 750–751, 1953
16. Burke DJ: Additive scales and statistics. Psychol Rev 60: 73–75, 1953
17. Gaito J: Nonparametric methods in psychological research. Psychol Rep 5: 115–125, 1959
18. Gaito J: Scale classification and statistics. Psychol Rev 67: 277–278, 1960
19. Gaito J: Measurement scales and statistics: resurgence of an old misconception. Psychol Bull 87: 564–567, 1980
20. Brown FG: Principles of Educational and Psychological Testing, ed 2. Hinsdale, IL, The Dryden Press Inc, 1976
21. Bolton B, Lawlis GF, Brown RH: Scores and Norms. In Bolton B (ed): Measurements and Evaluation in Rehabilitation. Baltimore, University Park Press, 1976
22. Style Manual, ed 4. Washington, American Physical Therapy Association, 1976
23. Schor SS: Fundamentals of Biostatistics. New York, GP Putnam's Sons, 1968
24. Edwards AL: Statistical Analysis, ed 4. New York, Holt, Reinhart and Winston, Inc, 1974
25. Weinberg GH, Schumaker JA: Statistics: An Intuitive Approach, ed 4. Belmont, CA, Brooks/Cole Publishing Co, 1980
26. Guilford JP, Fruchter B: Fundamental Statistics in Psychology and Education, ed 6. New York, McGraw–Hill Book Co, 1977
27. Horowitz LM: Elements of Statistics for Psychology and Education. New York, McGraw–Hill Book Co, 1974
28. Huntsberger DV, Leaverton PE: Statistical Inference in the Biomedical Sciences. Boston, Allyn and Bacon, Inc, 1970
29. Currier DP: Placement of recording electrode in median and peroneal nerve conduction studies. Phys Ther 55: 365–370, 1975

30. Remington RD, Schork, MA: Statistics with Applications to the Biological and Health Sciences. Englewood Cliffs, NJ, Prentice–Hall, Inc, 1970
31. Kerlinger FN: Foundations of Behavioral Research, ed 2. New York, Holt, Rinehart and Winston, Inc, 1973
32. Wilson EB, Jr: An Introduction to Scientific Research. New York, McGraw–Hill Book Co, 1952
33. Daniel WW, Coogler CE: Sampling in physical therapy research. Phys Ther 55: 1326–1331, 1975
34. Crocker LM: Let's reduce the communication gap. Guidelines for preparing a research article. Phys Ther 54: 971–976, 1974
35. Makrides L, Richman J: Research methodology and applied statistics, Part 5: Experimental design. Physiother Canada 33: 6–14, 1981
36. Dunn OJ: Basic Statistics: A Primer for the Biomedical Sciences, ed 2. New York, John Wiley & Sons, Inc, 1977
37. Montoye HJ: Collecting Data. In Hubbard AW (ed): Research Methods in Health, Physical Education, and Recreation, ed 3. Washington, Am Assoc Health Phys Educ Rec, 1973
38. Rosenthal R, Rosnow RL: The Volunteer Subject. New York, John Wiley & Sons, Inc, 1975

6

Nonexperimental Research

Research is a great adventure of the mind.
Gen. Dwight D. Eisenhower

Nonexperimental research is an endeavor that depicts and portrays traits and abilities of subjects; it shows the status of a group or organization; or it reveals trends or changes in characteristics of people. It may also describe conditions as they occur without the influence of the research.[1] Descriptive studies are called behavioral research if used to study the behavior or reactions of human beings,[2] or they are referred to as survey research if used to answer a question or depict opinions of subjects.[3] Nonexperimental research can satisfy curiosity, can solve a problem, and can be considered as any investigation not involving experimentation.[4] The data-gathering procedures of nonexperimental research enable the investigator to determine how facts relate to problems. Nonexperimental research is a process of systematic data collection.

Nonexperimental research in this book is an "umbrella" term to describe techniques that permit data collection without rigid controls, that do not involve experimentation, that measure behavioral characteristics with software and that are descriptive. Instruments used in nonexperimental research methods are generally less precise than those used in experimental investigation because of the evasive nature of the substance observed and studied. Software or paper instruments are the data-gathering tools of nonexperimental research. Statistical analyses can be applied to data gathered by software instruments because numerical values can be assigned to behaviors. A criticism of descriptive procedures is that they depend heavily on verbal behavior of respondents[6] and judgment of the observer.

Although nonexperimental procedures are commonly used in social sciences, psychology, education, and the humanities, they are also used in business and health fields. In health and medical research nonexperimental methods are used to study the nature and extent of illness, attitudes about use and receipt of health services, socioeconomic problems, growth

117

and development processes, and harmful factors in the physical environment.[7]

Nonexperimental research uses techniques for obtaining information directly or indirectly from the groups studied. Some specific instruments used in the direct technique are the oral interview, observations of behavior, rating scales, checklists, photographs, oral or practical tests, and case reports. The indirect technique employs questionnaires, attitude scales, classroom tests, and examinations of records. Depending on their use, some instruments are used for direct and indirect techniques. If the instrument is administered and recorded by an observer, the technique is direct. On the other hand, an instrument may be self–administered and recorded indirectly by the person being studied. Rating scales, checklists, questionnaires, and diaries can be interpreted as direct and indirect techniques of nonexperimental research.

Instruments are used in nonexperimental research to obtain standardized information from sampled persons or groups. The same instrument must be administered to all members of the sample, and conditions of administration must be similar. Information gathered from the sampling must be quantified (forced or multiple choice questions) or codified (open–ended questions) so that it can be analyzed and reported quantitatively. If the information is collected from a sample selected from a predetermined population and is gathered at one point or period in time, it is a cross-sectional survey. If the entire defined population is queried, the survey is called a census. When the data are gathered at different points in time to study time–ordered relations, the process is called a longitudinal survey.[8]

This chapter concentrates only on certain procedures and instruments used in nonexperimental research. These procedures and instruments represent direct and indirect approaches to data collection. The various instruments presented can operate in- and outside of laboratory situations. Instruments such as rating scales, checklists, and questionnaires can be used in experimental research. An investigator may want to compare behaviors of a group of subjects on two different occasions using rating scales. Whenever a method of comparison involving two or more groups, events, or quantities is used in a study, the process is an experiment. The experimental methods of research are discussed later in this book. The historical method is also discussed briefly. This method is performed outside the conventional laboratory setting. Although informative studies are descriptive and exploratory, they establish norms or baseline data.

DIRECT METHODS

Oral Interview

The oral interview is a way of involving the investigator or his assistants face–to–face with the subject to obtain information through conversation.

Types of Oral Interviews. The interview can be classified into one of two types, which are functions of their classifications.

1. Informal. This type of interview is used in reviewing applicants for employment or college admissions, or in counseling employees. Questions are usually devised during the actual process of the interview in accord with the spontaneous needs of the interviewer and direction of the conversation. The responses are free (open–ended); the interviewee responds spontaneously to questions or flow of conversation between the persons involved in the interview. The informal interview is flexible with the direction of conversation. The informality enables the respondent to relax and react as if the situation were taking place in a natural and commonplace fashion, an everyday situation. The informal interview can be held with the respondent and several interviewers, for example, while dining or during group dialogue.

Since the purpose of interviewing is to gather information that cannot be obtained in another manner, the interviewer forms impressions, and following the interviewing session, puts the impressions into some narrative form. A record of the conversation is made for later and acts as a source for comparing other respondents. The informal interview is not often used for research, however, because it lacks organization of specific and similar questions asked of all interviewees. In other words, the informal interview is not structured in advance and can change directions during conversation with regard to the needs, personalities, and responses of the interviewees. This form of interview is unlikely to be consistent when repeated. Occasionally the informal interview is used in pilot research when the researcher wants to determine the feasibility of a content area or ascertain the appropriateness of questions in advance of an actual study. As questions become more directed and organized in specific content areas, the informal interview loses some of its informality and approaches the formal interview.

2. Formal. The formal interview is used in research because questions can be organized in advance of the interview, questions are limited to specific content areas, and responses are controlled. In controlled responses, the respondent is given specific choices to answer each question and must select one answer. For example, the patient might be questioned about how many physical therapy treatments he or she received for a low back strain, but the choices of response may be "less than five," "five to ten," or "more than ten" treatments. The respondent then selects one answer as the controlled response to the question (forced choice). The formal interview has more uniformity and comparability than the informal interview because of its controlled structure. Responses to the formal interview are consistent and, therefore, may be used as a research instrument. Only the formal interview is discussed in detail.

Planning the Formal Interview. Questions are planned in some coordinated pattern before the interview is administered. Several questions may have to be devised to obtain the desired information about one content area. Changes in wording may be necessary when asking questions in sensitive areas. Respondents must understand the questions completely before correct or satisfactory responses can be expected. The questions must be structured effectively to ensure communication between the interviewer and the respondent. The entire interview sequence (guide or schedule) should be planned and organized in advance of the actual interviewing. In preparation of the interview, questions should be written and rewritten several times to obtain full information and to avoid ambiguity. The informal interview can be used to pretest questions among friends, experts in the content areas, or a few patients for whom the interview will be intended. This pilot (exploratory) approach provides the researcher with valuable information about the appropriateness of questions, reactions to questions, levels of understanding, and length of time needed for the interviews. Questions must be planned carefully and worded precisely.

Requirements for Successful Interviewing. Planning the questions carefully has already been mentioned. The selection and training of interviewers are important and will be discussed separately. The order of questioning is important; questions that seek priority information must be asked early in the interview in case the respondent becomes disinterested and refuses to answer any more questions. Controversial or sensitive questions should be saved until the end of the interview to avoid abrupt termination before the most important information has been obtained. Using several interviewers, each having small numbers of subjects to interview, reduces fatigue, interviewer bias, and length of time for the study.[9] A preface outlining the need, purpose, and use of the interview information is helpful in setting the tone of the interview and relieving any apprehension for the respondent. Assurance of anonymity is important. If a tape recorder is used, the respondent must be aware of and agree fully to its use. Taping or notetaking is advisable when the respondent provides nonconfidential, factual and statistical information; it is inadvisable if he or she is giving confidential matter.[10] Taping and notetaking may threaten the respondent in the latter situation. Nevertheless, the interviewer must choose one of these methods. The exact recording of responses as well as the exact questioning must be followed during interviews for preservation of the information.[11]

Job of the Interviewer. Once the interview plan has been determined, the interviewer must locate members of the sample. Sometimes locating members means traveling to different locations within or outside a city. Going house-to-house, or interviewing physical therapists while working may be examples of the traveling needs of a study. The interviewer must obtain the interview after locating a member of the sample.

The interviewer must gain the respondent's acceptance and gain access to the interview by being polite, friendly, and being considerate of the respondent's available time. The interviewer must ask questions with an acceptable tone of voice, interpret responses, and proportion the time of the interview, yet allow enough time for the respondent to respond as necessary. The interviewer's job has been estimated as one-third interviewing and two–thirds traveling, locating respondents, editing interviews, and performing required clerical tasks.[9]

Interviewer Training. Training each interviewer on interview proceedings will generally improve the quality of the study. Interviewers must have training, even for highly structured interviews, if dependable and objective information is to be gathered. The amount of training required rises as the extent of the interview increases and its structure decreases.[8] The interviewer(s) must be aware of what information is relevant to the study, what information is nonessential, and the difference between factual, opinion, and knowledge responses. Every interviewer should know the procedures for recording interviews and editing their contents. Some instruction on how to remain neutral to responses is essential. Training should consist of familiarization with the interview structure, conditions, logistics, and controls. Once these factors are learned, interviewers should conduct practice interviews and receive corrective feedback for improving their performances. When researchers and students work alone in studies using the interview training, tapes or films should be used for training. Videotape recordings of practice sessions are effective as corrective feedback.[8]

Sources of Error. Errors are ever present in research, and interviewing is no exception. Several sources can contribute to errors, for example:

1. Errors of Interviewer. In spite of the training given to each interviewer, errors will occur. Interviewers might not ask particular questions with the same voice inflections and this could cause different interpretations by respondents. The interviewer might probe differently using different questions with the same voice inflections and this could cause different interpretations by respondents.[11] The interviewer might probe differently using a variety of questions with different respondents which could result in errors of response. Errors can result from transforming responses of respondents to records, or in coding information. Interviewers can bias the results by interjecting opinions or making subtle remarks about questions or responses. If the interviewer does not understand the language or colloquial expressions of the respondents, wrong interpretations could be made.

2. Errors of Respondents. Not understanding the requirements of the question or a lack of knowledge about how to answer the question can lead respondents to lie or give fictitious responses. Respondents may not wish to cooperate once the interview begins or may give replies without thought to terminate the interview. Of course, the accuracy of the interview depends on the success of getting honest responses. The tendency of the respondent to give inaccurate responses is called the response effect.[12]

Sources of Refusals and Discrepancies. Interviewers who are trained poorly, faulty interviews,[13] and the process of the interview[14] are major contributors to refusals in interviews. Rates of refusal in interviews can vary between ethnic groups and ages. Older people are more reluctant to give interviews than people 45 years of age and younger; no distinct personality type has been associated with refusals.[15]

Inconsistencies among respondents seem to occur more often among men, older respondents, and people having less education than among women, younger respondents, and persons who have had some college education. Age of respondents is usually reported more reliably than educational levels of respondents. Women provide more inconsistencies about their real age than do men. Reduction in content error is attained when questions about the respondent's actual educational level are preceded by questions about whether the respondent had sufficient opportunity to obtain all the desired education.[16] No differences in the respondents' reporting psychiatric symptoms to men or women interviewers were found by Colombotos and coworkers.[17]

Inconsistencies can be caused when interviewers are embarrassed by certain topics, such as why women cannot have babies, income levels, whether families are receiving welfare, religious affiliations, and who friends are.[18]

Advantages of the Interview. Each survey instrument has its own uniqueness for gathering particular types of information. As a result of its uniqueness, each instrument has certain advantages. Some advantages of the interview are:

1. Collects Distinctive Information. The interview is used to gather information about opinions, attitudes, and beliefs on certain issues. People are less likely to reveal information of a confidential nature in other methods of data collection than in the interview, face–to–face with the interviewer. The interview tends to be a device for asking either general or specific questions. The respondents can react freely to its questions or can be given a choice of several responses to each question. The interview is used to seek information which cannot be obtained by other data–gathering instruments.

2. Enables Instant Interpretation of Responses. The interviewer can interpret a response to a question and then ask other questions to supplement replies or can alter the line of questioning to other topics. Most other instruments cannot redirect questioning according to responses given. If a respondent does not understand a question within the accepted predetermined guidelines for alternative wording, the interviewer can reword the question. Alternative wording may introduce a source of variance.

3. Establishes Rapport with Respondent. The personal contact with the respondent affords an opportunity for the respondent to obtain a clear understanding of the research. Although subjects are given some information about a study before participating, often they are not given an opportunity to ask questions about a project to any great extent. The interview permits the "personal touch" during the data-gathering process.

Disadvantages of the Interview.

1. Honesty. The interviewer must assume that the responses are given honestly. Respondents may answer a question in the manner they think the interviewer wants to hear, or they might not wish to divulge exact or real personal information about such things as income, religious beliefs, marital relations, tax returns, whether they have followed a therapist's recommendations for home care, and so forth.

2. Interviewer Bias. The interviewer often interjects personal influence into the conversation causing the respondents to react to specific questioning that may be contrary to their own beliefs or opinions. The interviewer may interpret such responses in a way that supports his own interpretations of the study.

3. Expensive. Oral interviews requiring large numbers of interviewers and respondents can be costly. Each interview may require only 30 minutes, but traveling and locating the same respondent may require an additional 30 to 60 minutes. Overhead expenses include labor, travel, and clerical costs.

Observations

Making observations of a person, groups of people, or events are direct methods of gathering information. Although some degree of observation is an essential ingredient in all research, various types of observations are used in descriptive approaches to research. Observation techniques are used to a large extent in educational and psychological research when children's behavior is studied. It is used in physical therapy during functional analyses when the therapist wants an impression of how the patient performs specific activities. Observational approaches to research are pre- *i* ferred over self–report data (indirect method) when prejudice or bias might occur. Observational methods usually yield more accurate quantitative data than that gathered from indirect or self–reporting methods.[8] The presence of the observer during a behavioral situation may alter the real situation, placing a constraint on the information collected. Repeated observations are time-consuming, but several sessions of a sufficiently large subject sampling are necessary for dependable information. Also, having two or more independent observers of a single event greatly improves the consistency of the data.

The major types of observations are participant, nonparticipant, and ethnographic.[19] Participant observation is the direct witnessing of some behavior and then the recording of that behavior on some software instrument for later interpretation. Nonparticipant observation might include simulations and case studies. Not all observations are done in naturalistic settings. Occasionally the researcher prefers simulated situations where some aspects of the activity are controlled or manipulated. In simulation observation, the situation is created by the researcher. Although the behavior exhibited by the subjects is not natural, the technique permits observations of behaviors or situations that are uncommon or complex. Role playing is an example of simulated observation. This approach has been used to determine the consistency of rating scales in assessing the clinical performance of students.

Ethnography is a "shot gun" approach in observational studies. It may involve participant, nonparticipant observations, or both. It is a qualitative form of research that studies and describes behavior which unfolds in the clinic; it reveals how we interact with our health care associates.[20] General questions rather than hypotheses guide the study and data may be represented by variables and review of the literature. The researcher uses a variety of data–gathering instruments or strategies along with observation. Data–gathering instruments include interviews, questionnaires, and attitude scales, but along with these instruments other data, such as portions of medical records (eg, progress reports), surveys, quality assurance reports, and review of literature are used.[20] Ethnography involves intensive information–gathering of several variables over an extended period of time and in a natural setting.[19]

Observational data are recorded by using a diary, checklist, rating scale, or case-study procedures. Each will be discussed briefly.

Diary

The diary requires recording information in narrative form at predetermined intervals. The intervals can be specific times during the day, daily, weekly, bi–weekly, or some other designated period. The researcher sets the times for observing the behavior, events, or items. For example, a physical therapist may want to study movements of a child with multiple handicaps and may make observations in the morning and evening for a period of days. (A study of a patients' behavioral activities or reactions to treatment sequences is another example.) The events of each observation are recorded as a chronology, or diary. A case study is a product of the diary. The diary is often a narrative summary of occurrences during the designated interval; anecdotes may be kept on the sequence of observations. Progress notes, a patient's record covering the course of hospitalization, or records of a series of treatments may be considered forms of the diary. Logs and journals are also forms of a diary and are considered indirect methods of nonexperimental research if they are self–reported.

Checklists

Checklists usually list specific behaviors, events, or traits which the observer then tallies as having or not having occurred during the period of observation. The numbers or types of responses are recorded in appropriate categories. If a therapist wants to research occurrences or presence of symptoms associated with a specific condition (low back strain) through assessment, a checklist is used to record the presence or absence of symptoms. The list of activities to be observed is preplanned before the observation. The researcher usually is interested in certain criteria or occurrences and prepares a list of things of interest to the study. Depending on how quantities are recorded, data can be analyzed by statistical methods: computations of means, percentages, relationships, and comparisons can be made.

Although numbers are assigned and statistical methods used, the underlying information is subjective, the result of the observer's judgment. Checklists are crude instruments when converted to quantitative values. Overinterpretation of data is a danger which must be guarded against. The researcher must constantly ask whether the checklist items are representative measures of what is being assessed. The value of the checklist can be increased by performing pilot studies to ensure that terms on the checklist are really similar to those the respondents would use in daily behavior. This device is suited to test hypotheses and operates at the conscious and overt levels. The checklist is a direct method of nonexperimental research if used by an observer to list behaviors of others; it becomes an indirect method if the respondent uses the instrument for self–assessment. Using the checklist as an indirect method of survey permits responses from the respondent without writing lengthy narratives (checking choices) or giving long verbal discourse (free responses). The checklist is suitable for a mail-type instrument for self-assessment or as a "door-to-door" type instrument for evaluation by an interviewer.[21] A profile or outline form can also be a form of checklist.

Rating Scales

A rating scale enables the researcher to observe the actual behavior or event and record what is observed or make judgment about interactions between events, traits, or behaviors. The observer records the occurrences by checking off items on a list or rates the object or behavior according to categories on a numbered scale. The scale measures a subject's behavior and permits an element of intensity in the responses.[9] Scaling is a procedure that attempts to determine quantitative measures of subjective abstract concepts.

Types of Scales. The kinds of scales used for recording occurrences may differ slightly.

1. Category. This form of rating scale is categorized into several behaviors which are then subdivided into levels of responses. The observer or judge checks an appropriate level of a particular category when the subject's behavior has been observed. The manual muscle test conforms to the category-type scale when the grading system uses "Normal," "Good," "Fair," "Poor," and "Trace." A rating scale variant for assessing the frequency of pain among patients having low back strains is illustrated:

How often do you have pain in your low back?
—Always present
—Often present
—Sometimes present
—Seldom present
—Never present

This is an ordinal scale providing a relative position or level of the patient's condition. Other examples of ordinal level evaluation forms are Disability Rating Scale, Physical Rehabilitation for Daily Living, and Maryland Disability Index.[22]

2. Numerical. Numbers are assigned to the levels of a category in place of or in addition to descriptive phrases. The numbers form a scale and provide equal intervals.

Appropriate statistics can be used in describing or analyzing numerical scales.[23] In the above example, the frequency of pain among low back strains can be evaluated by using a scale formed with numbered values:

5	4	3	2	1
Always Present	Often Present	Sometimes Present	Seldom Present	Never Present

The activities of a daily living scale of rehabilitation among nursing-home residents is an example of a numerical rating scale.[24]

The psychological factors associated with prolonged work are of interest to researchers studying physiological stress. The psychological factors of stress (prolonged work) can be studied by subjectively rating the intensity of the physical work; this is called perceived exertion. Physical work brings about certain sensory inputs (joint pain, muscular effort, breathing patterns, and sweat) that permit the participant to perceive exertion. Borg has developed a psychophysical numerical ratio scale for rating perceived exertion (RPE). His scale ranges from values of 6 to 20 allowing for a 15-point scale. The scale is both valid and reliable for many physiological variables such as perceived exertion. Heart rate and work intensity ratings are a linear function.[25,26]

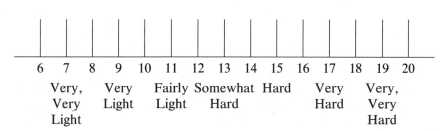

3. *Graphical.* This instrument combines the category and scale traits by forming equal-appearing intervals over descriptive phrases. The graphic instrument forms a continuum of equal intervals in the mind of the observer but does not assign numbers to the scale.[26] The example would then appear as:

Always	Often	Sometimes	Seldom	Never
Present	Present	Present	Present	Present

Advantages of Rating Scales. Rating scales are easy methods for recording information. These scales provide vivid concepts of what is being judged and are quick and easy to interpret. The scales offer variety in measuring data, and because intervals and numbers can be assigned, statistical analyses are possible. Additional advantages of the rating scales are that they require little time to use, are generally interesting, and have a wide range of use.[27]

Rating scales can also be constructed as indirect methods (self-assessment) of surveying subjects. The instrument is more sensitive and informative than merely "yes" or "no" answers. Scales actually encourage guessing on the part of the respondent, therefore impressions are projected.

Disadvantages of Rating Scales. These instruments are often abused because they are so easy to construct and use. People sometimes treat the information from scales as absolute or real, whereas the information is really subjective by nature and indicative of how a respondent wants to make judgments on a continuum.

Raters may rate hard or easy depending on the circumstances or questions of the scale. People have the tendency to rate persons whom they like higher than those they dislike. The tendency to rate hard or easy can be prevented by designing asymmetrical scales which have only one unfavorable descriptive term (poor) and four favorable terms (fair, good, very good, and excellent).[6]

The categories of a rating scale are subjective, and this can cause rater bias. Whenever a rater carries over a generalized impression of the scale's topic from question to question, a systematic bias occurs. Raters may systematically rate 50% or more of the questions above average, average, or below average.[4] This bias can be thwarted by rating one trait at a time for all topics, or by having one trait at a time for all topics, or by having one trait on a page rather than having one topic on a page.[6]

Construction of Rating Scales. In construction of scales consideration should be given to the number of intervals along the scale. If a scale is divided into a large number of intervals, the selection becomes so finely divided that the observer has difficulty in choosing a level and rating the event quickly. If a scale has only a small number of intervals, the scale will be coarse and will not differentiate between levels. Three to seven intervals are the numbers most often preferred;[6] occasionally, four to ten will be used.[9] If an odd number of intervals is used, the middle interval serves as a "neutral" zone, which forces ratings to either side of the neutral zone. Some observers do not like to use the neutral level; errors of central tendency can be avoided by using the odd-numbered intervals. Changing the position of the extreme favorable and unfavorable words can prevent systematic ratings, for example:

painful ＿＿＿＿＿＿＿＿＿＿＿＿＿ pleasant
well ＿＿＿＿＿＿＿＿＿＿＿＿＿ sick

Another concern about scales is that the two or three intervals between the extreme points are not identified as easily as the polar end points.[22]

The Case Report

The case study or report is usually a comprehensive account about a subject or a particular disease or condition. The details of the report are concerned with the unique or exceptional characteristics of a course of physical therapy, or the aspects of a rare condition. The case report may also focus on a family, unit of equipment, a community, or a hospital function with data being gathered over a period of time (weeks to years), making it longitudinal by design.[28] The purpose of a case report is to determine the logical interrelations of its components.[11] The details may provide valuable data for formulating tentative generalizations about patients who have similarities.

The case report is a kind of survey or profile because it encompasses observation; it is a record of behavioral responses, or shows various patterns of traits. The study may involve test scales for a number of traits or characteristics. The report must be presented in a clear, concise, narrative style.[29] Medicine, rehabilitation, law, clinical psychology, physiology, and education are fields that use the case study, whereas it has no advocates in physical education.[30]

Components of the Case Report. The report should have a title that briefly reveals what the study is about. The title should identify the disease, condition, or the treatment. Historical data covering the period of time leading to the presenting of the patient as well as demographic data (age, sex, occupation, and race) are considered important for background information.[29] This information could be obtained from records (files) or from the patient or a member of the family and includes details of onset and prior treatment. Complete and accurate medical and physical therapy procedures should be included in the report. A summary of diagnostic measures and physical therapy assessments, pertinent physiological and pathological findings, and unique devices yielding particular measurements are also included in the report. If follow–up information was not available when the case was reported, then statements about the prognosis are desirable. An appraisal of the effectiveness of recommendations is also helpful to readers.

Value and Limitations of the Case Report. The case report is "almost synonymous" with nonexperimental research because it describes in great detail the events, characteristics, and traits of an individual.[31] The case report is also effective in studying organizations, educational programs, or communities.[3] Because a case report relates the uniqueness of a treatment approach or a disease, the information supplied is sometimes generalized to provide increased understanding of a number of essential qualities.[30] The report provides insight into the factors associated with the unusual condition or treatment approach and can lead to further research. It permits the researcher to see a patient in his total relation to therapy, to the institution, or to the health care system. Both subjective and objective information is acceptable in the case report, as well as the study of variables that are troublesome to quantify. The case report allows the researcher freedom in how much data to collect and disseminate; the researcher can begin or end whenever he has sufficient data or when time becomes a critical factor.[4] Case reports provide readers with a source for hypothesis (proposition) testing. It is particularly amenable to clinicians who do not want to engage in experimental research but want to make valuable contributions to the physical therapy literature by reporting detailed descriptions of unique cases.

Because the case report represents a single and unique situation, caution must be exercised in making generalizations about a single subject. A datum may not be representative of a population or provide a firm basis for scientific prediction or inference. Randomization, replication, and control procedures are characteristics of research not typically used in case reports that make it possible to generalize about findings. The information supplied in the report may not be objective but selectively described and may include the researcher's prejudice from working closely with the subject.[4] Because the conclusions are based on a single and unique case, the conclusions of the report are difficult to verify without undertaking a controlled study.

Occasionally the single case or subject is used in experimental research when a variable is manipulated. The single subject (time series) experiment includes the collection of baseline data before and after replications of treatment. This approach is presented in Chapter 9 dealing with experimental designs.

INDIRECT METHODS

Questionnaire

The questionnaire, like the formal interview, is an instrument that uses a set of predetermined and prearranged questions given to respondents to obtain standardized, quantifiable data. The same questions are asked of all respondents so that comparable information can be gathered. Two types of questionnaires are commonly used, the self–administered and the group–administered questionnaire. In the self–administered questionnaire, the respondent is asked to complete and return it to the researcher. The mail questionnaire is the best example of this type and is discussed in greatest detail in this section. The group–administered questionnaire is given to a collection of subjects assembled who answer all the questions before being dismissed. An example is a group of physical therapists attending a meeting and who are given a questionnaire to complete; on completion, the members of the group depart.

Preparation. Theoretical guides for planning the questionnaire are generally lacking. The researcher using this instrument must rely on experiences, logical reasoning, and some general rules for assisting in its development. Defining the problem is the first step in planning research. Once the problem (question) is defined, aims and objectives are formed. Literature must be reviewed to aid in asking pertinent questions and assisting the researcher in planning the scope of questions. The researcher must decide whether a hypothesis will be tested or whether gathering general information will answer the question. If a hypothesis is to be tested, quantitative information will probably be required in the questionnaire (factual questions) and the method will be experimental rather than descriptive. Counts or values are obtained so that statistical analysis can be administered. If general information (opinion) is asked for, the data will be qualities. Statistics to be considered might be tallies, percentages, or correlation (Chapters 7 and 10).

Careful planning of the design helps in obtaining meaningful answers to the questions. Whatever the problem or objective in sampling, considerations must enter into the design. People who can supply the information desired must be selected as respondents (the sample). Certain problems require a representative sample of subjects to answer the questions. For example, if the problem concerns a particular hospital issue then physical therapists, nurses, social service workers, administrators and procurement personnel, housekeepers, physicians, and others must be included in the sample to fulfill the requirements of a cross–sectional design. Some problems are complex and require careful selection of subjects for the sample to disentangle complex interrelations among variables (factorial design). Perhaps a physical therapist wants to study the functional problems resulting from a specific type of hip surgery on patients having arthritis of the hip joint. The therapist wants to design a series of questionnaires and follow–ups over a period of years. The longitudinal design enables the therapist to determine cause–and–effect relations over a long period of time[18] (see designs, Chapter 9).

The design selected helps decide the type of question to ask. The open and forced–choice questions are used commonly in questionnaires. In the open question or free-response question, the respondent is free to provide the amount of detail he wishes to any or all questions. The respondent is also free to determine the form of answers (short answer or narrative discussions) to the questions. The forced–choice questions provide several answers and the respondent chooses the most appropriate answer. The question might ask: "How many classroom hours does your program devote to research instruction?"

      _____ less than 10, _____ 10 to 20, _____ 21 to 30,
      _____ 31 to 40, _____ over 40 hours

Writing Questions. The actual composing or wording of questions must receive great attention. Questions must be appropriate to the problem and aims of the study; they must provide the information necessary to test the hypothesis or provide information relevant to the general subject. Each question must be clearly written, contain a single idea, avoid negative wording, and be free of jargon and large technical terms. Some of the common concerns about writing questions are discussed briefly.

1. Direct and General. If factual information is necessary, the question must be worded so that the specific information is obtained. "How many licensed physical therapists are working full time in your department?" A general question can be constructed from the example by asking for information of a more general nature. "How many people do you have working in the department?" The two approaches should not be confused because responses will be mixed when respondents interpret a question having different meanings. The second question could be interpreted by some respondents as meaning licensed physical therapists or it could be asking for therapists, therapist assistants, aides, and clerical personnel. Ambiguity can be avoided by structuring questions in simple, easily understood forms. Avoid words that have more than one meaning when asking for specific information.

2. *Complex and Simple*. Questions that are very long or complex should be avoided. A respondent may be confused or not answer a complex question. "Have you treated many patients with brain damage over a long period of time, how were these patients handled, and were you successful in achieving desired treatment goals?" This particular question is vague, long, asks for too much detail, and is complex because of its ambiguity. Questions must be kept simple in construction and easy for the respondent to answer. If multiple answers are sought from questions, or if questions involve several variables, then several questions should be asked so that no overlap of information is being requested. Questions should be mutually exclusive:

"How many children having cerebral palsy and displaying spasticity of one limb did you treat in May?"

"Was passive exercise used as part of their treatment regimen?"

"Was the Bruiminks–Oseretsky Test of Motor Proficiency used to assess effects of treatment?"

Perhaps more questions could be asked to obtain the information requested in the original question. Questions must be sensitive to wording and emphasis. Leading questions or questions about memory are considered poor.[9]

3. *Examine Questions*. After writing questions, put them aside for a few days and then reread and rework them to improve quality and to eliminate ambiguity. When questions have been constructed to your satisfaction, administer them to friends or colleagues knowledgeable in the content area. Ask your colleagues to critique the style, wording, and meanings of the questions. You will be surprised to learn how many questions still need rewriting. Different people have different frames of references and will offer good ideas for improving the questions. Pilot work (pretesting) is a good idea in nonexperimental research for the improvement of the data–gathering instrument and method. Pretesting the questionnaire helps to identify instrument deficiencies; it also helps respondents make suggestions for improvement. Pilot work can assist the researcher in determining the accuracy of the responses. Some responses can be checked for accuracy (e.g., income) and if found to be inaccurate, questions can be reworded, or forced–choice questions can replace free–response questions. The researcher can determine which questions will be most successful, which questions are weak and vague. Additional questions may be suggested to the researcher by the pretest results.

Ordering Questions. The questions requiring the least thought or reasoning should occur first on the list. If the respondent is at ease and thinks the questions are simple and require little effort, then chances for completing the questionnaire are greatly improved. The more provocative questions should follow in a logical sequence if interrelated. The respondent will not mind putting a little thought into the answers, and as he gets into the "swing of things," he will want to finish. Questions of a sensitive or an embarrassing nature should occur last, if important enough to use, and be few in number to ensure completion of the questionnaire.

Length of Questionnaire. Setting the length of a questionnaire is a difficult task, but one which everyone must make. If the researcher knows the sample members being queried, then longer questionnaires may have a good chance of success; but if the researcher is unknown to the sample members, the success rate of the questionnaire will probably be low. People have a tendency to ignore questionnaires that are lengthy and require large amounts of time and effort to complete. If the questionnaire is of a timely and interesting nature, the success rate will, of course, be high. Students who want to use the mail questionnaire for class projects or for investigative studies should keep the length short, thirty questions or less. Sometimes just knowing that the questionnaire belongs to a student will "turn people off."

Uses of Questionnaires. The mail questionnaire is used to gather information about issues, opinions, or views. The executive body of an association might send questionnaires to a representative sample of its voting members to determine their wishes or beliefs, or to test the feasibility of the study before deciding to take a stand on certain policies or political matters. A physical therapist might pool chapter members before introducing a motion at the annual business meeting to change the name of the chapter's newsletter. The questionnaire is used to determine status of an issue. A politician might sample constituents concerning their views on a particular piece of pending legislation before he returns to his legislative body to vote on the issue. The politician is determining the status of the problem before committing himself on the issue.

Questionnaires are used in research to obtain facts and knowledge about a specific subject. They are used to determine how strongly held are the views on an issue, to determine reasons for a course of action, to determine general feelings on an issue, and to determine respondents' awareness of an issue.[9] The McGill pain questionnaire has been designed for clinical assessment of pain and can be analyzed statistically. It measures pain by a pain–rating index, number of words chosen, and intensity.[32]

Reasons for Rejection by Respondents. Responses to mail questionnaires are frequently meager, with returns of 40% to 50% or less being common,[32] whereas a response rate of 60% is good and 70% is very good.[11] If questions are poor, complex, long, or ambiguous, the respondent becomes discouraged or does not understand what is expected of him. Lengthy demands made on the respondent may prevent the questionnaire from being returned to the sender. Often questions are embarrassing or too personal for the respondent. If there is no relation between respondent and researcher, then chances of completing a lengthy questionnaire are extremely poor. Timing the questionnaire mailing is also important. A teacher who receives a questionnaire just prior to examination periods is not likely to respond; an administrator who receives a questionnaire when he is working on the annual report or budget may not respond; the physical therapist who is just returning from vacation and must get caught up on clinical work will also not respond. Perhaps you can think of other reasons; if so, consider those reasons when planning a survey. Responses may be extremely poor if respondents must incur personal costs for the return of the questionnaire, or if budget considerations dictate questionnaire information or mailings. The Readership Survey Results—1972 of **PHYSICAL THERAPY** is a good example where only 5% of readers responded to the questionnaire.[34] The researcher must decide whether anonymity on the questionnaire is important. Some questions, particularly those of a personal nature, may be threatening to respondents if they are asked to identify themselves. However, anonymity probably increases the honesty of responses and the number of returned questionnaires. Follow–ups are difficult and inefficient when the researcher does not know who did and did not respond.[19]

Aids for Improving Returns. All questionnaires must be accompanied by a self–addressed stamped envelope. Respondents refuse to cooperate when they must spend money to ensure the success of someone else's research. The questionnaire must be constructed for the convenience of the respondent: not too many questions, questions must be clear and not ambiguous, the questionnaire must be easy to respond to (forced choices are good), and questions should be impersonal. The questionnaire must be neat and organized and not contain too much reading. A letter must accompany the questionnaire explaining the purpose and providing clear instructions for completion. Authoritarian or excessively polite letters may be ignored. People forget or misplace questionnaires and need persuasion for completing and returning them, so follow–up mailings are recommended. Follow–up mailings increase return rates. Two to four weeks between mailings is a reasonable lapse of time. Follow–up mailings can be improved by rewording the cover letter and sending another questionnaire along with another self–addressed stamped envelope. A reminder to complete and return the questionnaire is worthless if the original questionnaire has been destroyed (filed). Persistance often pays dividends. If the return rate is low enough to jeopardize the study, a second or third follow–up may be necessary, but the researcher must decide when the returns no longer justify the expense of sending out more questionnaires. Members of a sample who are not interested, have little education, or represent an economically poor social class may contribute to poor response rates.[8] Sample selection is important for ensuring responses.

The Cover Letter. A cover letter must accompany all mailed questionnaires. It briefly explains the purpose and significance of the study and helps motivate the completion and return of the questionnaire. Cover letters should be addressed specifically to the potential respondent (Dear Ms. (name), not Dear Ms. or Sir). The "personal touch" helps to improve the percentage of returns. If possible, some reference to association (professional ties) is desirable. Endorsement by a respected, well–known member of the association (group, institution) improves responses, particularly if the researcher is a student. Respondents should be given a deadline for returning the completed questionnaire (2 to 4 weeks). Neatness and composition of the letter and questionnaire are important. Offset duplication on letterhead improves appearance of material as well as the image and value of the responses. A sample letter is shown in Figure 6.1

Presenting Results. The total sample size, the percentage of returns, and the rate of response for each question should be presented in the results of

Letterhead paper	Program of Physical Therapy University of Null Blackbird, PA 17261
	March 14, 1990
Use sample matching → in cutting offset stencil	Ms. Mary Doe Department of Physical Therapy Null Hospital Blackbird, PA 17261
Use offset process for appearance of individually typed → letter when duplicating	Dear Miss Doe:
Purpose → Importance →	The enclosed questionnaire concerned with procedures used in selecting physical therapy students is part of a statewide study being conducted by the Program of Physical Therapy at the University of Null. The results of this study will help to provide criteria to be used for improving present selection procedures and determining the administrative status of the selection process. The selection process affects the caliber of students that you receive for clerkship.
Reasonable time → limit Offer results → Thank respondent →	Your cooperation in completing the enclosed questionnaire by April 5 will be greatly appreciated. Each return ensures a more accurate assessment of the selection process. Your comments concerning any aspect of the present selection process not covered in the questionnaire would be welcomed. A copy summarizing the survey results will be mailed if you desire. Thank you for your cooperation.
	Sincerely yours,
Different color → to appear personally signed	I. M. Smith, Dean

Figure 6.1. Sample cover letter for questionnaires.

a questionnaire survey. Presenting the percentage of respondents choosing alternatives to each question is one approach to reporting results.

Advantages of Questionnaires. The mail questionnaire has several advantages for the researcher. Some of these advantages are:

1. Low Cost. When compared with the interview, the mail questionnaire is inexpensive. Costs involve supplies, postage fees, and clerical assistance and are dependent on the size of the sample and the number of follow-up mailings.

2. Sampling Representation. If time to complete the study is unimportant, a good representation of a sample can be obtained. Follow–ups can be continued or additional subjects can be sampled until a good sized sample is reached. The questionnaires can be mailed and additional work or research can take place during the interim between mailings and returns. This type of survey often requires months to complete.

3. Low Personal Error. Errors which occur when repeating a question many times in an interview are nonexistent on a questionnaire because exact copies of the questionnaire are mailed to all members of the sample. The data are computed easily because tallies and simple statistical methods are used in analysis. Since the respondents do not have access to results of the survey or to interviewers, they cannot then influence answers recorded by an observer.

4. Data Verification. Sometimes factual information can be verified by comparing data supplied by respondents with that of other known sources. Respondents' ages or positions may be verified by obtaining files or records if they are members of an organization, employees of a hospital, or students enrolled in a university. This advantage is important because researchers need to defend the accuracy of their data.

Disadvantages of Questionnaires.

1. Ambiguity of Questions. Despite rewriting questions several times and subjecting them to pilot work, ambiguity can creep into the questionnaire. Ambiguity may occur in the technical detail of the question if the respondent's level of understanding is less than expected.

2. Finality of Responses. Once the questionnaire is returned, the responses are final. The researcher cannot ask the respondent what was meant by a certain reply. No rechecking, no further probing, or no asking of additional questions is possible after the questionnaire has been mailed.

3. Alteration of Questions. Even when forced–choice answers are supplied along with questions, respondents often alter the answers to suit their convenience. The questions may not fit the respondents' situation exactly, thus they may alter the question or the response. Respondents see the entire questionnaire before responding to the first question, therefore, responses to one question are not always independent of responses to other questions.[9]

4. Identity of Respondent. Questions are usually designed for a particular group of people by occupation, membership, patronage, or experience. The researcher, however, is never sure that the respondent is actually the person for whom the questions are intended. A physical therapy administrator might be asked about administrative procedures used in his clinic, but a secretary might be asked to complete the questionnaire. The researcher has limited control over who the respondents actually are.

Attitude Scales

An attitude is a state of mind regarding some event or person. The mind may be in a quiescent or active state concerning an attitude expressed through behavior. Attitudes have cognitive components (beliefs), emotional components (feelings), and action components (behavior). Attitudes can be weak (no identified conviction), strong (firm conviction), abstract (theoretical), intense (tender, violent), and enduring or transient (exist over a long or short period of time).[11,21] A scale is a collection of phrases or numbers placed on a continuum (linear sequence) for weighing or measuring values. Thus, an attitude scale is a device for assessing the predisposition toward an event or person.

An attitude scale consists of a series of statements reflecting the cognitive, emotional, and action components of attitude. The subject is given a series of statements and is asked to respond by agreeing or disagreeing with the assertions. Since statements are structured to represent various levels or degrees of a particular component, the subject's response will be dependent on the wording of the statement. The device is a crude measuring instrument, but of all the survey instruments, the attitude scale is probably the most sophisticated. The attitude scale has acquired the highest technical development among nonexperimental research instruments.[21]

The purpose of the attitude scale is to divide people into broad categories (partitions) based on their attitudes toward some stated object or situation. The scale is designed to determine physical therapists' attitudes toward their jobs or professional scopes, practices, or opportunities. Patients are assessed to determine their attitudes about their physical therapy. Attitude scales have been used to a great extent in sociological, educational, and psychological studies. Searches of the physical therapy literature have not revealed frequent use of attitude scales. These devices yield important information about public or professional reaction to physical therapy, or physical therapists' satisfaction with academic preparation for meeting the demands of clinical work, or physical therapists' reactions toward their associations' activities. Many relevant questions can be asked about any one of these suggested topics. In practice, more statements can be made about a topic than can actually be used in the scale form.

Although attitude scales have received much technical attention (outside of physical therapy), the contents of measurement are subjective and are not inclusive. As stated earlier about rating scales, the device is subject to error and only indicates the numbers of subjects expressing certain states of mind about a situation or person. Analysis of scale values of data can, however, yield considerable information about attitudes. The information can serve as an indicator or guide in establishing policies or procedures, approaches to treatment, curricular changes, and many other applied interests. A single statement or reaction to a single statement cannot be regarded with much authenticity. Reactions to many statements must be averaged before meaning can be extracted from the scaling devices. The device is valuable if administered to a group of subjects or administered to a single subject when normative values are available for comparison.

Researchers planning to measure how one or more subjects feel about a specific topic should first search the literature to ascertain whether an attitude scale has been constructed to meet their needs. Most likely an attitude scale that has been published and found suitable for the student's or clinician's purpose measures what it was developed to measure, and the results it obtains are repeatable if measured on another occasion. These assurances of a scale can save the researcher a tremendous amount of time and effort. If a suitable scale is not available, it will be necessary to develop one.

Careful attention must be given to the construction of the scale so that the respondent's choices are presented to the respondent in a way that indicates the researcher's neutrality. Moser has cited three steps for assuring success of an attitude scale: (1) identify statements which are appropriate and logically related to the attitude dimension being considered; (2) put the statements together in a meaningful fashion so that there is representativeness of the attitude dimension; and (3) perform pilot work on the device to establish baselines for assisting interpretations of the responses.[9]

Considerations of Measurement. Certain features of the scale must be built into the instrument to ensure success. These features must be considered when preparing the scale and when modifying the instrument following a pilot test.

1. Homogeneity. All statements in the scale must relate to a single topic or attitude component. If beliefs toward a particular issue are to be assessed, then statements involving emotional aspects of the topic should be excluded. For example, if the instrument is to measure the patients' beliefs about the benefits of physical therapy, then statements about difficulties concerning transportation to the clinic should be excluded.

2. Equal Intervals. Although units of value and intervals are assigned arbitrarily, the units should maintain equality or at least appear to be equally distant between intervals. Equal–appearing distances on the scale make the data easier to handle than if the scale was not linear. Linearity relates to a bivariate distribution, which means that as the quantity of one variable increases (or decreases) the quantity of the other variable increases (or decreases) also. One variable can decrease as the other variable increases and still be linearly related. In an attitude scale, the most favorable statements should hold the highest weights to maintain linearity, or be constructed so that a straight-line relationship is maintained. For example, if three statements are made, they should be graduated in value so that the stronger statements have more (or less) value than the weaker statements.

"Physical therapists make good citizens."	0.15
"I find physical therapists are vigorous people."	0.48
"I think physical therapists are conceited."	0.50

The difficulty comes in equating the proper weights to the particular attitude. Techniques have been devised, however, to measure different aspects of attitudes and take into account the problems of linearity.

3. Repeatability. Scales should be designed so that if a particular attitude scale is administered to a group of subjects today, it should have similar values or scores if administered tomorrow. The difficulty with attitude measurements is that subjects do change their attitudes about conditions frequently. For example, the boss may reprimand you about a certain administrative error you committed yesterday. You believe that the boss was unfair or that the reprimand was unnecessary; therefore your attitude may be guarded or negative toward the boss. If the boss takes you to dinner the following week and the event is very satisfying, you may then believe that the boss is not such a "rotten egg" after all; your attitude has changed. The outcome of the attitude scale may change between two administrations because of the occurrences taking place between measurements (temporal effect of internal difficulty). Repeatability of attitude scales is quite high. The illustration is an isolated instance of an attitude change in a transient issue, but repeatability is more lasting on many issues: political, religious, professional, and educational views. A graduated scale or continuum where higher values (6 and 5) are equated in size to differences occurring elsewhere on the scale (2 and 1) assists greatly in the repeatability of the instrument.

Types of Attitude Scales. Only the two most commonly used scales will be presented, but these will provide differences in approaches to measuring different components of attitudes; these scales represent equal–appearing (Thurstone) and summated (Likert) scales.

1. Thurstone Scale. Thurstone was a pioneer in attitude scaling and his scale is one of the best known methods of measuring attitudes. The scale is an attempt to assess the strength of an attitude by an agreement-disagreement continuum in which each item is assigned a scale value. The scale value indicates the strength of the attitude and differentiates strength by means of equal–appearing intervals.[33] Thurstone attempted to assess attitudes by comparing statements in pairs and then judging which statement was more positive (or more negative) than the other statement. His work in experimental psychophysics led to equal-appearing intervals.[21]

The procedure begins by forming a large pool of graduated statements ranging from least to most favorable. The pool of statements is written on separate strips of paper and edited for ambiguity, duplication, grammar, and sentence structure. Editing reduces the number of statements in the pool. A group of people are selected as judges to assess each item in the pool by its degree of favorableness. Judges ideally are those who are knowledgeable in the content area of the attitude under consideration. Careful instructions are given to the judges so that each has a complete understanding of how to rank and evaluate the statements. Groups of judges differing widely in views usually have good agreement when assessing attitude statements.[21] The judges assess each statement and place it in a pile according to its degree of favorableness. Judging is performed independently. The number of piles are predetermined as 7, 9, or 11. Odd numbers of intervals provide a "neutral" position or value of the statements. Each statement receives a ranking by each judge according to the pile in which it was placed.

The median and interquartile deviation for each statement are then determined. The interquartile deviation and median measure the variation and central tendency, respectively.[5] These statistics enable the researcher to further reduce the pool. Statements in each pile are examined for their interquartile deviations. Those statements having the highest deviations indicate ambiguity and are eliminated. The medians for each statement pile are examined; the medians may be unevenly distributed along the scale, but they represent distinguishable differences among statements resulting from the judging. The medians, for example, may be 9.0, 8.4, 8.1, 7.5, 6.9, 6.7, and so forth.

The desired number of statements, 20 to 30, is selected for the instrument. In the Thurstone method the higher the scale value, the less positive the attitude toward a situation or person.[35] The mean of the scores obtained from an administration of the instrument indicates the respondents' attitude grouping. The mean computed for a group of respondents will determine the attitude for a particular group, class, or organization of people. For example, an attitude scale administered to physical therapists attending an annual conference will indicate the group's attitude toward increasing the membership fees of the association. The attitude of one subject can be compared to a group's attitude by comparing means obtained from the group and the subject. Some criticisms of the Thurstone scale have been the characteristics and attitudes of the judges (ages, sex, and skill). The Thurstone scaling process is laborious.[9] Table 6.1 provides a partial example of a Thurstone scale.

Table 6.1
Example of a Partial Attitude Scale: Attitudes Toward Physical Therapy*

Check (   ) every statement below that expresses your feeling toward physical therapy. Interpret the statements in accordance with your own experience.

1. When I receive physical therapy I enjoy the atmosphere of the clinic.	(4.0)
2. I believe in what the physical therapist tells me, but I have some reservations.	(4.5)
3. Sometimes I feel that physical therapy and the therapist are necessary and sometimes I doubt them.	(5.6)
4. I believe in physical therapy and its benefits because I have been accustomed to good treatment.	(4.0)
5. I believe physical therapy is losing ground as a science.	(7.4)
6. Physical therapy is needed in health care; it has always provided benefits and good feelings.	(1.4)
7. I like physical therapy, but do not miss it much when I miss a treatment.	(5.1)
8. I believe physical therapy is a powerful form of medicine for rehabilitating the sick and injured.	(1.2)

* Respondent's attitude grouping is the mean. $\bar{X} = 33.2 \div 8 = 4.2$ on a 9-point scale.

2. Likert Scale. The Likert scale is a summated rating scale or set of statements considered to be of equal value in describing the attitude. Respondents choose between the degrees of agreement or disagreement associated with each statement. The sum of the scores represents attitude.

Construction of the Likert scale is less laborious than construction of the Thurstone scale, but the results of the two scales closely agree.[20] The Likert scale is concerned mostly with homogeneity, making sure that all statements center on one topic or attitude. No judges are needed in its construction.

Five levels or degrees of agreement–disagreement are used for each statement. The levels are "strongly agree," "agree," "neutral," "disagree," and "strongly disagree." Weights are assigned to each level (numerical rating scale) for scoring and analysis. The ordering of weights may have to be reversed according to whether the statement is stated positively or negatively; scores may be 5, 4, 3, 2, and 1, respectively. In the process of score reversal, "neutral" level is always number three.

The writing and collection of statements form the initial process of constructing a Likert scale. Statements are composed for the "agree" and "disagree" levels only because subjects respond to extreme statements in similar fashion; that is, there is very little disagreement about extreme statements. Experience has shown that statements of neutrality do not function well.[9] Since only two levels of statements are used, an equal number of "agree" and "disagree" statements can be constructed. All statements are scored from 1 to 5 arbitrarily and then all scores are summed to determine the range. If 100 statements have been written and scored, the lowest sum in the range is 100 and the highest sum possible in the range is 500. The scale is administered to a selected sample of subjects.

Agreement about scoring the statements must be made before administration of the instrument. If a positive attitude toward job satisfaction means a high score, then agreement with statements like "The chance to do research" or "The association with good people" should be scored as 4 or 5.

In the example given in Table 6.2, suppose two statements were scored as 3, three statements as 2, three statements as 4, and two as 5. A cursory inspection of Table 6.2 might give the impression that the exemplary respondent neither enjoyed nor disliked his job.

When scores are summed the total is 34.

Statement	Score (x)
1	5
2	2
3	3
4	4
5	2
6	4
7	2
8	4
9	3
10	5
	$\Sigma x = 34$

The maximum score possible on the ten statements is 50 ($10 \times 5 = 50$) and the neutral position totals 30 (10×3). The score of 34 is slightly above the neutral attitude and in the direction of a positive attitude toward job satisfaction; the agreement before administering the scale was to label positive statements with values of 5 and 4. Further inspection of Table 6.2 shows that the respondent has a somewhat negative attitude about the opportunities the job has to offer, since five responses were in the "neutral" or "disagree" levels (statements 2, 3, 5, 7, and 9). The respondent seems to enjoy working with and associating with patients and hospital employees but does not believe that the type of work he or she is doing offers a challenge or provides status. Caution in over-interpretation of the responses must, however, be exercised.

No conclusions can be made about the meaning of distances between scale positions because the instrument is not an interval scale. The Likert scale is an ordinal measuring device. Repeatability is good for the Likert scale; the number of statements is arbitrary but should total at least 20. One problem with this scale is that the total score can be obtained in a number of ways. Scores checked for each statement can change between 1 and 5 on varied administrations, yet the total scores of the scale can be

Table 6.2
Example of a Physical Therapy Job Satisfaction Scale

Read each statement carefully; decide how satisfied you feel about that particular aspect of your present job described by each statement; be honest; check the appropriate score that best describes your feelings. Check ( ) all statements.

	Strongly Agree 5	Agree 4	Neutral 3	Disagree 2	Strongly Disagree 1
1. An opportunity to help the sick and disabled.					
2. My job offers variety.					
3. The job offers few opportunities to grow.					
4. The opportunity to be responsible for the outcome of treatment.					
5. The chance to do research.					
6. The routine in my job.					
7. The status which my job offers.					
8. An opportunity to meet important people.					
9. The challenge of the work.					
10. The association of good people.					

exactly the same or similar in value. When large numbers of subjects are administered to, the Likert attitude scale, percentiles, and standard deviations can be computed.

HISTORICAL METHOD

Historical research is critical investigation of accounts of the past, careful weighing of the validity of accounts and their sources, and interpretation of the accounts after their weighing.[33] Some early historians preserved tales and accounts of the past for entertaining or provoking readers, but most used historical information to praise the state or church or to promote an issue.[36] Modern historians have attempted to bring historical methods in line with scientific methods by establishing procedures for investigation.

Historical research differs from the scientific method because of its elusive subject matter. The historian uncovers data through a search of accounts of the past such as documents, relics, and diaries, whereas the scientist creates data by making observations and measurements to describe events and performance.[8] Modern historians contend that within limits the historical method is scientific.[36] The method enables the historian to investigate subject matter and source materials critically and objectively.[4] Suppositions are established and then data which confirm or contradict the suppositions are collected; historians, however, cannot employ controlled observations or make repeat measurements.[30]

Identifying the problems to be investigated, locating sources of past facts, evaluating these sources, and summarizing and interpreting the gathered historical information are basic steps in the conduct of historical research. Each step is discussed briefly.

Identifying a Problem

As in other research, one of the first considerations in historical research is to identify the problem. As outlined in Chapter 2, a thorough review of the literature is important in identifying a problem. Discussing the problem, topic, or hypothesis with experienced historians is also useful for initiating the research process. Since the purpose of historical research is to discover new knowledge, explain, or predict, the availability of resources to study a well-defined problem must be known prior to the investigation.

Source of Investigation

In their attempt to collect information and increase understanding about the past, historians search for historical roots. The two sources of materials used in historical research are primary and secondary sources.

Primary Sources. The historian locates and examines original materials of the past. Primary sources may be located at repositories of historical information, may still be in existence at their original locations, or may be owned and maintained by persons, groups, or organizations. Primary sources consist of official (state, church, minutes of organizations) or personal (letters, speeches, articles, diaries, diplomas) records, eye witness accounts, photographs or illustrations (drawings, paintings), published or printed materials (textbooks, certificates, contracts, accounts, articles), physical remains (ruins, equipment, relics, clothing, artifacts), and mechanical records (tapes or video recordings of interviews, meetings and speeches). Once the historian has located and collected data, he must validate it. Although the data may be original, the historical researcher must verify and ensure that the data are trustworthy and representative of the true account. Sometimes the process of validating primary sources is not easy and gaps must be filled by the researcher, or the sources must be accepted without verification.[30,36]

Secondary Sources. A secondary source is an account, description, or reproduction of the original by persons who did not see, hear, or live the past accounts or experiences.

Information contained by secondary sources may have been changed or distorted through transmission. Primary sources are always best and must be sought by the researcher for obvious reasons. Secondary sources, however, have definite value to the researcher because: (1) primary sources are not always available; (2) secondary sources help as an introduction to the subject area; (3) secondary sources provide an overview of the subject; and (4) secondary sources help the researcher form suppositions. Secondary sources of historical information may include abstracts, newspapers, encyclopedias, periodicals or interviews, as well as accounts based on secondhand information.[30,36]

Evaluation of Sources

The existence or collection of data from primary or secondary sources does not guarantee the researcher of their validity, authenticity, or accuracy.[35] Historians have established two standards for evaluating materials collected before the research is reported.

External Criticism. This form of evaluation is preoccupied with the validity of the source. The source might be in existence and be original, but the historian must verify whether the data are real; the intent or frame of reference in which the account took place, was written, or was given. Perhaps the author's original statement is located and verified as being the statement made by the author, but the researcher must determine whether the author was competent when making the statement.[30,36]

Internal Criticism. This form of evaluation is concerned mostly with the content of the source or statement and its meaning. The researcher may verify that the statement can be attributed to a certain author and that the author was competent, but the statement still remains suspect until the truth of the statement is determined.[33] The evaluation of the source is thus transferred from authenticity of the statement to the trustworthiness of its contents.[36]

The historical research method, unlike the scientific method, does not contain precise technical vocabulary and terms often have different meanings. Despite established procedures, historical research has apparently declined in some disciplines. The decline has been attributed to the universal acceptance of the scientific method.[33]

Physical therapists can use the historical method to preserve the rich history of their profession.

Interpretation

Summarization and interpretation are integral parts of historical research. These activities involve logical analysis, therefore the researcher must be as objective as possible. The researcher cannot confirm that one event in the past caused another but must make assumptions or inferences that assign causality to historical events. The researcher must be careful with the language used in the interpretation to avoid the wrong interpretation. The more information uncovered about a historical event, the more likely the cause of the event will become known or at least be defensible.

In no form of research can the researcher study or examine the entire population of events or phenomena. The researcher, therefore, usually samples a portion of events or is limited by the availability of past documents and relics and then makes generalizations based on the sample of information. The researcher's findings are always strengthened by increasing the sample size or the amount of available data on which inferences are based. As many primary and secondary sources relating to the event as possible are needed to make correct interpretations. The researcher is cautioned to restrict interpretations about causes and generalization of interpretations to the evidence gathered.

SUMMARY

Descriptive or survey methods are logical and specific approaches to nonexperimental research and can provide considerable understanding from a small number of variables.[11] Nonexperimental research provides information about what respondents are thinking and feeling and how they are reacting to some stimulus. Information gathered can be broad, detailed, and specific. Because of the elusive nature of some types of data, nonexperimental research exerts little control over variables involved in an investigation.[4] Lack of controls in research leads to inconsistency. The software used to collect data may not be as accurate and precise as the hardware used in experimentation. Despite its weaknesses, nonexperimental research enables an investigator to study areas in which controlled experimentation may be impossible.

The historical method is performed outside the conventional laboratory and is quasi–scientific in technique. This nonexperimental method can, however, make valuable contributions to physical therapy. However important, it has seldom been used in studies reported in the physical therapy literature. Using this method, physical therapists could preserve the history and examine questions vital to the well–being of the profession. Table 6.3 summarizes the research process presented thus far.

Table 6.3
Cumulative Summary of the Research Processes Presented

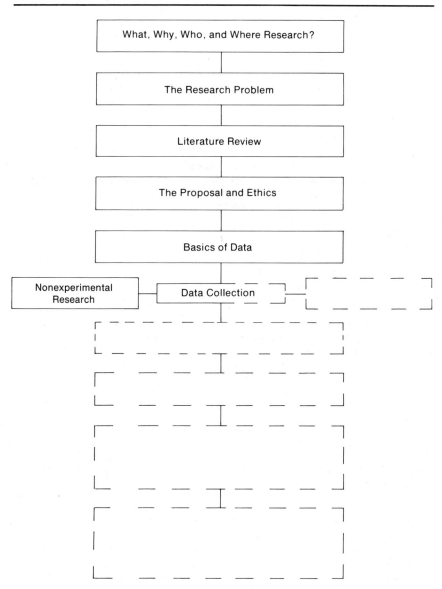

REFERENCES

1. Ethridge DA, McSweeney M: Research in occupational therapy. 1. Introduction. Am J Occup Ther 24: 490–494, 1970
2. Meyers LS, Grossen NE: Behavioral Research: Theory, Procedure, and Design, ed 2. San Francisco, WH Freeman and Co, 1978
3. Espenschade AS, Rarick GL: Descriptive Research. In Hubbard AW (ed): Research Methods in Health, Physical Education, and Recreation, ed 3. Washington, Am Assoc Health Phys Educ Rec 1973
4. Treece EW, Treece JW Jr: Elements of Research in Nursing, ed 3. St. Louis, The CV Mosby Co, 1982
5. Scott MG: Instrumentation: Software. In Hubbard AW (ed): Research Methods in Health, Physical Education, and Recreation, ed 3. Washington, Am Assoc Health Phys Educ Rec 1973
6. Emory CW: Business Research Methods. Homewood, IL, Richard D Irwin, Inc, 1980
7. Suchman EA: The Survey Method Applied to Public Health and Medicine. In Glock CY (ed): Survey Research in the Social Sciences. New York, Russell Sage Foundation, 1967
8. Borg WR, Gall MD: Educational Research: An Introduction, ed 3. New York, Longman, 1979
9. Moser CA, Kalton G: Survey Methods in Social Investigation, ed 2. London, Heinemann Educational Books, 1972
10. Gordon RL: Interviewing Strategy, Techniques and Factors, ed 2. Homewood IL, Dorsey Press, 1975
11. Babbie ER: Survey Research Methods. Belmont, CA, Wadsworth Publishing Co, Inc, 1973
12. Sundman S, Bradburn NM: Response Effects of Surveys. Chicago, Aldine, 1974
13. Pomeroy WB: The reluctant respondent. Public Opinion Quarterly 27: 287–293, 1963
14. Schwartz A: Interviewing and the public. Public Opinion Quarterly 28: 135–142, 1964
15. Dohrenwend BS, Dohrenwend BP: Sources of Refusals in Surveys. In McKinlay JB (ed): Research Methods in Health Care. New York, Prodist, 1973
16. Haberman PW, Scheenberg J: Education Reported in Interviews. In McKinlay JB (ed): Research Methods in Health Care. New York, Prodist, 1973
17. Colombotos J, Elison J, Loewenstein R: Effect of interviewers sex on interview responses. Public Heatlh Rep 83: 685–690, 1968
18. Dohrenwend BS, Colombotos J, Dohrenwend BP: Social Distance and Interviewer Effects. In McKinlay JB (ed): Research Methods in Health Care. New York, Prodist, 1973.
19. Gay LR: Educational Research: Competencies for Analysis and Application, ed 2. Columbus OH, Charles E Merrill, 1981
20. Schmoll BJ: Ethnographic inquiry in clinical settings. Phys Ther 67: 1895–1897, 1987
21. Oppenheim AN: Questionnaire Design and Attitude Measurement, London, Heinemann Educational Books, Inc, 1966
22. Bruett TL, Overs RP: A critical review of 12 ADL scales. Phys Ther 49: 857–862, 1969
23. Gaito J: Measurement scales and statistics: resurgence of an old misconception. Psychol Bull 8: 564–567, 1980
24. Sokolow J, Silson JE, Taylor EG, et al: A new approach to the objective evaluation of physical disability. J Chronic Dis 15: 105–112, 1962
25. Borg G: Perceived exertion: a note on history and methods. Med Sci Sports 5: 90–93, 1973
26. Borg GA: Psychological bases of perceived exertion. Med Sci Sports Exer 14: 377–381, 1982
27. Guilford J: Psychometric Methods, ed 2. New York, McGraw–Hill Book Co, 1954

28. Cox RC, West WL: Fundamentals of Research for Health Professionals. Laurel MD, RAMSCO Pub Co, 1982

29. Style Manual, ed 3. Washington, Am Phys Ther Assoc, 1970

30. Clarke DH, Clarke HH: Research Processes in Physical Education, Recreation, and Health. Englewood Cliffs, NJ, Prentice–Hall, Inc, 1970

31. Simon JL: Basic Research Methods in Social Science. ed 2. New York, Random House, Inc, 1978

32. Melzack R: The McGill pain questionnaire: major properties and scoring methods. Pain 1: 277–299, 1975

33. Kerlinger TN: Foundations of Behavioral Research, ed 2. New York, Holt, Rinehart, and Winston, Inc, 1973

34. Readership survey results—1972. Phys Ther 53: 293–299, 1973

35. Thurstone LL, Chave EJ: The Measurement of Attitude. Chicago, University of Chicago Press, 1929

36. Van Dalen DB: The Historical Method. In Hubbard AW (ed): Research Methods in Health, Physical Education, and Recreation, ed 3. Washington, Am Assoc Health Phys Educ Rec 1973

7

Confidence in Research and Instruments

For what a man had rather were true;
he more readily believes.

Francis Bacon

Research is undertaken to determine relations or differences between two or more variables and to seek good scientific results. Good scientific results are not necessarily supportive of the researcher's desired outcome, but imply freedom from errors and prejudices. The research process includes measurement, which, in turn, involves instruments, procedures, and people. Measurements are subject to many kinds of error, which may limit the effectiveness of the research findings and destroy credibility for the consumer. The consumer is the reader of a research report, a practitioner attempting to implement research findings, or a teacher conveying new theories to students. Accuracy and consistency of instruments, procedures, and people involved with research are important for instilling confidence in and giving credibility to research. Confidence is the assurance placed in the theory and in the capabilities of its practitioners, as well as in the findings of a particular clinical investigation. "It ain't so much the things we don't know that get us in trouble. It's the things we know that ain't so."[1] We must have confidence in what we do and know that the way it is done is correct.

The concepts of sampling technique and variation were discussed earlier. Subjects in our study samples exhibit a variety of individual differences; age, sex, color of hair, body weight, height, skills, personality, and interest. Researchers can consequently expect different probabilities of outcome on individual scores. The consistency of the final score depends on the freedom from errors and biases. Errors are fallacies, untruths, and inaccuracies which occur in the research process unless they are recognized and prevented by the investigator. Biases are prejudices or influences introduced by the researcher, or by using certain techniques and instrumentation. The design, statistical analyses, or the statistician can assist in eliminating error and bias in sampling and measurement, but only the researcher can perceive how varied the conditions can really be in any given study. An instrument can be highly accurate and dependable, but if the researcher has not identified the problem specifically, has not designed the study well, and has not taken appropriate steps to prevent, control, or correct for error in measurements, the study will be worthless.

The degree of accuracy that an instrument has is referred to as validity, whereas the degree of consistency or dependability of an instrument is called reliability. Both research and measuring instruments must possess validity and reliability.

Accuracy and consistency in measurement are not faultless. Measuring devices are devised to measure what we think is being measured and humans must take, read, and interpret the measurements. The true quantity or dimension of a characteristic is rarely, if ever, known in perfect (absolute) terms or values. The difference between a true measurement (X_T) and an observed measurement (X) is called error and can be formulated, $X_E = X - X_T$,[2–4] where X is the combined score (recorded score), T is the true proportion of the combined score, and E is the error component or proportion of the recorded score. Measurements taken over or through the skin, for instance, to investigate some biological organ or structure are estimates, since more accurate measurements could be taken if the organ or structure was removed and measured. Social customs sometimes insist on estimates of phenomena. An awareness of the limitations of the method for obtaining information must be given consideration when planning research studies. Some of the more common classes of error are discussed in the following section.

ERRORS

Sampling, random, and systematic errors are inaccuracies that occur by chance during a study or experiment and are often synonymous in meaning. A common definition of these errors is the deviation of a sample result from its expected outcome.

Sampling Errors

If we treated a group of patients having similar soft tissue injuries of the ankle (severity, location) by appropriate methods of physical therapy (**ICERS**—ice, compression, elevation, rest, support), we would expect the patients to show some definite improvement within 3 to 4 days. If a few of the patients did not respond favorably in the expected time, the deviations could be due to chance and are called sampling errors. We should not be surprised that not all of the patients reacted favorably to the treatment, because different persons exposed to similar conditions behave differently. The variances might be explained by physiological differences of protoplasm or age. Variation plays a heavy role in the theory of scientific inquiry and measurement; variability is the central theme of research. The researcher is faced with the insurmountable task of controlling the events in the research process, so that the outcome of the experiment can be interpreted. Since error is forever present in the life and behavioral sciences, the researcher must be willing to take risks and accept some error. In the formula, $X = X_T + X_E$, the measured score is assumed to be a function of the true quantity related to the population trait and of the experimental error. The true quantity (X_T) of the overall observed score is related to the population trait through the design of the study.

Sampling error is the difference between a parameter (true value) and a statistic. In the concept of error, a statistic is an estimate of a parameter and can depart from the true value.

Random Errors

Random errors are the inconsistent discrepancies that occur by chance. Random errors do not exhibit any trend above or below the mean, which assumes the value of zero if a large number of repeated measurements are taken of the same quantity or trait. Random errors are not related to the individual observations or to the true score. In statistical theory, the true value is the boundary approached by the arithmetic mean as the number of measurements are repeated an infinite number of times. An infinite number of measurements is not usually possible when dealing with human subjects because of tolerance, fatigue, time, and availability. The researcher takes consolation in assuming control over as many factors as possible in the research process and by assuming that measurement errors are slight and distributed randomly. Such random errors do not form a bias but increase the value of the computed variance or standard deviation, which then is compounded with effect and error. The researcher has the difficulty of deciding whether the recorded values suffice for making conclusions.

Equivocal decisions in which the observer is not sure of the value or the event can lead to random error. In some studies, multiple readings or duplicate responses are made so that the mean of the recorded scores is used as the true value. The lack of practice or standardization of testing procedures before the research data are collected can induce error at the beginning of the data collecting process, but these errors tend to disappear once the observer acquires experience and finesse in measuring the trait. If different equipment is used to record values, some of the differences occurring between values can be attributed to the idiosyncrasies of the equipment. In the study by Stewart and coworkers, inconsistencies were found in the timers and in the dosages per unit displayed on the meters; leakages were also found in the electrode cables of different ultrasound units.[5] Different units of equipment performing the same function fluctuate according to the unit, or, like people, they have their own personalities.

If you ever have measured the width of a closet to construct shelving, you, no doubt, found that your measurement was either slightly less or slightly more than the actual width after cutting the wood. The slight difference may not have caused any practical difficulty and the shelf may fit into place. The board was not precise in measurement. If you measure the width of the closet several times you might notice that each measurement differs slightly (depending on the precision of the tape measure), such as: 60.8, 61.2, 61.1, and 60.9 centimeters, respectively.The lack of a precise measurement is a random error. If you were recording the isokinetic strength of a subject's elbow extensors and then asked the subject to repeat the effort several times after adequate periods of rest, you would notice that each recorded value differed somewhat (30.5, 30.7, 30.4, 30.6, and 30.5 cm-kg) at a particular point of measurement. Several factors influence the measurements and this only complicates the situation. The subject could have become fatigued, may not have given maximum effort each time, may have altered the position of the body between measurements, or the researcher may not have read the recording instrument correctly each time. These kinds of situations detract from the precision of the measurement or study. On the other hand, the researcher could have taken several measurements of the event in question and then found the mean of the distribution of measurements; the mean would have been an accurate indicator of the true measurement because events, traits, or variations of the event would be distributed uniformly above and below the mean. Random errors are distributed similarly to naturally occurring phenomena in accordance with the normal curve.

Error can be computational, such as the misplacement of a decimal point in recording numbers or calculating results, the transportation of digits, recording the wrong number, or even using the wrong scale in conversion or reading a meter. If personal judgment enters into reading a scale, then different observers obtain different readings, or the same person might be inconsistent in rendering judgments. In nerve conduction measurements, the greatest error occurs when the examiner reads the values from the oscilloscope or photograph or takes measurements of the length of the nerve segment under study.[6] A method has been devised to exclude judgment in nerve conduction measurements by recording the value and readout electronically.[7] Clinical electromyographic units use this approach routinely today.

Systematic Errors

Systematic errors are constant errors that persist until discovered and are corrected. If the tape measure used to measure the width of the closet was inaccurate because of the marked units, or if the tape measure had some spacing before the first unit began (metal tip) and this space was inadvertently ignored, then all subsequent measurements would be incorrect by that amount of built–in error. These errors are systematic errors.

If the researcher perceives the pointer on the dial of a meter as a whole for every measurement read, when in fact, the pointer indicates a value slightly less than the whole unit, the errors will be systematic. Systematic errors are the same for each observation, procedure, or quantity measured. If the errors are consistent and of the same magnitude, the standard deviation remains unchanged because the error becomes a constant and is added to all observations. If, however, the constant error is somehow multiplied by each measurement, the standard deviation will be multiplied by the magnitude of the constant error.[2]

Biases of various types can contribute to systematic error. A bias is a systematic deviation of the expected outcome of a measurement or of a study and is caused by factors other than those resulting from the manipulated variable (treatment).[8] The researcher can systematically bias data by rounding off scores. Anytime a raw number is changed for the convenience of the researcher (rounding), some systematic error is introduced. The error will be greater when tenths are rounded to whole numbers than when thousandths are rounded to hundredths for example. Bias can be present in selecting subjects, instruments, and treatment methods. In Chapter 5, several methods of sampling were presented; any deviation from a random selection of subjects can cause bias, because prejudice is introduced when one item of the population has a greater chance of being selected than other items. This type of selection occurs when different methods are used or subjects are treated differently. Suppose you are interested in studying the effects of exercise on subjects. If well-trained subjects (for example, athletes) are selected to study conditioning in an experimental exercise, the gains will be less than if sedentary subjects were selected for the conditioning program. If the researcher is aware of these differences between subjects before beginning and decides to select only sedentary subjects because they will show greater gains than athletes, then bias is introduced through selection. If the effects of physical therapy on edematous soft tissue injuries are studied and heat and cold therapies are selected for treating patients with acute ankle sprains, then bias is introduced because heat causes increased edema if used earlier then 2 to 3 days following the injury. Again, this is an example of selection bias or systematic error.

Perhaps motivation is being studied as a factor in the therapy of patients with meniscectomies. If football players are selected as one sample and soldiers and government employees are selected as other samples, bias may have been introduced because differences in motivating factors are evident before the study has begun. Similar differences might occur between private patients and ward patients. If a researcher elects to study only patients having minimum medical involvement, rather than those severely involved so that improvement can be demonstrated, then bias has been introduced.

By this time, the reader probably thinks that errors can never be overcome in research. On the contrary, well planned studies can prevent or control variables sufficiently so that errors are not present or are reduced to a minimum. Biases are often introduced purposefully so that differences can be demonstrated for specific reasons. If the researcher is aware of and can defend biases in the study, critics are usually tolerant and will accept the biases if properly selected, controlled, and designed. Defining a sample and particular characteristics of the sample, as opposed to other characteristics, is considered a form of desired bias.

In research that requires human subjects to perform while being measured for data, the outcome can be influenced by the subject's cooperation, willingness and interest in participating, and knowledge of the research. If the subject must repeat the performance several times, the results or values should be withheld from the subject until the test is completed. The subject could place more or less skill or effort into the performance once knowledge of the values is known.

Researchers usually have some internal feelings about the outcome of the study. They hope the results will verify some hunch, opinion, belief, or hypothesis, and they may exert some influence when taking measurements. The recorded values perhaps will be rounded off systematically to the next highest value on all measures greater than the whole unit, thereby making the statistical values larger. The researcher could even encourage subjects to perform better in one task than in another.

Researcher Errors

Other analytical errors relate to the researcher who uses inappropriate statistical analyses: using the median when the mean is appropriate, using the t test for multiple comparisons of several variables when analysis of variance is appropriate, or comparing standard deviations of several samples having dissimilar test conditions for example. Even selecting the wrong instrument or the wrong method for measuring data can contribute to error in the study. If for some reason we were interested in measuring accurately the reaction time of a group of children with cerebral palsy before and after teaching them a particular motor skill and we used a wristwatch instead of a chronometer, the instrument selected may be inappropriate. Some colleagues advocate using only simple, unsophisticated equipment for clinical research. The results obtained from this approach would be suspect according to the theory of measurement because of the amount of error introduced by the measuring instrument. Since scientific inquiry seeks truth, the question arises as to whether a physical therapist is justified in using crude devices for measuring an existing phenomenon when refined devices might provide more accurate information and be available to the researcher if more effort had been expended. Different treatments have specific effects and comparisons among them might be hazardous. Isometric exercise is specific to the point (position) in the range of motion for developing strength. If the patient exercises only in full elbow extension, the triceps brachii muscle will be strongest in full extension and will not exhibit proportional increments of strength at other points along the range of motion unless also exercised at those specific points. The initial effects of heat and cold on the skin are different and cannot be compared if only initial effects are studied. The problem and aim of the study should indicate an awareness of the specificities of different methods. The examples cited may not have any influence on the outcome of your particular study, but you must be aware of their possible influence on data and take appropriate precautions.

Errors are increased if the reader must read the meaning into the data or must interpret each reading during the occurrence of the data. In clinical electromyography, the examiner makes visual measurements and interpretations of the data as they appear on the oscilloscope screen. Nonnumerical recordings can lead to faulty observations and interpretations.

Eliminating observer error is important for ensuring accuracy and dependability. Unless practice and standardization of the test procedure are enforced before the data are collected, observers cannot become more competent with practice and, if maximum competency is not obtained for each datum collected, then scores will fluctuate throughout the testing procedure. Delays in collecting data can contribute to error because learning (experience), environment (seasons), and aging effects influence scores taken at different times. Handling of subjects, data, and equipment may possibly contribute to error. Having several therapists collect data for a collaborative study and having the data collected with different instruments at different facilities can undermine a well-planned study because too many uncontrolled variables exist.

Parallax is another type of personal error which occurs when taking nonnumerical recordings from an oscilloscope or meter. Parallax is the apparent displacement of an object, line, or figure by (random) change in the observer's position. The errors may be subconscious. Unless the person reading the information on the oscilloscope screen is looking directly (straight line) at the images on the screen, the information contained in the images can be distorted, causing erroneous values. Angles of eye focus other than a straight line will cause this distortion. Figure 7.1 illustrates this situation.

Figure 7.1.   Parallax resulting from different sightings of an object or scale.

SAMPLE SIZE

Ideal accuracy in research is achieved when all members of a population are tested under controlled conditions. Because of cost, inaccessibility, and limited time, all members of a population usually cannot be tested. Samples are therefore drawn from the population and are tested; computed statistics then are used to estimate the values of the population. An estimate of how many subjects or observations will be acceptable in a study interests researchers when accuracy is considered. If variation exists in a characteristic, the accuracy of any estimate of the parameter will be reduced as the size of the sample is decreased. This relation is clearly shown in this chapter's discussion on reliability and also in Chapters 10 and 11.

The student conducting a research project for the first time frequently asks his adviser, "How many subjects must I have?" or "How many places must I survey?" The answer is use the largest sample possible. Since a researcher is interested in learning about a population, the larger the sample studied, the more likely the measured findings will be representative of the population parameters. The researcher is less likely to obtain negative results or to make incorrect inferences about the collected data when samples are large. In research relations (correlation) at least 30 subjects are advisable, whereas in experimental studies involving comparisons of groups, a minimum of 15 are desirable. The numbers are arbitrary and not well founded; each study should be considered on its own merit and the decision becomes a judgment (yours and the adviser's or an advisory committee). Several factors should be considered in making the decision about sample size:

1. Definition of Variable. If the trait and method of gathering data are so well defined that each datum possesses the same value or trait as the next datum being measured, the answer is one datum. In physical therapy no variable seems to be such that every member in the population possesses the same amount of the variable. Human and animal subjects seem to have considerable variation among their members, and studying the variations involves the theory of probability. Information is available for estimating sample sizes when responses are to treatments qualitative[9] and when responses are quantitative.[10]

Researchers can choose the same sample size used in a closely related study that has been published. Knowledge about the standard deviations from previously reported studies can be used in estimating your sample size. For example, suppose you located two reported studies in which standard deviations were cited for the dependent variable. The mean of the two standard deviations or data gathered from your pilot work can be used for estimating the sample size. Borg and Gall have offered the formula $N = (2s^2 \times t^2)/D^2$ for estimating the sample size (N) for two groups. They assume that the groups are of equal size and that the standard deviations are similar.[11]

N = number of cases needed in each group to achieve a significant difference at the 0.05 level (Table C, Appendix)

s = hypothetical mean standard deviation, 12

t = t test value, 2–tailed, for 0.05 significance level for 20 cases, 2.086

D = half of the mean standard deviation which is the estimated difference between the means of the two groups, 6

$$\text{e.g., } N = \frac{(2 \times 12^2) \times 2.086^2}{6^2} = \frac{288 \times 4.35}{36} = 35$$

The formula estimates that 35 cases will be needed in each of the two groups.

2. Assurance of Representation. Because of sampling variations, the researcher cannot be absolutely sure that the sample data is representative of the population. This difficulty increases when samples of convenience are used; however variations occur with other types of sampling also. The population must be defined clearly so that no doubt exists about who or what is represented. If a population is sampled, data must provide the most representative information for answering the question. Defining the problem provides answers and insight for selecting the sample most representative of the population. In the end, however, the defined population determines the size of the sample. If therapists in San Francisco are defined as a population, measuring each therapist would not be too difficult and the question about representation is solved.

3. Time and Costs. Meeting the needs of the pocketbook probably determines the size of the sample quicker than most other factors. If the researcher has unlimited time and funds, great pains can be taken to ensure a representative sample. Assistance can be obtained for a price and this reduces time in gathering data. The sample of convenience is most often used in practice because of constraints imposed by time and costs. The general rule of thumb is to include as many numbers in a sample as practical for answering the question.

Some beginning researchers think that a large number of subjects is needed to convince readers or critics of the outcome of the study: yes, if statistical analyses are not being used to analyze the data and only counts or percentages are used as the best representation of the parameters; no, if parametric statistical tests are used to analyze measurements. Statistical tests of significance are rugged and take into account the number of data in a sample. Such tests assist in making the appropriate conclusion based on the number of data collected. Small numbers of data obtained from a well-planned and controlled study and analyzed properly usually yield more accurate information than large numbers of data handled and analyzed poorly. If expected differences between treatments are large, small numbers of subjects are appropriate; however, if differences are expected to be small or are unknown, then large numbers of subjects are needed.

4. Criterion for Publication. Research is never complete until the results have been published. Referees of some journals are impressed by large sample sizes; however, statistics applied properly may negate use of large samples. Of course, statistics are based on sets of standards and norms which take into account the size of the sample. Surveys or relation studies do not have similarly established standards. The latter usually contain large numbers in the selected samples, because the closer the sample size is to the true size of the population, the more accurate the conclusions. Statistics are not needed when the entire population has been measured; since no probability is present, the values are then true.

Some colleagues maintain that more than 30 data constitute a large sample in experimental studies whereas others state that more than 50 constitute a large sample. Alder has defined a small sample as being less than 30 variates and a large sample as more than 30 variates.[12] Small sample sizes are used in research involving animals because of costs and the ultimate loss of the subject.

5. Large samples are needed when:

a. Many variables are uncontrolled. If the researcher cannot control the important variables in the study, large samples are needed to achieve confidence in the results.

b. Small changes are expected. Sometimes differences between group means or associations between groups will be small because of the nature of the measurement. Large samples are desirable in these situations.

c. Groups are subdivided. Occasionally the researcher must subdivide cases into small groups because of the design of the study. To prevent very small numbers of cases appearing in each subgroup, increased numbers are desirable.

d. Dependable scores on the dependent variable are not available. If data are inconsistent because of the elusive nature of the dependent variable, a greater number of cases or measurements should be included in the study. This situation may apply more in research using software instruments for measurement.[11]

RELIABILITY

Suppose a physical therapist determined the heart rate of a subject by counting the pulses of the radial artery in a unit of time. The same procedure of palpating the artery, counting the pulses, and measuring the time with a stopwatch was repeated several times. The closeness of the measured outcomes would then indicate the dependability of the procedure. Reliability is the dependability, repeatability, or reproducibility of research or a measuring instrument. Whenever close agreement of the same phenomenon exists among several measurements, the reliability of the procedure, instrument, or research will be high. Under conditions of minimal error, the researcher and consumer can interpret the results of a single study with confidence.[13]

Several instruments used in nonexperimental research were discussed in Chapter 6; experimental research instruments are discussed in Chapter 8. The concept of reliability applies to both methods of research and is presented so that the reader can develop an awareness of the importance of precision in research.

Definitions of Reliability

Several synonyms for reliability have been used earlier. Some additional synonyms used commonly to define reliability are stability, consistency, and predictability.[14] An instrument is reliable if it consistently measures similar values in the same quantities or qualities with repeated application. Reliability refers to the extent to which an instrument agrees with itself, a relation index.[15] A reliable instrument is capable of displaying similar scores when the same instrument is used for a second administration of the same quantity; the instrument should give constant values for a constant quantity being measured. In measuring muscular performance of a group, random errors may be present because of transient effects of fatigue, motivation, parallax of the instrument's indicator, learning, or other factors that are temporary or changeable. An instrument may be reliable, but the study is not because of errors. Precision also describes reliability. High values of reliability are indicative of the relative absence of errors in experimentation and sampling.

Theory of Reliability

We know that measures of values (scores) are confounded with errors. The theory of measurement takes into account that all scores of human behavior contain amounts of the variable being measured in addition to the error component. The true amount of the variable (or person's trait) is reflected by measured values, and that amount of the trait should be constant when measured repeatedly under similar conditions. We know that variation occurs among subjects, and we know that the amounts of the trait (dependent variable) vary when conditions vary. Suppose we assess the amount of a patient's injured soft tissue by measuring the heat emission of the injured area. We assume that the measure (degrees Celcius) remains constant until healing begins, and after healing begins, the recorded temperatures will change in proportion to the healing. We also assume that part of the recorded temperature is due to error (measuring) and that part is due to the amount of soft tissue injury (true value). Since errors of measurement are random or occur by chance in different directions (e.g., self–compensating),[14] each occurrence of error is independent of all other errors of measurement.[15] Random errors follow the probability curve of distribution.

Let us examine the reliability of the mean, which we respect highly in research and science. This examination of the concept of reliability from a theoretical approach will increase your understanding of measurement and the concepts of central tendency.

Reliability of the Mean. We know that in order to study the heat produced by injured soft tissues, we cannot measure all patients in the world having injured soft tissues. We must take a sample sufficiently large and representative of patients having injured soft tissues of the type we want to study. To be representative, we must select patients from varied sources. The computed mean of our sample data will depend on the number of patients in the sample and the variability of the measures being recorded (degrees Celcius for electromagnetic radiation). Examination of any number of data clearly shows that the addition of one (or more) datum (data) to the sample will alter the original mean. The additional datum affects change more in a sample with 16 data than in a sample with 64 data. The reliability of a statistic increases in proportion to the square root of the number of additional data. The mean obtained from 16 data is four times more reliable than a single datum ($\sqrt{16} = 4$). The mean obtained from 64 data is eight times more reliable than a single additional datum ($\sqrt{64} \div \sqrt{1} = 8$), but only twice as reliable as the mean from 16 data ($\sqrt{64} \div \sqrt{16} = 2$). We also know that if the variance or standard deviation of a sample of data is large, the individual data tend to scatter widely. The opposite effect of scatter among data occurs when the measure of variation is small. Scatter of data influences the mean (extreme scores).

The reliability of the mean is measured by its standard error. The standard error of the mean (**SEM**) is the standard deviation of a distribution of means taken from all possible samples of a population. If a variable, X, is distributed in a population with a mean, μ, and standard deviation, σ, and if all possible samples are taken from the population, then the sample mean, $\overline{X}$, will be distributed so that as the sample size increases in numbers, the standard deviation (standard error) of the mean will be $s_{\overline{x}}$.[16] The formula for the **SEM**

$$s_{\overline{x}} = \frac{s}{\sqrt{n}}$$

where s is the standard deviation and $\sqrt{n}$ is the square root of the number of subjects in the sample. The **SEM** is influenced then by the standard deviation and the square of the size of the sample. A decrease in the standard deviation or an increase in the sample size results in a small **SEM** or an increased reliability of the mean.[17] Sample size is an important consideration in planning research.

If we wanted to measure the functional lung capacity of a patient having emphysema before beginning a therapeutic program to increase the functional expiratory capacity, we could ask the patient to breathe into a respirometer. The value recorded would give us an indication of the patient's functional lung capacity for that particular effort. Remember that the score recorded is combined with the true measure (capacity) and error. If we ask the patient to repeat the effort, rest, repeat, rest, repeat, and continue many more times without causing fatigue, the recorded scores will not be exact. With repeated efforts and recordings, we assume that the range of capacities has been recorded and that the mean of all the scores is the best estimate of the patient's true capacity and can be used to predict the patient's next score. If the recordings are repeated many times, the distribution of scores should form a normal distribution when frequency and magnitude of scores are plotted. The first value recorded is not as reliable a measure of the patient's true capacity as the mean of scores from many repeated efforts.

Each recorded measure of capacity contains a true value and an error value. The situation is represented by the formula:

$$X = X_T + X_E.$$

If the mean is the true score of the patient's capacity, then the variation in scores can be represented by the standard deviation of the mean (**SEM**).

Reliability of the Variance. Scores can be discussed in terms of variance (standard deviation squared) by using a formula similar to the one above, that is, $S_x^2 = S_T^2 + S_E^2$ where S_x^2 is the variance of the observed scores, S_T^2 is the true proportion, and S_E^2 is the error proportion. In practice we cannot separate the true proportion and error proportion from a recorded score. The theory of measurement circumvents this dilemma by assuming that two equivalent measures of the same trait can be measured and their relation studied (correlation).[18] The reliability of a measuring instrument can then be stated as the proportion of the true variance to the combined variance of the recorded scores.

Factors Influencing Reliability of Instruments for Nonexperimental Research

Since most of the instruments used in nonexperimental research are paper instruments (questionnaire, scales, written tests, and checklists), certain factors influence the dependability of the measured scores. These factors are not necessarily unique to the paper instruments. They can also influence some of the mechanical and electronic instruments when subjects must cooperate in the execution of the measuring process.

In taking measurements with paper instruments, errors or variations result if subjects do not understand or cannot follow the directions for performance. Personality characteristics can interfere with the scores or responses provided on the instruments. Attitudes or degrees of motivation can be influencing factors on one instrument but not on another. The presence of these factors depends on the instrument and the subject's behavior and reaction to the instrument or specific items or questions on the instrument. A subject's ability to respond to certain questions or items varies according to skill or knowledge of the topic. A subject may respond truthfully to some questions because he or she knows the correct response or true situation, whereas at other times he or she creates responses to appease the examiner or to complete the questions on the instrument. Physical or mental conditions at a given time vary according to moods, health, fatigue, interests, or feelings. The person conducting the measurement could be another influencing factor. Different administrators or researchers can influence responses by their degree of enthusiasm, delivery of instructions, voice, personality, and ability to handle the environment in which data are collected. Environmental fluctuations can influence information gathered by paper instruments. Distractions can disturb respondents concentrating on responses to the instruments. Distractions include noises and interruptions.

Determining Reliability of Software Instruments

Standard error of measurement provides an index of the stability of a score. The reliability (correlation) coefficient is the most frequently used index for determining the internal consistency of instruments, but it is a measure of relative stability.[15] Several varieties of designs for obtaining reliability are available; some are suited for paper instruments only.

Split–Half Method. This method is also referred to as an immediately equivalent form method.[15] The split–half method is used when construction of an alternate or equivalent form of the instrument (classroom test, attitude scale) is not feasible; that is, the administration of the instrument twice is unwise. In the split–half method, questions or items on the instrument are divided (split) into two equivalent parts (halves); the single form of the instrument is then treated as two. The division into two groups can be made before the instrument is administered, or the instrument can be scored after administration with scores of off-numbered items going to one group and scores of even-numbered items going to the other group. This method is likely to be used when testing the reliability of certain questionnaires, such as measuring personality traits, attitude scales, and performance tests (written or skilled types, such as motor or dexterity tests given to children with developmental disabilities). Repeated measurements using these kinds of instruments can be difficult because familiarity of content increases skill of performance. The split–half method reduces the need to repeat the administration of the instrument, because all data essential for computing the reliability are gathered during the one administration. Chance errors can affect the scores on both halves of the instrument in a similar fashion. This causes a trend for inflation of the reliability coefficient. The instrument designed for determining reliability should be longer than other instruments (numbers of items) so that relatively few items on either half present any problems of influencing reliability. When an instrument is split in half, the correlation between scores tends to underestimate the reliability. The Spearman–Brown formula can be used to correct for the reduction in length of an instrument and for the lowered correlation coefficient.[19]

$$r_D = \frac{N r_{12}}{1 + (N - 1) r_{12}}$$

where r_D is the correction correlation coefficient to be estimated, r_{12} is the split–half correlation coefficient computed on data, and N is the proportional increase and is always 2 for split–half. Using data for the Attitude Toward Physical Therapy, Table 6.1 of Chapter 6, the split–half correlation was 0.75. Substituting values into the Spearman–Brown formula, we have:

$$r_D = \frac{2(0.75)}{1 + (2 - 1)0.75} = \frac{1.50}{1.75} = 0.86$$

The correlation coefficient for the instrument, if it was full length, is estimated to be 0.86, a reliable attitude scale. (Discussion of the theory and computation of the correlation coefficient will follow later in this chapter.)

When planning an attitude scale, the statements are generally distributed randomly rather than according to their weighted value on a scale. The reason for this is to prevent the respondent from responding systematically to only a cluster of statements in one portion of the instrument. When testing the instrument for reliability, the odd–even arrangement will be a mixture of weighted values unless statements are arranged according to their level of difficulty or are of similar weights. No rule exists for approaches to obtaining two equivalent halves and, therefore, the reliability of the split–half method varies according to the researcher's arrangement of the odd-even statements. In the example cited and computed for split–half ($r_D = 0.75$), the reliability can be as high as 0.97 when the right items are arranged in a certain way (e.g., odd = 1, 2, 5, and 6; even = 3, 4, 7, and 8). An r_D of 0.11 represents a great difference (0.86 vs 0.97) in reliability, and the researcher must decide whether this method is the best approach for testing the reliability of this instrument.

Alternate Forms Method. This approach is also known as parallel forms method. The amount of agreement between two separate forms of an instrument is used by many psychologists to test reliability. The idea is to compose two separate instruments measuring the same content but not have them be so identical as to be revealing, and to administer them on separate occasions. A difficulty arises, however, if the instruments are administered too close together in time, because respondents may remember items. When two different forms are administered, the danger of respondent memory is eliminated because respondents have not seen the second form. Because alternate forms are different in appearance, they are often administered immediately after the first form. The instrument then can be administered without any effects from learning entering into the responses. Since little time intervenes between administrations of the instrument, a measure of stability is reflected in the coefficient.[20] Reliability coefficients will be inflated if the forms are identical and underestimated if the forms are too dissimilar.[17] The product moment method of correlation can be used to determine the reliability coefficient of alternate forms. Alternate forms can be easily constructed from the Thurstone scale because items are worded similarly and have similar weightings. Reliability is also good on the Likert scale because range of answers permits variation for the respondent. A reliability of 0.85 is common on Likert scales.[21]

Test–Retest Method. Repeating the administration of a test to measure the same quantity under similar conditions is an easy method of determining dependability of the instrument. Repetition of measurement is made on the same group of subjects and under similar testing conditions to ensure duplication. Test–retest reliability is the degree to which scores are stable or consistent over time. This approach provides evidence that a score measured at one time will be the same or very similar if the same instrument was used to measure the quality or quantity at another time. Analysis of variance is used to determine the index of reliability (intraclass correlation).

Using this method for determining reliability of paper instruments can cause some difficulty if the tests are administered too closely together. If sufficient time has not elapsed to erase memory and reduce recall, then respondents quickly mark the responses they recognize. Respondents concentrate on the areas of the instrument which they had difficulty with or were unable to complete earlier. Concentrating most of the test time on a small area can result in increased score values or altered responses, which might then cause a lowered coefficient of reliability for the instrument. A sufficient lapse in time between the first and repeated administrations of the instrument is essential to reduce or prevent the effects of memory, practice, and contact with other respondents. If sufficient time passes between administrations of the instrument, a reliable index of consistency can be obtained.

This approach is used in checking reliability of paper instruments because it negates the need for an alternate measuring instrument or for splitting a group of measures into halves for comparison. The alternate form and split–half methods are, however, preferred to the test–retest method for determining reliability of paper instruments because of the uncertainty of memory effects on the retest form.[17]

Determining Reliability of Hardware Instruments

The test–retest method is an excellent way to assess the reliability of mechanical or electronic instruments used in experimental research. The interval of time between measurements is usually not as important with hardware instruments as with paper instruments because the subject does not apply memory. What is important, however, is that measurements using hardware be recorded at similar times if physiological traits are being recorded to avoid undue influence of diurnal and circadian rhythms. Physiological traits can change in one person at different times of the day, month, or year because of influences of activity (wakefulness, fatigue, experiences, postures), environment (climatic factors such as temperature, humidity, terrain, lightness, darkness, seasons), and menstruation in women. Most body systems are affected to a certain degree by events throughout the day. The alterations in scores caused by these physiological changes may or may not affect the outcome of the experiment, but they certainly must be taken into consideration when planning the study procedures and the interpretation of the data.

Suppose you were interested in checking the consistency of an electrogoniometer. You could measure a series of specified angles along a range of motion in random fashion and note the markings on the recording paper. Another series of angles along a range of motion can be measured and recorded with the same electrogoniometer, again measuring each specified angle at random so that no systematic arrangement of angles is selected. The two sets of scores constitute a bivariate distribution and can be compared for their degree of consistency by the product moment method of correlation.

The researcher must decide what level of reliability is required of the instrument or measurement method in the measurement of the dependent variable. No universally accepted correlation values have been established for reliability coefficients; however, two schemes for consideration are offered:

A[19]		B[22]	
0.90 to 0.99	High reliability	0.80 to 1.0	Very reliable
0.80 to 0.89	Good reliability	0.60 to 0.79	Moderately reliable
0.70 to 0.79	Fair reliability	0.60 and below	Questionable reliability
0.69 and below	Poor reliability		

Inter–Rater Reliability

We have been discussing reliability in research and in instruments used in gathering data. Obtaining consistent results or readings from an instrument read by different individuals is also important. When two or more examiners measure some quantity, the consistency of their recorded values should be similar. Different observers should be able to record the same value, but this is not always the case. The amount or degree of agreement between observers is called inter–rater reliability. Earlier, the term parallax was discussed. If observers are positioned differently from an oscilloscope or meter, they could perceive the quantities displayed differently, which would then detract from the consistency, dependability, or reliability of the readings.

The common approach to assessing inter–rater reliability is to test and retest and then calculate the reliability coefficient for the two distributions of scores. Inter–rater reliability must be high or the instrument is considered ineffective. Sometimes personnel must be trained to read a particular instrument. If the observers are familiar with the instrument and units of measurement and measuring techniques are standardized, then the correlation coefficient between scores observed by different observers is usually high. The researcher must be aware of inter–rater reliability if the gathering of data is delegated to assistants. The collected data and results of the study might be erroneous if high agreement between observers does not exist. Inter–rater reliability may be poor when many persons are involved in gathering data (reading instruments); for example, several therapists gathering data at different facilities and using different instruments.

Intra–Rater Reliability

In practice, physical therapists like to believe they are consistent in the way they administer each measurement; they also believe that the scores obtained are dependable. Intra–rater reliability is the degree to which a practitioner can replicate his or her measurements of a variable and obtain similar outcomes repeatedly. Reliability measures obtained by replicating measurements of the same variable by the same person have less variability than those obtained by different observers. Consequently intra–rater reliability is more consistent than inter–rater reliability.[23] A person apparently has the ability to measure consistently because he or she repeats the conditions that are most familiar. Different raters may measure under dissimilar conditions. For example, physical therapists do not agree on a single method of manual muscle testing and, consequently, they teach different approaches in the educational programs. Two observers do not take measurements in the same way, even when conditions are similar.

Such factors as dexterity, parallax, motivation, learning-and-practice experience, inattention, contrivances of the test environment, and hand–held instruments interact to diminish controls and effect the measurement outcome.[24] Performance stability is a factor in replication of measurements and a single practitioner can apparently do this task better than two or more practitioners. Visual inspection and judgment enter into so many measurements that they preclude error–free outcomes. Practitioners can increase agreement of measures by repeating measurement trials and following standard procedures. Stratford and colleagues have suggested several strategies for improving measurement.[25]

Calculating the Reliability Coefficient

Many statistical techniques for estimating reliability, such as the Spearman–Brown formula, the standard error of measurement, Pearson's product–moment correlation, and analysis of variance, have been used in research.

The test–retest method has been used extensively for estimating the consistency with which a measure assesses a given trait or characteristic, or the amount of error attributable to two observers performing the measurements. The Pearson product–moment correlation method (presented in Chapter 10) has been commonly used to determine the degree of agreement in each situation. This method calculates an interclass coefficient and has several limitations.[22,26]

Testing subjects or making observations on two different occasions is a common procedure with the test–retest approach. Two sets of scores are obtained; however, only one variable is measured, which requires a univariate, not a bivariate statistic. The product–moment correlation is limited to two scores per subject (univariate situation) and cannot differentiate among several possible sources of error. The product–moment correlation coefficient (r) is high when scores are inconsistent; systematic increases or decreases in one set of scores occur while the scores of the other set do not vary. The product-moment correlation method is unable to identify portions of the variance attributable to systematic and random influences.[26] Systematic increases and decreases are treated as reliability, when, in fact, these changes reflect familiarization, learning fatigue, or disinterest among subjects.[27]

Because reliability is concerned with consistency over time, several remeasurements are considered a better index of stability than only two measurements. Analysis of variance (**ANOVA**) procedures are appropriate for determining reliability involving several trials[26] and whenever one variable is measured on two occasions (inter– or intra–rater reliability). Although computational and theoretical details of one–way **ANOVA** are covered in Chapter 10, a brief discussion of **ANOVA** as it relates to reliability is included in this chapter.

Analysis of variance has an advantage over the product–moment correlation method in that it examines the sources of variability between and within scores. The symbol for the reliability coefficient is R when **ANOVA** is used in its estimation. The coefficient is a ratio representing specific components of score variation and can offer separate estimates of the relative size of each component. The **ANOVA** and R coefficient are considered more accurate than the product–moment method.[28]

Since the test–retest approach to reliability examines variability of measurements on repeated trials, it measures only one variable. The coefficient R examines a single variable and is appropriate when used with **ANOVA**. R is an index of the relative homogeneity of scores within the groups or trials in relation to the total variation among all scores. The computed R value decreases in magnitude as the heterogeneity of the intraclass scores increases, and R increases as all intraclass scores become more homogeneous.[27] Interpretation of the R coefficient is similar to that of r, product-moment correlation. Maximum negative association with R occurs whenever the heterogeneity of the intraclass scores is maximum and trial means are similar.

The R coefficient is determined from variance scores in **ANOVA** but the variance terms (mean square) used in the calculation of R vary with the different **ANOVA** designs. For example, in the one–way **ANOVA** design, R is determined by using between–subjects and within–subjects variation. The more complex **ANOVA** designs, in addition to the variances used for the one–way **ANOVA,** use subject–by–trial interaction as a source of variation to compute R. Between–subjects variation is considered true score variance whereas interaction, or within–subject variance, is considered a measurement error. Reliability using **ANOVA** can be estimated by the formula:

$$R = \frac{MS \text{ between} - MS \text{ within or } MS \text{ interaction}}{MS \text{ between}}$$

where R is the reliability coefficient, MS between is the ratio of sum of squares between trials (SS_B) divided by degrees of freedom (df) between, and MS within (or MS interaction, depending on **ANOVA** design) is the ratio of sum of squares within trials (SS_W) divided by df within.

Using the theory and the computation for one–way **ANOVA** found in Chapter 10, an example can be given: Let us assume that we want to determine the reliability of a method of holding a Doppler flow meter probe manually to measure blood flow velocity effects of electrical stimulation to a particular muscle. Five subjects are selected and three measurements are taken from each subject undergoing similar test conditions on the same day. Summary of the measurements and computation are shown in Table 7.1. A one–way **ANOVA** random design is applied to the data as if each score was randomly obtained rather than being a repeated measurement. The **ANOVA** computation of Table 7.1 follows that illustrated in Table 10.5. The obtained R coefficient is 0.84, which is interpreted as good reliability for the method of measuring blood flow. For a more complex **ANOVA** design, for example a two–way **ANOVA**, the MS

Table 7.1
Computation of the R Coefficient of Intraclass Correlation as an Estimate of Reliability (Fictitious Data in Cm/Sec)

Subjects	Trials			ΣX	$(\Sigma X)^2$	ΣX^2
A	36	35	38	109	11881	3965
B	35	35	37	107	11449	3819
C	36	36	36	108	11664	3888
D	33	32	34	99	9801	3269
E	37	36	38	111	12321	4109
	Totals ($\Sigma\Sigma$)			534	57116	19050

$$n = \text{number of subjects} = 5 \qquad N = \text{subjects} \times \text{trials} = 15$$

$$SS \text{ total} = \Sigma\Sigma X^2 - \frac{(\Sigma\Sigma X)^2}{N} = 19050 - \frac{534^2}{15} = 39.60$$

$$SS \text{ between trials} = \Sigma \text{ samples} \frac{(\Sigma X)^2}{n} - \frac{(\Sigma X)^2}{N} = \frac{57116}{3} - \frac{534^2}{15} = 28.27$$

$$MS \text{ between} = \frac{SS \text{ within}}{\text{subjects} - 1} = \frac{28.27}{4} = 7.07$$

$$MS \text{ within} = \frac{SS \text{ within}}{N - n} = \frac{11.33}{10} = 1.33$$

$$R = \frac{MS \text{ between} - MS \text{ within}}{MS \text{ between}} = \frac{7.07 - 1.33}{7.07} = 0.84$$

interaction term for determining the F ratio is used as the source of measurement error in the numerator of the formula for finding R (designs are discussed in Chapter 9).

The interclass correlation coefficient is used to determine reliability of dichotomous data and two raters, but it is most appropriate for polychotomous data and more than two raters (or one rater over several trials).[28] The calculation of the intraclass correlation coefficient (R) is preferred over the product–moment correlation coefficient (r) for estimating reliability.[28–32]

VALIDITY

Suppose a physical therapist repeated an experiment several times in which the heart rate of subjects was measured by counting pulses of the radial artery in a unit of time. If the mean heart rate from experiments did not agree closely with the mean heart rate recorded simultaneously by a cardiac catheterization method, then their relation is suspect. Assuming that the cardiac catheterization measure (criterion) is the more accurate method, then the amount of agreement between the two constitutes the degree of validity of the palpation technique. The criterion measure is considered a standard because it is the most accurate method for measuring heart rate; all other methods are compared with it for accuracy. If errors or biases are nonexistent or minimal in research, the accuracy of the investigation will be high.

The accuracy of an instrument or a research study is essential for reasons which should now be obvious. Systematic error was discussed as contributing to the inaccuracy of an instrument or study; the lack of systematic error helps to increase accuracy. Validity constitutes the degree to which an instrument measures what it is supposed to measure. This definition limits the scope of an instrument to measuring only that unit which it is designed to measure; validity is specific to each instrument or to each study. Validity of one type of strength–measuring instrument does not guarantee validity of a similar instrument. A tensiometer may be valid for assessing forces, but a strain gauge (which appears to be very expensive, sophisticated, and valid looking) may not necessarily be a valid instrument. Certainly the instrument is capable of measuring kilograms but, if checked with known forces and found to be measuring values higher or lower than the known forces, the instrument is not accurate (valid). Sometimes the instrument can be adjusted or corrected for this systematic error and then becomes more valid than before the corrections. We must have some assurance that we are measuring what we are supposed to be measuring. Validity is less of a problem in the physical sciences than in the behavioral sciences when measuring instruments are involved. When the measure or quantity is relatively stable or constant, the quantities can be measured easily by specific mechanical and electronic instruments. For example, many instruments are designed simply to measure accurately distance, mass, electricity, and time; measuring the behavior of a human, however, is more complex because of the elusiveness of behavior. More methods are available for assessing the validity of paper instruments than for assessing hardware instruments; the need is greater for assessing paper instruments than mechanical or electronic instruments. This discussion covers concerns about validity of instruments in experimental and nonexperimental research.

Validity of Software Instruments

In Chapter 6 several instruments for measuring qualities and quantities directly or indirectly were discussed. How do we know that an instrument will measure what we think when we design it for our research? Survey instruments are designed for the purpose and use of the user. The type of validity is dependent on the intended use. Specific types of validity assessments must be available to determine the degree to which an instrument measures what it is designed to measure. The American Psychological Association has identified three types of validity (content, criterion–related, and construct) for tests and survey instruments.[27]

Content Validity. Content validity is a measure of how well an instrument measures the content of a particular trait or body of knowledge. Content validity is the representativeness of the subject by the items selected to measure a trait or characteristic; it describes how well the instrument reflects information about a particular phenomenon in the universe or about a population.[14] If a therapist wants to study the attitudes of patients toward a specific form of mobilization, a pool of items or statements is compiled. When the instrument has been constructed and the 20 or 30 items have been selected, the researcher assesses the content validity of the instrument.

Content validation is essentially judgmental. The statements in the attitude scale are examined individually for their representativeness of the attitude to be measured. The relevance of each statement to the attitude must be considered, as well as the assigned weighted values. The researcher might ask colleagues who are knowledgeable about the process or about the attitude to be measured to evaluate the appropriateness of the statements for representing the content. The Thurstone scaling method does this when judges are asked to order items. If the judges do not comment on the representativeness of the statements but only order them according to the continuum, then content validation is not provided. When the particular trait or attitude to be measured is clearly defined by the researcher, then the associated content of the trait or attitude can be established. Judges who can relate the statements to the defined trait have a good grasp of the contents included in the instrument, and thus make good judgments. The statements are judged for representativeness of the identified content. The process of using judgments to determine representativeness is, of course, subjective. Using several different judges helps to determine which statements are consistently rated high or low. The instrument must be reliable to be valid. The split–half method of reliability can be used to determine the internal consistency of the instrument and is more objective than judgments. A high correlation coefficient tells the researcher that the statements are measuring the same variable. If an instrument measures one variable or factor and if it is identified as being representative of a certain content area, then the instrument has content validity.

Criterion–Related Validity. If an instrument demonstrates a close relation to another instrument (criterion) when measuring some known quantity or quality, the instrument is said to be valid. The criterion is an already well-established, well-accepted instrument considered to be the best of its kind. Because of this high degree of acceptance, new instruments are compared with it for determining criterion–related validity.

Suppose a therapist wants to measure the job satisfaction of colleagues working in general hospitals in Dallas. A new instrument is designed and constructed. The instrument is tested as a pilot project by being administered to a group of therapists. The Minnesota Satisfaction Questionnaire (a normative instrument) is administered to the same group of therapists. The scores obtained on the two instruments form a bivariate distribution and are analyzed for their degree of association by the product–moment method of correlation. If the correlation coefficient is high, the new instrument is valid for measuring job satisfaction because it agrees with the criterion. If the two instruments are administered at the same time, the validity is concurrent. Concurrent validity is criterion–related validity and is measured when the predictor instrument (the one being tested) and the criterion instrument are administered concurrently. The extent of the relation of the two instruments, or the degree to which the two instruments measure the same trait or quantity of a variable, reflects accuracy. Predictive validity is another type of criterion–related validity and is measured when the criterion measurement is made after the predictor instrument (new) has measured data. If the personnel director of a large hospital administered a job satisfaction questionnaire (new instrument) to all new physical therapy employees after 1 to 2 months of employment and then administered the questionnaire 1 year later, the first set of scores administered will predict the employee's satisfaction. If the two sets of scores are closely related after the second administration of the questionnaire, then the instrument has good predictive validity.

The two types of validity are similar; time is the only difference. Instruments possessing predictive validity are often used to solve problems. In education, an aptitude test is used to predict success in college or in some vocations. Intelligence tests in psychology predict a person's ability to learn or to cope with technology. Faculty members of physical therapy programs are greatly concerned about admitting only those students who will make the best therapists. If "best therapists" could be defined and then an instrument developed to measure the desired traits, then the instrument could predict candidates who would make good therapists. The instrument could be tested for its predictive qualities by measuring a group of successful therapists who had been measured before admission to the program and had graduated; scores for determining predictive validity could then be compared. A validated instrument like this would be helpful in selecting future students; perhaps research ability could be one content measure.

The degree of association or difference between two variables provides evidence to support criterion–related validity. Statistical methods can be used to provide a relative measure of association (correlational) and difference (mean differences between groups). In the correlational approach, the students are grouped into categories—"successful" or "unsuccessful." The coefficient is computed to predict from a test score to a measured criterion of success on a job sometime later. The measurements taken later can then be compared with those obtained earlier to determine relations by the product moment method of correlation. Degrees of job success can be determined in this way. Correlation does not imply causation or effect; that is, the reason for the outcomes. Studies in relations measure only the degree in which variables differ. A positive correlation implies that variables tend to vary in the same direction, higher scores on one variable tend to relate or vary with higher scores on the other variable. Low correlation values indicate that there is little association between the variables. Small sample findings can lead to false information because coefficients obtained from small samples tend to be inflated.

Another way of establishing criterion–related validity is to test the differences between means obtained from different samples. If the difference between means is great, the instrument differentiates between groups. If the admissions instrument could discriminate between good and unsatisfactory candidates for becoming physical therapy students or if it could predict on-the-job success, the instrument would predict accurately and would be desirable for student selection.

Construct Validity. Construct validity is concerned with identifying the concept (construct) that accounts for the variance of the survey or test, or for explaining the differences in the measured scores by the instrument. In addition, construct validity addresses the validation of the theory behind an instrument. When concepts are identified for explaining the variance, then hypotheses can be formed for testing the construct. The results derived from testing hypotheses determine the acceptance of the identified concept. This particular procedure raises the determination process to a higher level of scientific inquiry (hypothesis testing) and gains acceptance for the process in the scientific community.

Construct validity cannot be determined by statistical analysis because it is a judgment on the theoretical aspects of a concept or measure based on research findings involving the concept or measure itself. Rothstein has identified the manual muscle test, muscle strength, and muscle endurance as examples of implied construct validity (all in need, however, of solid footing).[33]

Validity of Hardware Instruments

Error is not the same problem to physical scientists as it is to behavioral and life scientists. In the physical sciences, error is minimal or, if error exists, it is corrected or eliminated. If a device does not measure what it is supposed to, it is eliminated, reconstructed, or adjusted and the experiment goes forward. No matter what scientists do in the behavioral and life sciences, error and variation exist. Validity is less of a problem than reliability when using mechanical or electronic instruments. When test instruments are new or constitute new approaches to old instruments, the researcher or manufacturer wants to know if the instruments achieve their claims. Often the researcher is faced with defending the validity of the instrument in a research study. The next section discusses the validity of hardware instruments.

Face Validity. Some instruments are one of a kind, the only instrument that measures the phenomenon. Face validity merely defends the extent to which the instrument appears to measure what it claims. This validity merely provides a narrative or verbal defense of the instrument. Suppose a manufacturer markets a device to measure the speed of electrons and it is the only instrument capable of measuring electrons. If the particular instrument is the only one of its kind, then it cannot be compared to another measure; it is defended on faith, or face value. The instrument measures what the manufacturer states. Face validity is an accurate measure of what a device is supposed to measure after it is constructed.[25] Face validity is used in the physical sciences and is not a major concern in the life sciences. In experimental research where comparison type studies are performed, the researcher may or may not be concerned with the measurement validity of the instrument. This may be accepted on face value and used appropriately for measuring the data. Experimental research often involves the customized construction of instruments not available commercially, creating a one-of-a-kind device for defined measure.

Criterion–Related Validity. This approach is similar to that used in nonexperimental research. If a newly contrived instrument or a new approach to measuring a known phenomenon is improved but another measuring device is available and accurate, the researcher can use the criterion–related approach for determining validity of the new tool. The older, established instrument is used as the criterion measure and the degree of agreement with the new instrument is determined by the correlation method. Each instrument measures several quantities of the known unit, and the bivariate distribution formed by the scores obtained by each instrument is determined for degrees of relation. An example of this is the Scholander apparatus used to measure quantities of P_{CO_2} and P_{O_2} from the expired air of subjects during exercise. The Scholander apparatus is simply constructed, accurate, and inexpensive, but it is tedious to operate. Electronic devices available commercially measure quantities easily and rapidly. Researchers who want to know how closely a commercial apparatus agrees with the standard Scholander unit often determine the criterion–related validity of the commercial unit in exercise research.

Another form of criterion–related validity more commonly used than that discussed in the previous example is calibration. Calibration is the determination of an instrument's accuracy to a known scale or standard unit. An oscilloscope is calibrated by comparing a deflected unit of voltage with the grid on the face and, if perfect agreement is not obtained, the oscilloscope is "trimmed" until the displayed quantity corresponds with the standard scale or unit. Calibration is a relative approach or an approximation to the unit believed to be real. The irony of calibration (criterion-related validity) is that determinations are occasionally objective for subjective values. If interval level measurements are being performed and the instrument is calibrated, the zero point on the interval scale is arbitrary, not absolute, as in ratio measurements. Because good research results are dependent on minimizing error, great efforts are made to calibrate instruments for accuracy before gathering data. This procedure of validating instruments gives readers and the researcher confidence in the outcome of the study.

The instrument's measuring ability can drift from accuracy because of constant use, age, handling, abuse by users, maintenance, and environmental conditions surrounding the instrument during operation.

Calculating the Validity Coefficient. Criterion–related validity is the degree to which scores on one instrument are related to those on another. The coefficient is determined by establishing the relation. The Pearson product–moment correlation technique (Chapter 10) has been used for determining association, but because a single variable is being assessed, this approach is dubious. When the correlation technique is used, however, measurements are taken from a defined group of subjects by administering the new instrument followed by the established instrument (criterion measure). The two sets of scores are then correlated. The resulting coefficient indicates the criterion–related validity of the new instrument. The scheme for comparing reliability coefficients of instruments is similar for interpreting the validity index.

The paired *t* test (Chapter 10) also is appropriate for testing two groups of scores on a single variable. The *t* test determines whether there are additive effects or bias present between the two groups of scores. The coefficient of variation (Chapter 5) is used to show the relative degree of variability for the two groups; this approach is less desirable than the other two suggested for determining validity.

SUMMARY

Sampling, random, systematic, and researcher errors are inaccuracies that can occur during an investigation. Research must be consistent and accurate if it is to be useful to the practitioner.

Error affects both reliability and validity. Reliability is the degree to which research and instruments are consistent or dependable; validity is the degree to which research and instruments do what they are supposed to do. The test–retest method is a common means of determining reliability and requires that a project or measurement be administered two or more times to the same subjects. The criterion–related method of determining validity requires that measurements taken with a new or unestablished instrument be compared with those gathered from an established (criterion) instrument.

Calculation of **ANOVA** and *R* provide an index for reliability, whereas other methods are used for validity. Table 7.2 provides a summary of research processes presented thus far.

Table 7.2
Cumulative Summary of the Research Processes Presented

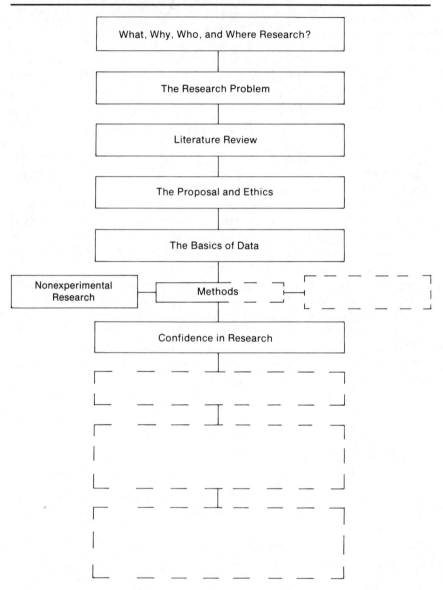

REFERENCES

1. Cox KR: Planning Clinical Experiments. Springfield, Charles C Thomas Pub, 1968
2. Ferguson GA: Statistical Analysis in Psychology and Education, ed 5. New York, McGraw–Hill Book Co, 1981
3. Wilson EB, Jr: An Introduction to Scientific Research. New York, McGraw–Hill Book Co, 1952
4. Guilford JP, Fruchter B: Fundamental Statistics in Psychology and Education, ed 6. New York, McGraw–Hill Book Co, 1977
5. Stewart HF, Harris GR, Herman BA, et al: Survey of use and performance of ultrasonic therapy equipment in Pinellas County, Florida. Phys Ther 54: 707–715, 1974
6. Honet JC, Jebsen RH, Perrin EB: Variability of nerve conduction velocity determinations in normal persons. Arch Phys Med Rehab 49: 650–654, 1968
7. Nelson RM, Brooks R, Currier DP: An automated method to determine the conduction time of peripheral motor nerves. Proc World Confed Phys Ther 7: 140–146, 1974
8. Cain RB: Elementary Statistical Concepts. Philadelphia, WB Saunders Co, 1972
9. Cochran WG, Cox GM: Experimental Designs, ed 2. New York, Wiley, 1957
10. Cochran WG, Snedecor GW: Statistical Methods, ed 6, Ames, Iowa, Iowa State University, 1967
11. Borg WR, Gall MD: Educational Research: An Introduction, ed. 3. New York, Longman, 1979
12. Alder HL, Roessler EB: Introduction to Probability and Statistics, ed 6. San Francisco, WH Freeman and Co, 1977
13. Schor S: Fundamentals of Biostatistics. New York, BP Putnam's Sons, 1968
14. Kerlinger FN: Foundations of Behavioral Research, ed 2. New York, Holt Rinehart and Winston, Inc, 1973
15. Thorndike RM: Reliability. In Bolton B (ed): Handbook of Measurement and Evaluation in Rehabilitation. Baltimore, Universtiy Park Press, 1976
16. Morehouse CA, Stull GA: Statistical Principles and Procedures with Applications for Physical Education. Philadelphia, Lea & Febiger, 1975
17. Garrett HE: Statistics in Psychology and Education, ed 5. New York, Longmans, Green and Co, 1958
18. Gulliksen H: Theory of Mental Tests. New York, Wiley & Sons, 1950
19. Blesh TE: Measurement in Physical Education, ed 2. New York, The Ronald Press Co, 1974
20. Moser CA, Kalton G: Survey Methods in Social Investigation, ed 2. London, Heinemann, 1972
21. Oppenheim AN: Questionnaire Design and Attitude Measurement. London, Heinemann, 1966
22. Richman J, Madrides L, Prince B: Research methodology and applied statistics, Part 3: Measurement procedures in research. Physiother Canada 32: 253–257, 1980
23. Gajdosik RL, Bohannon RW: Clinical measurement of range of motion: review of goniometry emphasizing reliability and validity. Phys Ther 67: 1867–1872, 1987
24. Krebs DE: Measurement theory. Phys Ther 67: 1834–1839, 1987
25. Stratford P, Agostino V, Brazeau C, et al: Reliability of joint angle measurement: a discussion of methodology issues. Physiother Canada 36: 5–9, 1984
26. Roscoe JT: Fundamental Research Statistics for the Behavioral Sciences, ed 2. New York, Holt, Rinehart and Winston, Inc, 1975
27. Standards for Educational and Psychological Tests. Washington, Am Psych Assoc, 1974
28. Bartko JJ, Carpenter WT: On the methods and theory of reliability. J Nerv Ment Dis 163: 307–317, 1976
29. Safrit MJ (ed): Reliability Theory. Washington DC, Am Alliance Health Phys Educ Rec, 1976

30. Kroll W: A note on the coefficient of intraclass correlation as an estimate of reliability. Res Q Am Assoc Health Phys Educ 33: 313–316, 1962
31. Safrit MJ: Evaluation in Physical Education: Assessing Motor Behavior. Englewood Cliffs, NJ, Prentice-Hall, 1973
32. Lahey MA, Downey RG, Saal FE: Intraclass correlations: There's more there than meets the eye. Psychol Bull 93: 586–595, 1983
33. Rothstein JM: Measurement and Clinical Practice: Theory and Application. In Rothstein JM (ed): Measurement in Physical Therapy, New York, NY, Churchill Livingstone Inc, 1985

8

Experimental Research

I have formerly lived by hearsay, and faith,
but now I go where I shall live by sight. . .
John Bunyan

The ultimate in scientific inquiry is experimentation. Through experimentation, it is possible to test hypotheses, to question authority, and to classify and differentiate traits or variables. An experiment is the manipulation of some variable or variables (independent) under rigidly controlled conditions to observe the effects of the manipulation. Experimentation enables the researcher to compare two or more variables to determine whether the effects (dependent variables) are equal, unequal, larger, or smaller than the other variables. The unique feature of experiments and comparative research is hypothesis testing. The experimental method is the only approach of truly testing hypotheses as they concern cause and effect relations. Testing hypotheses in research experiments is characterized by measuring, recording, analyzing, and interpreting data by manipulating at least one variable under investigation. Experimental and comparative research are synonymous in meaning and, therefore, are used interchangeably in this book.

Hardware instruments are metal implements, devices, equipment, or machines used in the research process and consume a proportion of the discussion in this chapter. Although hardware instruments are commonly associated with experimental research, software instruments may be used in experimental research to compare behaviors of a group of subjects on two different occasions. Discussion in this chapter concentrates on the what and where of experimental research, the research process, control in research, its limitations, and general considerations of instruments.

DEFINITIONS AND PURPOSES

Experimental research is the process of testing hypotheses or principles. It involves the manipulation of a controlled variable(s) and the observation of the effect of such skilled handling on a predetermined vari-

181

able.[1] Experimental research can be further defined as observation under controlled conditions in which software and hardware instruments are used to measure responses resulting from the controlled conditions. In experimental methods of research, controlled conditions (also called norms, models, or baselines) are standardized procedures used to assess the effects of the experimental treatment or manipulation.

In experimental research, the investigator manipulates one or more independent variables while observing the effect on one dependent variable and controlling other appropriate variables. The researcher's manipulating of the independent variable is a characteristic that separates experimental research from other forms of research. The independent variable is what causes the difference between the variables being tested. The independent variable is also referred to as the experimental or the treatment variable. The outcome or posttest result of an experiment is the dependent variable or the experimental effect. The dependent variable is sometimes called the criterion variable and accounts for the change occurring between groups or events as a result of manipulating the independent variable(s). In other words, the dependent variable is contingent on the independent variable(s); it is the measureable outcome. The dependent variable may be measured by hardware or software instruments.

The purpose of experimental research is to observe behavioral or physiological characteristics that change with various treatments or controlled conditions and to compare observed differences. It permits researchers to make comparisons between different approaches to treatment and to establish cause-and-effect relations between two or more variables.[1] In experimental research the researcher creates the cause by deliberately making the independent variables or groups different and then by observing the effect that this difference has on the dependent variable.[2] The researcher judges the effectiveness of a particular method by observing the difference occurring between pretest and posttest measurements. The pretest scores serve as the control against the outcome of the study.

Experimental research occupies the highest position on the hierarchial scale of investigative methods. It is the most demanding and most productive research method. If properly managed, it produces the best evidence about the cause-and-effect relations of hypotheses.[2] Experimental research makes inference and prediction possible. It comprises several operations that already have been presented and some processes still to be discussed. Such operations include identifying and delimiting the problem, the literature review, approval of the proposal containing the method of the study (design in Chapter 9 and analysis in Chapters 10 and 11), sampling data, controlling variables, and reporting the findings (Chapter 12). Experimental research provides the scientist with the opportunity to measure quantities, to determine causes or effects of measured quantities, and as a result of findings, to question authority. Oyster and colleagues attributed the tightest, most precise form of research to experiments which permit the researcher to trust the outcome of experimentation.[3]

Experimentation in physical therapy uses designs which enable control of certain variables and also enable certain interpretations to be made. The experiment is a scientific way of determining cause-and-effect relations quantitatively. Comparative studies usually involve statistical analyses that determine differences between two or more means. The experiment is designed in such a way that the factor(s) causing the difference between means has been isolated and is identifiable. Chapters 10 and 11 discuss statistical methods for determining differences in comparative research.

THE SETTING

Scientific research can be conducted in many settings, ranging from simple observations of a child's behavior during a specified activity (case study of child behavior) to a rigidly controlled complex experiment (comparative study). A laboratory is often the setting for experimental studies that remove human subjects or animals from their natural environment to manipulate treatments or variables. Some authors make a distinction between laboratory and field settings.[4] The laboratory setting is usually a room or suite where extensive equipment is available to measure and control conditions. The laboratory is considered an artificial setting because it takes subjects away from their natural settings for observation. An example is the energy cost studies of walking performed in a laboratory (as opposed to performing the measurements in a natural environment where individuals walk and engage in normal work activities). The latter situation would be considered a field setting. The field setting is one in which the researcher goes to the natural environment to take the measurements or to observe behavior under certain conditions. No distinction between the two settings will be made hereafter, because the laboratory is defined as the environment in which the researcher and subjects operate to gather data for the study. Distinction is made in this book, however, between descriptive and comparative research methods. In nonexperimental research, the investigator is interested in describing the project status, whereas in experimental research, he or she is interested in uncovering the cause-and-effect relations. The experimental methods involve micro- and macroresearch.

THE PROCESS

The steps in experimental research are similar to those in other types of research. The researcher chooses and defines the problem, chooses subjects and measurement tools, selects the appropriate experimental design, collects data by following specific procedures, analyzes data, and makes predictions or inferences.[2] The experiment is conducted to confirm or refute the hypothesis. Experimental investigations are directed by one or more hypotheses that state the expected outcome between variables.

Group–comparison Experiments

The scientific method, when used in clinical research, usually involves two or more groups, an experimental and a control group. Basically in group–comparison experiments, the experimental group(s) receives a specific treatment for testing, whereas the control group receives no treatment other than measurements. Treatment in the experimental group is a manipulated variable serving as an independent causal agent or effect. The two groups of subjects are compared to determine differences. Withholding treatment from the control group presents an ethical issue in health disciplines. In effect, the group–comparison experiments usually involve an experimental group(s) that receives a new or experimental treatment concomitantly with a conventional form of intervention. The control group receives only the conventional form of treatment. Both groups are then similarly measured and treated with accepted procedures. Comparison is possible when responses to the manipulated variables are measured for each group. An example of a group–comparison experiment is a study of treatment effectiveness during the six weeks immediately following knee surgery for anterior cruciate ligament repair. The control group receives muscle setting and constant passive motion exercise; the experimental group receives vigorous isometric exercise through electrical stimulation, in addition to the same exercise regimen as the control group. The two groups of patients are compared for different effects caused by the electrical stimulation.

Assuming that pretest measurements are similar among groups, the various forms of treatment are administered to the experimental group(s). Following sufficient time for the treatments to take effect (if possible), the researcher remeasures the groups on posttest. If the groups change on posttest measurements, the researcher determines by statistical methods whether the change is significant, and if so, the researcher decides that the intervention was a success or a failure. The outcome can be generalized (prediction, inference) for situations with similar conditions to permit judicious approaches to patient care.

Group comparison permits the testing of hypotheses relevant to causal relations based on three factors: (1) concomitant variation, (2) occurrence of cause and effect, and (3) control of influencing internal agents.[5,6] Measurement of the dependent variable in each group before and after treatment usually determines the concomitant variation of the dependent measure occurring in each group. If knee torque is assessed before surgery and six weeks after intervention, the influence of electrical stimulation on preventing muscle wasting and weakness can be compared between the two groups of patients having anterior cruciate ligament repair. Comparing the two groups determines whether the dependent variable (torque) is equal or not between the experimental and control groups. Statistical tests are usually used in physical therapy experiments to determine whether different amounts of dependent variable exist between groups of subjects (patients).[6] The occurrence of cause and effect here depends on timing. The researcher must realize that the effect did not exist prior to the causal event. Researchers test the two groups before treatment to discern that each group possesses the same amount of dependent variable (for example, knee torque) prior to the intervention. The independent t–test is used to test for equality before intervention. In the event that the dependent variables between groups are unequal prior to treatment, the analysis of covariance may be used to assess and adjust the collected data after treatment (Chapter 10). Controlling the influencing internal agents concerns extraneous variables that might contribute to outcome measurements. This involves internal validity (Chapter 9).

Although the group–comparison experimental design is traditionally considered the most powerful and effective research approach to hypothesis testing, some limitations have been suggested. Gathering large numbers of homogeneous subjects for experiments presents difficulties: for example, obscuring individual data when reporting descriptive statistics (means, standard deviations); and trying to generalize group research findings to fit the single subject. In addition, proponents of single–case experiments worry about the wide range of subject characteristics and how these things influence the project.[7]

CONTROL IN EXPERIMENTATION

Control is central to scientific inquiry and experimentation because it serves as a baseline for comparing the effects of the manipulated variable(s). Experimental designs require a special control group of subjects for comparison against the effects of experimentation, or sometimes each subject serves as his or her own control. Experimental designs incorporate controls when several variables are involved; no variable is allowed to operate in the control group. Zero values or placebos are used as baselines whenever the characteristics under study are measured on all subjects of each group. One group's measurements are used as the baseline for later determination of the effects of the manipulated variable (difference between means may be claimed as the effects).

Controls in experiments also relate to factors other than the effects of a certain treatment. If two or more groups of subjects are used in the experiment, selection of subjects conforming to specified criteria can serve as a control to eliminate error, to enhance precision and accuracy of the experiment, and to standardize the testing procedures. Selection of subjects based on a narrow range of ages, same sex, similar occupational activities or physical life styles, severity of diseases, or similar body weights and heights, can serve as controls. If most variables are controlled by selection of subjects, standardized testing procedures, the same measuring instrumentation, and the same operator to take all data measurements, then error is reduced and variables are controlled so that differences in means can be attributed only to treatment effects. Experiment designs account for certain changes in the experimental variable, but the researcher must control all aspects of the experiment which can be controlled. Testing must adhere to rigorous procedures to ensure proficiency; using control groups helps when maturation and learning factors might influence results.[8–10]

Certain experimental factors can be controlled during the experiment as routine procedures to reduce error and permit only the effects variable to operate in the experiment. The control group in the group–comparison experiment provides the baseline for comparison to determine amounts of dependent variable in each group. Control of experimental factors increases the credibility of generalizations from experiments.

The researcher must choose all subjects with care. Sampling procedures already have been discussed in Chapter 5. Other factors must be considered when selecting subjects. Age is an important factor if the problem centers on a particular variable influenced by age. If the researcher is interested in the conduction velocities of a certain nerve, age could influence results. Studies have been reported in which results were analyzed on the basis of velocities for certain ages.[11,12] A specific age or range of ages such as the physical working capacity of sedentary men between the ages of 40 and 45 years might be of interest. The decision must be made whether homogeneity or heterogeneity of age is the important factor in the experiment. The sex of the subjects must be considered. In some studies, gender is not an important factor, whereas in others, it is. Motivation and interest factors are important in studies in which the measured data depend on the cooperation of the subjects. Strength measurements depend on the motivation and interest of the subject, whereas nerve conduction values are independent of the subject's motivation or interest. The occupations or physical activities of subjects in a sample may be important for physiological measurements. The contention is that active subjects can be expected to achieve better scores than sedentary or passive subjects in tests in which conditioning factors influence the scores.

Cox and West[13] have offered other controls for enhancing the validity of experimental research. Random assignment of subjects to groups prior to treatment eliminates bias by making the groups as equal as possible. Matching subjects by extraneous variables (variables of no interest but which may influence the outcome, e.g., sex or age) and then assigning one member of each pair randomly to the experimental group is a useful technique for obtaining equivalent groups prior to administering treatment. Another approach is to eliminate an influencing variable from the study by holding it constant. An example is to have the same observer take all measurements so that differences caused by different observers will be eliminated. Using a placebo to let subjects think they are receiving the experimental treatment and using analysis of covariance, a statistical method, to adjust scores on the dependent variable for pretest differences between groups are two other ways of obtaining equivalent groups to improve control in experimental research.[13]

The use of proper controls in comparative research produces more convincing results than if controls were lacking. An irrefutable answer to an important research question is the basis for expanding the body of knowledge of physical therapy. Control in experimentation is a measure of the researcher's ability to prevent extraneous influences from entering into the investigation and prejudicing the outcome.[3]

LIMITATIONS

Although it is the best approach to conducting research experimental research has limitations. Randomization is an excellent way to obtain equivalent groups and eliminate bias prior to administering experimental treatments; it may, however, be impossible to apply. In health research, subjects are not commonly members of intact groups, a condition required for applying the randomization process. Experimental treatments frequently are applied to subjects for a period of time insufficient for an effect to take place. For example, exercising trained subjects for only 1 or 2 weeks with a new approach may be insufficient time for the new treatment to take effect. Likewise, the intensity or the difference of the treatments may be so subtle that any change between pretest and posttest is not measurable. If electrical stimulation is applied to a muscle with an intensity equal to 15% of maximum voluntary contraction of the muscle, the difference of 15% from 0% may be insufficient to show a treatment effect. Withholding treatment or using a placebo with a group of patients is unethical and unacceptable for experimental research. Control over extraneous variables and the maintenance of a constant environment during the experiment may be impossible.[13] Researchers must be aware of such limitations and make every effort to avoid, prevent, or eliminate as many of them as possible.

HARDWARE INSTRUMENTS

Research must be objective and objectivity implies that data must be measured quantitatively (Chapter 5). A variety of instruments, both old and new, are available for measuring and recording the quantities physical therapists deal with constantly. Applied research assists the practitioner by validating those things used in patient management. The researcher measures forces, motion, temperature, light, sound, gas volumes and contents, respiratory functions, action potentials, currents, and cardiac functions.[14] The researcher must, therefore, be acquainted with instruments available to assist in objective measurements. Only brief and superficial coverage of instrumentation will be covered in this chapter; the student is advised to seek appropriate details about instruments through other sources: manufacturers' catalogues in purchasing departments of hospitals, universities, or research centers; visiting laboratories, workshops, local, state, and national conferences; writing to authors who have used particular instruments in their studies; and other resources such as:

RESOURCE AND BUYER'S GUIDE. This annual guide is a supplement to CLINICAL MANAGEMENT IN PHYSICAL THERAPY, published by the American Physical Therapy Association. It contains a detailed listing of manufacturers and distributors (with a brief description of their products), a product listing by category, and information about membership in the **APTA**. The company contact information is practical and helpful.

BIOMEDICAL PRODUCTS. This is a monthly paper for life science researchers. Published by Biomedical Products (PO Box 359, Dover, NJ 07801–9990); the subscription is free. About 600 product profiles are highlighted, each a number for identifying detailed information and for requesting catalogs about product information. The paper provides a postcard for obtaining this information.

SCIENTIFIC COMPUTING & AUTOMATION. This is a bi–monthly paper free to anyone interested in laboratory technology. Each issue contains more than 200 product profiles. There is an enclosed postcard available to obtain additional information about products. Write in care of the paper (Box 1952, Dover, NJ 07801–0952).

INDUSTRIAL HYGIENE NEWS. This paper is published seven times each year and has a format similar to that of the other listed newspapers. Each issue contains about 500 industrial hygiene, occupational health, and high-tech safety product profiles. There is an enclosed postcard for additional information about products. The newspaper is free by writing to INDUSTRIAL HYGIENE NEWS (Computer Center, 8650 Babcock Boulevard, Pittsburgh, PA 15237–9978). A catalog and buyer's guide is available for additional information.

SCIENCE GUIDE TO SCIENTIFIC INSTRUMENTS. This guide is published annually as a supplement to the journal, SCIENCE. Thousands of instruments and manufacturers are listed.

USES OF SCIENTIFIC INSTRUMENTS

Quantitative measurements are important in experimental (comparative) research. Much of the data gathered in comparative research concerns either human subjects or animals. Clinical research constitutes perhaps the greatest portion of comparative research methods and deals only with human subjects. Instrument systems are necessary for gathering quantitative data, which may encompass interactions with electrical, acoustical, chemical, thermal, mechanical, hydraulic, pneumatic, or optical phenomena. In physical therapy, instruments are used for:

1. Patient Assessment. Before treatment or patient management can be planned intelligently, clarifying examinations must be given. Improvement of existing tests and measurements are needed, as well as the development of new tests. Procedures are needed for accurately measuring quantitative values of strength, motion, gait, and the effects of a given therapy. Instruments used for these purposes must be economical, convenient to apply or operate, safe, and able to provide information expeditiously. Once baseline data are gathered about the weaknesses and strengths of a condition or problem, the therapeutic program can be planned and executed.
2. Monitoring. Instruments are used to monitor ongoing events or treatment and measure effects of a given treatment or procedure. Continuous or periodic information is essential to the therapist for modifying the therapeutic program or supplying information about the status of the patient undergoing therapy.
3. Control. Sometimes instruments are used in physical therapy to control an operation or provide support to a patient.
4. Research. Instruments are needed in research for gathering information. Variables must be measured in quantitative terms to assist the researcher in analysis and interpretation of the experimental effects. Sometimes clinical and research instrumentation are the same. Generally, clinical instruments are used to assess and treat, whereas research instruments are used primarily to gather precise information about effects of treatment, validity of treatment, and new knowledge pertaining to problems in physical therapy.

GENERAL CONSIDERATIONS OF INSTRUMENTATION

An experiment is the manipulation of independent variables under controlled conditions for the purpose of observing the effects of the manipulated variables. Instruments are necessary to assist in measuring and gathering data. Instruments are used in experiments to manipulate variables (provide a specific treatment or condition and to stabilize subjects) and to hold some variables constant while changing other variables in a fashion necessary to conduct the experiment.[15]

Instruments are adjunctive rather than central to physical therapy research. The study must be designed to seek certain information; the instrument selected must fit the design and fulfill the requirements needed to gather quantitative data.

The laboratory provides a facility to measure techniques and their effects and responses to treatment. By using standard laboratory techniques, clinical assessment and treatment procedures can be developed or verified and controls can be recorded. Clinical practice relies on laboratory methods, instruments, and findings. Although some persons are reluctant to accept gadgetry to achieve the goals of patient rehabilitation, instrumentation is recognized by most for its precision of measurement and quantitative delivery of physical phenomena. Instruments (gadgetry) of measurement are extremely important to physical therapists for measuring and assessing responses to treatment.[14]

Whatever the instrument used in research, the setup must be planned and designed with the purpose and research problem in mind. The researcher is advised to use established instruments because they usually are valid and reliable. Imperfections are likely to have already been removed from established instruments, so that the researcher saves important time by not having to develop a new instrument. Results obtained in the study using established measuring instruments can be compared with those of previous studies using the same instrument.[16]

Manufacturers

Instruments for measuring a particular phenomenon are available through several manufacturing sources. Some manufacturers provide good value for the cost of the instrument, whereas others provide overpriced instruments of limited value. Most manufacturers give specifications for their product, and specifications vary among models, brands, and costs. The researcher must know specifically what specifications of an instrument are needed for measuring the phenomena under investigation. A researcher may have to accept equipment that is available, but in the event that equipment must be purchased, he must study the instrument's specifications, talk to the manufacturer's representative and even request demonstrations, examine closely the availability and policies for repair services, and then decide which brand and model to buy. Discussing equipment with colleagues is very helpful and can prevent mistakes in selection. Most manufacturers offer warranties as protection to buyers against failure of equipment operation within a specified period of time from purchase.

Specifications

Equipment specifications must be known to the researcher before purchase. Specifications pertain to the particular instrument's features, characteristics, and functions. The researcher selects an instrument on the basis of its function and specifications. Instruments are selected for their capabilities and precision within the buying power of the researcher's money. Everyone is entitled to receive the best value for his dollar and, therefore, the importance of studying specifications of instruments, talking to colleagues about them, seeing the instruments in operation, and planning thoroughly before purchase cannot be overemphasized.

The researcher must plan or establish specifications for the instrument or equipment used in the investigation. A certain type of instrument needed to measure dependent variables may vary from source to source, qualitatively and quantitatively. The variations in specifications from different sources warrant planning and consideration by the researcher. Table 8.1 provides a list of general considerations for purchasing or custom-manufacturing research instruments, which are relatively straightforward. A few illustrations of problems are presented which may be encountered by the researcher if the above considerations are not taken into account.

A researcher may want to study exercise effects on the cardiopulmonary system of a group of subjects. An electrically operated treadmill is purchased within the allotted budget, but, on delivery, the door of the laboratory is found to be too narrow to accommodate the treadmill. Because of this lack of insight, additional money may be necessary to alter the doorframe. Suppose the treadmill is very heavy and mechanical assistance is required to carry and lift it to the laboratory located on the second floor of the building and no elevator is available. Also, the treadmill may require 220–volt **AC** current but 115–volt **AC** current may be all that is available in the space allotted for the treadmill. Perhaps the respiratory assessing device is not appropriate for providing oxygen to the subject performing the exercise. In this case, the subject could collapse shortly after beginning the exercise when his nose is blocked and his mouth is filled with a gas–collecting piece. This situation illustrates what could happen if the researcher has not planned properly and has not studied the

Table 8.1
List of Considerations When Purchasing or Custom-Manufacturing Research Instruments

Cost	Ease of manufacture
Size	Maintenance, repair servicing
Weight	Availability, delivery time
Material	Flexibility, adaptability
Strength	Validity, reliability, calibration
Durability	Ease of operation
Properties (chemical, electrical, mechanical)	Range, sensitivity, frequency response, noise level
Accompanying instructions	Method of recording, display (manual or automatic)
Trial loan, demonstraton	Safety

specifications of the instruments or facilities prior to purchasing research equipment. Suppose a tensiometer with a range between 0 and 500 kg has been purchased, but most subjects selected for a study can only exert 50 kg of force. The possibility exists that the instrument will not be sensitive in the 0–kg to 20–kg range because of the wide range incorporated in the design and the response of the materials used in its construction.

Cost must be a major concern to researchers. Funds may be available for equipment purchase, but suppose the costs of operating the equipment are very expensive. Supplies like film and film processing or special recording paper may be very costly, for example.

The versatility of the instruments must also be considered. Perhaps several studies can be conducted while using the same instrument. Limitations of an instrument, however, can prevent its use in other applications of study, or instruments may not be compatible with other equipment manufactured by different firms.

The complexity of operating an instrument will depend on the function of the instrument, the mode or form of the instrument (console or modular), and the knowledge of the operator about instrumentation. Researchers should read the instrument manuals that accompany instruments and learn to operate, calibrate, and make minor adjustments as needed.[17]

Measurements form an essential part of any quantitative investigation in the life sciences, and, for a measurement to be useful, the results must be understood properly by the researcher. Quantitative measurements improve our understanding of phenomena and enable us to control a process or system.[18] Certain features of any instrument should be considered; some of these considerations follow:

Accuracy. With hardware instruments, accuracy is the degree of systematic error. Cromwell and coauthors[19] have suggested several errors of instruments which interfere with accuracy. These errors are attributed to operational deficiencies of the instrument (1) because of design or materials of construction; (2) because of mechanical errors of meter movements; (3) because of component drift or temperature variations; (4) a result of poor frequency response of an electronic instrument; or (5) because of reading variations of parallax, inadequate lighting, or excessively wide ink traces on a pen recording. A calibration check of an instrument before each series of measurements is important to ensure that the baseline reading (zero) is correct. Among other causes of instrument error are laxity in quality control during construction, mishandling during shipping, incorrect assembly and use, accidental injury to the instrument, deterioration caused by wear, improper maintenance, and faulty repair.[20]

Linearity. Linearity is the degree to which the output variations agree with the input variations of an instrument.[19] The amount a measurement deviates from the calibration curve is important when taking precision recordings. The amount of deviation can be expressed by the full–scale input of the instrument. If the researcher determines the straight-line relationship (linear regression in Chapter 10) for input at several calibration readings and then forms a distribution of scores from various input quantities (measurement readings), another regression line can be formed for comparison of slope with the line formed by scores from calibration readings (Fig. 8.1).[18]

Hysteresis. Hysteresis is a characteristic of some electrical and mechanical instruments: when readings of known quantities are taken in descending order, they deviate somewhat from the readings taken in ascending order.[18,19] In mechanical systems, hysteresis is the result of energy being absorbed by the system during the loading (ascending readings) and not being recovered during the unloading (descending readings).[18] This characteristic is illustrated (Fig. 8.2) by a cable tensiometer. If a cable and an attached weight–pan are suspended from an anchoring point on the ceiling and weights of known quantity are added in gradations and corresponding readings are taken, the observer will note deviations in readings when corresponding quantities are removed in a gradated fashion.

Range. Recording instruments have a span in which readings may be taken. The span or range is usually referred to as the full–scale reading of a meter. The range begins at the lowest number or point on the scale and ends at the highest number or point. The range is sometimes referred to as full-scale. An example is the range of a cable tensiometer, which spans from 0 kg to 100 kg. The instrument selected for a particular investigation must be capable of measuring all quantities varying within a group of subjects or measurements.

Sensitivity. This characteristic of an instrument determines the degree or amount of variation that the device is capable of measuring. Sensitivity is considered in terms of its ability to detect the smallest variation in quantities. An amplifier for recording bioelectric potentials of muscular activity

$$\text{Percent Linearity} = \frac{\text{Maximum Input Deviation}}{\text{Full–scale Input}} \times 100$$

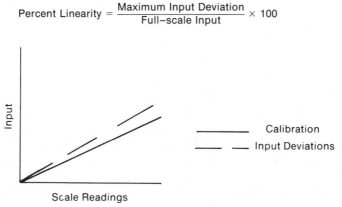

Figure 8.1. Hypothetical calculation lines for calibration and input deviations.

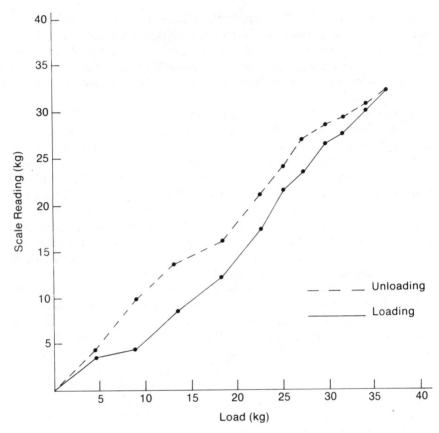

Figure 8.2.   Hysteresis loop of a cable tensiometer.

during contraction might have a sensitivity of 5.0 microvolts (μV) per millimeter of pen excursion, or 5.0 μV per major division on an oscilloscope screen.

Frequency Response. This condition deals with measurement of quantities that vary with time. In an electronic amplifier the frequency response is its variation in sensitivity over its range of detecting electrical signals. An amplifier is limited to its highest frequency that can be reproduced. The limitation of the frequency range is expressed by its bandwidth. The bandwidth is proportional to its gain (sensitivity) in handling certain frequencies:[21] for example, the frequency response of an electromyographic amplifier may be 2 Hz to 10,000 Hz, and that of an electroencephalographic amplifier may be 0.02 Hz to 100 Hz.[22] The instruments used in a study must provide faithful reproduction of the original physiological signal when recorded for measurement. Therefore, it is important to anticipate the upper and lower limits of the time–course of the response you want to record and then to use a recording system capable of sensing and displaying the responses faithfully.

Stability. The researcher wants instruments that provide constant baseline values, such as meters or components which do not constantly drift or vary from the starting point or standard baseline during the course of an experiment.[19] A competent investigator incorporates into the experimental protocol a regular test of baseline and a stable calibration factor for all instruments used in the study.

Although this concept has been introduced in the discussion of console and modular instrument forms, all systems and instruments should be designed to be operated and controlled as simply as possible. Instrument simplicity for operator control eliminates human error. Each component of a measuring instrument or system is calibrated individually at the factory against a standard, but the researcher must recalibrate the system once assembled, and this should always be done by using error–free methods or devices of the simplest kind.[19]

Electronic and mechanical instruments are expected to comply with the predetermined specifications of the manufacturer. The degree to which instruments consistently meet established values is important in research and clinical applications.[20]

MACHINE ANALYSIS OF DATA

For large studies or studies using complex statistical analyses (analysis of covariance or multivariate analysis), the computer can save the researcher computing and rechecking time. Analysis of research data requires planning, time, and the appropriate machine selection. If group sizes are small, the number of variables is limited, and the statistical analyses are simple. A calculator is a logical choice for the researcher.

Computer facilities which offer personnel services, instruction, and equipment are available at most universities and many large hospitals. Small hospitals or small towns may not have computer capabilities for processing research data. This situation may dictate the use of a calculator for handling data analysis.

Computers require that the researcher learn about facilities, services, and equipment. In some situations, these requirements are unnecessary because all facilities and services are available for a price. Both approaches should be investigated by the researcher prior to beginning a research project.

Preparing data for computers not only requires time but also costs money for processing. Generally, costs associated with computer analysis are for programming, keypunching, and operation or computer time.

Computers, like the library, are a friend to the researcher because they may be used in literature retrieval, data gathering, data analysis, and preparing the study for publication. Computers vary in size and costs, but as their capabilities, accessibility, and operations improve, their size and costs decrease. Hardware is the actual computer equipment, the physical and mechanical components of the unit. The mainframe computer is the largest in size and most costly. It is located in a computer center where specialists are available. It can handle the largest requirements for computerization and offers a wide variety of statistical software. Mainframe costs are continuous and, because of its popular service, the mainframe may be difficult to access. Larger and older computers use cards or tapes to input data, but other computers are often interfaced with the mainframe and these smaller units use keyboards. The mini computer is also capable of handling the largest computerization needs and has all the statistical software available. The initial costs of a mini computer are high and a computer specialist may be needed to maintain the system. The smallest and least expensive computer is the microcomputer (personal computer). The microcomputer can be used for particular as well as general purposes. The microcomputer is limited in its capabilities, but its use of magnetic disks (floppy and hard) as software increases its value. Software includes the computer programs that provide commands and communication capabilities. Researchers often do not have to write programs for their data analysis because programs for standard statistical analyses have been written and are available for the researcher. These prepared programs for standard statistical analyses are referred to as statistical packages. Each program in a particular package contains instructions for operating the program. The instructions are available at computer facilities or university book stores. Packages commonly used are **SPSS** (Statistical Package for the Social Sciences), **SAS** (Statistical Analysis System), and **BMD** (Biomedical Data Processing). **SPSS** includes programs for statistics frequently used in social sciences, whereas **BMD** provides a wide variety of statistical analyses used in educational research.

The actual data analysis requires little time on a computer, and the cost of computer time is usually reasonable. Costs for data analyses are often defrayed by grant funding, by some employers, or are sometimes free to students.

A major advantage of the computer in research, regardless of the size of the data set, is that data need to be entered only once. Once data are entered, they may be stored for future retrieval and manipulated at the researcher's convenience.

SUMMARY

An introduction to experimental research has been given here, with emphasis on control, fields of study, and instruments used in experiments.

Experimental research tests hypotheses of causal relations among variables and permits the investigator to maintain rigorous control over manipulated variables. It can be conducted in a laboratory or field setting. Experimental research is considered the most powerful of all research methods. Table 8.2 provides a summary of the research processes presented thus far.

Table 8.2
Cumulative Summary of the Research Processes Presented

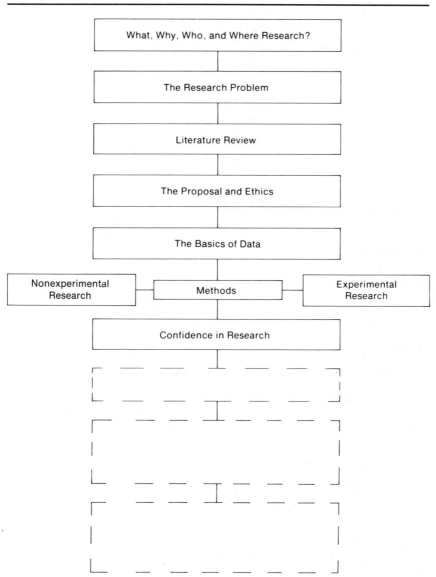

REFERENCES

1. Makrides L, Richman J: Research methodology and applied statistics, Part 1: General principles and basic concepts. Physiother Canada 32: 135–139, 1980
2. Gay LR: Educational Research: Competencies for Analysis and Application, ed 2. Columbus OH, Charles E. Merrill Pub Co, 1981
3. Oyster LK, Hanten WP, Llorens LA: Introduction to Research: A Guide for the Health Science Professional. Philadelphia, JB Lippincott Co, 1987
4. Meyers LS, Grossen NE: Behavioral Research Theory, Procedure, and Design, ed 2. San Francisco, WH Freeman and Co, 1978
5. Cook TD, Campbell DT: Quasi–experimentation Design & Analysis Issues for Field Settings. Boston, Houghton–Mifflin, 1979
6. Ottenbacker KJ: Evaluating Clinical Change: Strategies for Occupational and Physical Therapists. Baltimore, Williams & Wilkins, 1986
7. Barlow DH, Hersen M: Single Case Experimental Designs: Strategies for Studying Behavior Change, ed 2. New York, Pergamon Press, 1984
8. Clarke DH, Clarke HH: Research Processes in Physical Education, Recreation, and Health. Englewood Cliffs, NJ, Prentice–Hall, Inc, 1970
9. Gonnella C: Designs for clinical research. Phys Ther 53: 1276–1283, 1973
10. Lehmkuhl D: Let's reduce the understanding gap. 3: Experimental design: what and why? Phys Ther 50: 1716–1720, 1970
11. Wagman IH, Lesse H: Maximum conduction velocities of motor fibers of ulnar nerve in human subjects of various ages and sizes. N Neurophysiol 15: 235–244, 1952
12. Wagner AL, Buchthal F: Motor and sensory conduction in infancy and childhood: Reappraisal. Devel Med Child Neurol 14: 189–216, 1972
13. Cox RC, West WL: Fundamentals of Research for Health Professionals. Laurel MD, RAMSCO Pub Co, 1982
14. Hislop HJ: Modern instrumentation and its implications in physical therapy. Phys Ther 43: 257–262, 1963
15. Wilson EB, Jr: An Introduction to Scientific Research. New York, McGraw–Hill Book Co, 1952
16. Richman J, Makrides L, Prince B: Research methodology and applied statistics, Part 3: Measurement procedures in research. Physiother Canada 32: 253–257, 1980
17. Van Huss WD: Instrumentation Hardware. In Hubbard AW (ed): Research Methods in Health, Physical Education, and Recreation, ed 3. Washington, Am Assoc Health, Phys Ed, Rec, 1973
18. Cobbold RSC: Biomedical Measurement Systems. In Ray CD (ed): Medical Engineering. Chicago, Year Book Medical Publishers, Inc, 1974
19. Cromwell L, Weibell FJ, Pfeiffer EA, et al: Biomedical Instrumentation and Measurements. Englewood Cliffs, NJ, Prentice–Hall, Inc, 1973
20. Hanley TD, Peters R: The Speech and Hearing Laboratory. In Travers LE (ed): Handbook of Speech Pathology and Audiology. New York, Appleton–Century–Crofts, 1971
21. Dewhurst DJ: An Introduction to Biomedical Instrumentation. New York, Pergamon Press, 1976
22. Goodgold J, Eberstein A: Electrodiagnosis of Neuromuscular Diseases, ed 3. Baltimore, Williams & Wilkins Co, 1983

9

Experimental Designs

A conclusion based upon a badly conceived
experiment is usually further from the truth
than one based on clinical observation.
Sir Robert Platt
Universities Quarterly 17: 327, 1963

The ultimate form of research design is the experiment. The experiment provides the most rigorous test of hypotheses available to the researcher. It determines whether the relation between variables is one of cause–and–effect.[1]

The need for controlling variables and variable factors in research has been discussed on several occasions. Experimental designs are contrived, like instruments, to prevent or minimize the effects of bias (systematic error) and random error, and to maximize the measurement of the true quantity or quality. A proper design is supposed to enable the researcher to answer all questions without violating principles of scientific inquiry.[2] In comparative research appropriate designs maximize efficiency, control, and validity.[3]

The design of an experiment is the planned course of action for gathering, controlling, and analyzing the data. Gonnella[4] has defined design as the assignment of subjects to different treatments, the controlling of variables, and the ordering of the testing. The design incorporates the terms defined in the experiment or study, specifies the treatment plan, and determines the way subjects will be assigned to treatment groups.[5] Design of the research procedures is given utmost consideration during the planning and writing of the research proposal. Methods of analyses appropriate for the design must be made. Statistical procedures have been created to handle data gathered by certain designs or strategies. The concepts of validity and reliability must enter into the planning of the experiment also.

In nonexperimental research, designs involve the logic and technique of gathering data and making appropriate interpretations from the data. In experimental research, designs involve the selection of the appropriate statistical methods and strategies for analyzing data and then making appropriate interpretations from the data analyses. Most designs presented in this chapter are concerned with comparative research; that is, the comparison between two or more variables for determination of the difference between means of the dependent variables under investigation. Good designs will assist the researcher to eliminate systematic error, maintain precision and validity, incorporate simplicity for extraction of information from data, and help to calculate the uncertainties of treatment differences.[6]

EXPERIMENTAL VALIDITY

Earlier discussion has indicated that control of extraneous variables is of great concern in experimental research. Uncontrolled extraneous variables threaten the validity of an investigation because they can affect performance on the dependent variable. Validity is upheld if the experimental findings result only from the manipulated independent variable(s), and if these findings can be generalized to situations removed from the research setting but with similar conditions. The concern about experimental findings or observed differences on the dependent variable resulting only from the manipulated independent variable is referred to as internal validity. External validity concerns the ability to generalize situations removed from the research setting.[7] Some sources of variables which could invalidate the researcher's discussion of cause and effect have been identified and discussed.[4,8-10]

Internal Sources

These sources confuse the association between independent and dependent variables:

1. History. Studies in which measurements of the dependent variable (variable measured) are recorded before and after some form of experiment or event may result in contamination of the data. The uncontrolled events occurring between measurements might influence and confuse the information contained in the data gathered from the repeated measurements. The researcher must be concerned with the influence of events occurring between measurements. If human subjects are used, interest, motivation, and physical (injury) changes can occur to influence recorded scores on maximal muscular force. This source of contamination is prevented by methods of sampling, control of the subject's activities during the study, and methods of random testing.[4,9]

2. Maturation. This is also a time–related difficulty when measurements are taken over long intervals of time. The effects are directly related to the element of time rather than to the events occurring between measurements. Subjects grow, develop, or change over time. If the measurements are taken within a relatively short period of time, that time span can produce spurious results. For example, if measurements of muscular force are recorded in sequences too short to prevent fatigue, then the data are contaminated with the effects of fatigue. On the other hand, if measurements of maximal muscular force are taken at 1–year intervals to ascertain strength retention among children from some previous program of exercise, the results may be confused because the children have grown during the interval of testing.[4,9]

3. Attrition. The best laid plans cannot always prevent the loss of subjects in a study. Ample numbers of subjects should be included, with allowances for attrition built into the size of the sample. Some statistical designs call for pairs of data and if one of the pair drops out of the study, then the complete pair must be sacrificed to the study.

4. Testing. If the testing sequence affects the scores of the subjects, the values of the scores will be affected. Schenck and Forward found increased strength in subsequent single measurements of maximal isometric strength in their subjects.[11] This raises the question about the learning effects that might have occurred with repeated measurements. Subjects become test-wise when exposed to repeated testing or practice.

5. Instrumentation. The state of the instrument being used can influence scores. The instruments may not be calibrated properly; age, hysteresis, or sensitivity may influence recorded values. In paper instruments such as attitude scales or mail questionnaires, cultural, racial, or intelligence factors can influence the results of the survey. Different observers can also influence scores.

6. Statistical Regression. Although this threat to internal validity is only possible when subjects are selected on the basis of extreme scores (very low or very high), it can account for observed gains in learning during post-test measurements. Repeated testing of a variable tends to influence the outcome. Subject scores tend to shift (regress) toward the mean; that is, subjects scoring higher on the pretest tend to score lower on a posttest, whereas the opposite is true for those scoring lower on the pretest.[8] This threat to internal validity can be avoided by not selecting subjects on the basis of extreme scores.[12]

7. Selection. Volunteer subjects are probably different from nonvolunteers and, therefore, can be a source of bias. Nevertheless, required consent makes all subjects into volunteers in health research. To avoid selected samples that might bias the results, the researcher can control for the effect of selection by using more than a single group and by randomly assigning subjects to the groups.[12]

External Sources

The researcher is concerned about threats to generalizing as well as the problems of internal validity. As more stringent controls are applied to the experiment, less realism can be achieved or be expected between the findings and situations outside the experimental setting. The researcher is faced with losing scientific rigor in his experiment, so that realistic findings may not readily be transferred into clinical application. Compromise is the solution; maintain acceptable controls to make reasonable inferences.[12]

These sources of difficulty in the research method are hard to remedy, especially since they deal with representativeness and generalization of the data to the population. Testing subjects in a controlled environment and then making inferences about what is to be expected outside the environment is an example. Measuring a patient who believes the measuring process is a form of therapy is another example of something which could invalidate the interpretation of the findings.[4,9]

Researchers in the fields of psychology and education are most concerned about these sources of difficulty in their methods of gathering data. Although these difficulties are always present, the physical therapy researcher can usually avoid such pitfalls by random data collection and, whenever possible, by exerting rigid control over the independent variables and by proper statistical design.

Bracht and Glass have cited specific sources of external validity.[13]

1. Sample to Population Effect. This concerns the extent to which the researcher can generalize from the sample results to the defined population. Does the sample being studied really represent the true population? The researcher is usually safe by generalizing the experimental results from the sample to the experimentally accessible population. Also of concern is the extent to which characteristics of the subject interact with the dependent variables or treatment effects. Such factors as general skills, level of ability on traits needed in the research procedure, attitudes, emotional reaction, sex, and rapport with the researcher are examples of these characteristics.

2. Description of the Experimental Treatment. In reporting research, the author must describe the experimental treatment in sufficient detail so that other investigators can replicate the study if they choose.

3. Exposure to Multitreatments. Sometimes subjects are exposed to more than one manipulated independent variable. Because of this circumstance, the researcher cannot safely generalize his results to a situation in which variable X is administered alone. The effectiveness of any one of the variables depends on the presence of the manipulated variables.

4. Hawthorne Effect. Whenever subjects participate in research, they receive special attention. The special attention (Hawthorne or placebo effect) may alter subject behavior enough so that subjects perform better during the experimental measurements than they otherwise would.

5. Unusual Conditions. The experimental outcome may be effective because the research procedure is novel or unusual. The unusual condition can cause special effects rather than illustrate the treatment's real effectiveness. Fortunately most unusual effects usually wear off rapidly.

6. Researcher Effect. Subjects may react differently to the particular operator administering the experimental procedure.

7. Pretest Effects. The initial test or measurement session can serve as part of the treatment effect, causing different results than if the experiment was repeated without a pretest.

8. Posttest Effect. The posttest serves as a learning experience in which subjects become "test wise" as a result of the repeated measurements.

9. Interaction of Time and Experimental Effects. Experimental effects cannot always be generalized beyond the time period in which the experiment took place. Attitudes and emotional responses of the researcher and the subjects can change between pretest and posttest, and this can effect the outcome of the measurements.

10. Measurement of the Dependent Variable. The pretest and posttest measurements may be so similar to the treatment that generalization of the experimental findings is limited.

11. Interaction of Treatment Effects and Time of Measurement. If a posttest is administered on two different occasions, the posttest measurements can differ. The usual custom is to measure treatment effects immediately after ending the experimental procedure or training. Retention of treatment effects usually constitutes the difference between the first posttest and second posttest scores when some time has elapsed between measurements.

Although the outlined effects can influence the external validity of the experiment, the researcher usually reports limitations on the generalization of the research results. Selection of appropriate experimental designs and adequate control of extraneous variables usually enable the researcher to make inferences based on valid experimentation.

The appropriate selection of an experimental design is important. The design selected should be consistent with the objectives of the study and should control for various threats of invalidity, so that observed differences between pretest and posttest can be attributed with confidence to the experimental treatment. Most experiments in physical therapy use some form of single–variable design involving the manipulation of a single treatment variable followed by observation of the effects of the manipulation on one dependent variable.

Most of the designs discussed in this section can be used with statistical methods capable of dealing with groups of either equal or unequal size. The calculation procedures take into account groups of unequal size so that their sizes have proportional weightings. Thus, a large group of subjects cannot carry more weight than a smaller group.

STATISTICAL ANALYSIS AND DESIGNS

Analysis of data is an essential part of experimental design. Descriptive and inferential statistics are the two types of statistics commonly used in analysis of experimental data.

Descriptive statistics describes, organizes, and summarizes data. Measures of central tendency (mean and median), measures of relation (correlation coefficient), and measures of relative position (range, standard deviation, and coefficient of variation) are types of descriptive statistics. They permit the researcher to describe all individual scores in a sample by using one or two numbers (mean and standard deviation). Descriptive statistics is used if the recorded scores include all of the interesting observations to the researcher, or if the observations are inadequately gathered or too comprehensive to be representative of a larger group. That is, descriptive statistics should be used to describe the situation of each dependent variable, the location of central or key values in each group studied, and the variation or spread of the scores within each group.[12]

Inferential statistics enables the researcher to conclude, to speculate, to reason, and to generalize the results of the study from the sample to the populations, permitting generalizations from sample statistics (small and random portion of all observations of interest) to the larger population under similar observations.[12] These types of statistics (t, F, and r) are important in experimental research, especially since the researcher rarely measures statements that help the researcher conclude about differences between means. For example, if a difference between means is determined for two groups at the end of an experiment, the researcher infers whether a similar difference exists in the population from which the samples were selected. Presenting both descriptive and inferential statistics in the report of a study is an effective way of representing the results.

A distinction is frequently made between parametric and nonparametric statistics. Parametric statistics (Chapter 10) includes procedures that meet certain strict mathematical assumptions, whereas nonparametric statistics (Chapter 11) does not meet or approximate the rigid assumptions.

The choice of suitable statistical procedures is determined to a great extent by the design of the experiment and by the type of data to be gathered. The design and statistical procedures should be identified and described briefly in the research proposal, because different designs and research objectives require that data be gathered in different forms. The method of data analysis is very important in the research process. Statistical procedures help make maximum use of gathered data. Familiarization of many statistical techniques enables the researcher to vary analyses to extract maximum amounts of information from the data. Inappropriate analyses can cause misinterpretations. In the event that the researcher is not well acquainted with a variety of statistical procedures, a statistician should be consulted about the experimental design and the data analysis.

Inferential statistics and tests of significance play an important role in research designs. Tests of significance are used to test hypotheses. Their proper use is important for the success of the analysis and interpretation. Table 9.1 provides a summary of a few examples of tests of significance and their purposes.

Table 9.1
Tests of Significance, Inferential Statistics

Tests of Statistical Significance	Purpose
Parametric	
t test	To determine whether two means differ significantly from each other
Analysis of variance	To determine whether means on one or more factors differ or interact significantly from each other
Post hoc tests	To determine which pairwise mean comparisons are significant in analysis of variance when the *F* ratio is significant
Nonparametric	
Chi–square tests	To determine whether two frequency distributions differ significantly from each other
Mann–Whitney tests	To determine whether two uncorrelated means differ significantly from each other
Kruskal–Wallis tests	To determine whether means on one factor differ significantly from each other

DESIGNS FOR EXPERIMENTAL RESEARCH

Longitudinal Design

This type of design was briefly mentioned in Chapter 6. Longitudinal designs attempt to examine events or traits of a variable over a prolonged period of time.[14] Since most research is performed over time (all measurements are not made simultaneously), the amount of time between measurements is important. A study in which measurements are recorded during infancy and then repeated when the subject is an adult is a longitudinal study. All the influences of experience, growth, and environment are confounded into the measured scores. This type of study risks a high drop–out rate of subjects because of death, geographical relocations, and refusals. The information gathered is of great value when interest is centered on the changes which occur over time.

Cross–Sectional Design

This design meets the ideal sample when all possible classes of a trait, event, or subjects are represented in the sample. The stratified random sampling technique and the systematic sampling technique can both be used to provide a representative sample of a population. In random sampling, the possibility exists for exclusion of certain types or classes of things, but if the types or classes are known and can be located, random proportions of the classes can be made so that no classes are unrepresented. Cross–sectional designs enable the researcher to gather information from a manageable number of subjects and to draw inferences about the population from which the sample was drawn.

Prospective Design

This design is used most frequently in research. In the prospective design, the variable and sample are defined first and then data are gathered to determine incidences or magnitudes for comparing the experimental variable with other variables or known facts. This design gives the researcher the opportunity to plan the study around any factor, to study relations between two variables, and to determine effectiveness or differences between two or more variables. This design provides great flexibility, and time factors can be established and controlled in both experimental and nonexperimental research. A treatment can be given and then the effects can be observed following the manipulation or concomitant with the manipulation process.

Retrospective Design

The purpose of this approach is to uncover facts or information already existing. Historical research uses this approach. Different treatment methods can be administered and then their efficacy can be obtained, measured, and compared. Information can be extracted from files and records and then analyzed.

Retrospective comparisons of data in clinical trials are risky. The researcher has no assurance that the outcome is not seriously affected by differences in the makeup of the samples[15] and by effects of maturation when samples are compared over extended time sequences (e.g., 1 to 2 years). Patients composing two separate samples may have been treated by different therapists, different instruments may have been involved in the treatment processes, or improved methods of treatment delivery may have since been developed.

Blind Designs

The single–blind design tends to eliminate bias from the subject by not permitting the subject any knowledge of what he is receiving. The double–blind method is an approach to prevent bias from both patient and observer. In this method, knowledge of the conditions are withheld from both the subject and the observer. In drug studies, neither the subject nor the observer is told what ingredient is in a particular capsule. The capsules are coded for identification and recorded when given to a patient. The contents of the capsule might be the experimental drug or a placebo, but the contents are known only to someone not participating in the research. The double–blind approach also prevents the observer from scheduling favorite patients at times when he knows what the elements of the treatment regimen will be.

Suppose a therapist wants to study the effects of ultrasonic dosage on a certain condition using the double–blind approach: the ultrasonic generator is kept behind a screen and the controls are managed by a person behind the screen so that the therapist giving the treatment and the patient receiving the treatment are unaware of the dosage. This situation represents one use of a double-blind design in physical therapy research.

One–Group Pretest–Posttest Design

This design uses one group of subjects. Measurements are taken before any treatment is given to a group of subjects. Treatment is given to the subjects and then measurements are again taken following the treatment or experimental procedure. Designs are symbolized by letters where O is a measurement (pretest or posttest of the dependent variable) and X is the experimental treatment. The one–group pretest–posttest design is thus symbolized:

O   X   O

The differences between means of the two series of scores are compared to determine the effects of treatment. This design has been criticized for being unstable.[3,8,9,16] The arguments against the design are based on the uncontrolled temporal effects occurring between test administrations. Temporal effects are considered uncontrolled because no comparison is made between an experimental group of subjects and an equivalent untreated or control group, so that history and maturation factors are not measured or stabilized. The time occurring between pretest and posttest measurements (temporal effect) can contaminate the measurements so that the real effects of treatment are indistinguishable from the effects of the passage of time. In certain studies, growth and developmental factors (maturation effect) taking place in subjects between the pretest and posttest measurements sometimes contaminate treatment effects.[3] An example might be a study of children who exhibit growth and developmental changes in relatively short periods of time.

Cox,[17] a life scientist, has given a reasonable argument in defense of this design. If a method or treatment is tested which has already provided desirable effects (for example, dynamic resistance exercise increases muscular strength), then controls are not needed if the researcher is interested in determining how much of the effect is taking place.[17] A person performing dynamic exercises daily for several weeks should not demonstrate learning effects if he is measured for strength by movements similar to those performed in the strengthening program. Another example might be when ice massage and ice packs are being studied to determine which is superior for cooling muscle tissue. Both methods cool soft tissue, but the researcher wants to determine if any difference exists and how much. Having a control group may not be necessary when treatment effects are known from previous research. The measurements in these situations can be taken during one setting with minimum elapsed time occurring (temporal and maturation effects are minimized). The elapsed time between pretest and posttest measurements is the actual treatment time. Randomizing the order of pretest and posttest measurements among subjects (eliminating any set pattern) helps to eliminate contaminants from learning, temporal, and maturation factors.[6] Reliability of pretest and posttest data can be increased when more than one measurement is taken at each point in time. The different measurements can be compared to determine difference and, if no significant difference occurs statistically, the researcher is assured that history and maturation have not influenced the treatment effects.[18] The faults of history and maturation effects leveled at this design come mostly from psychology, education, and sociology.

The pretest and posttest means are compared for statistical significance using the paired *t* test. The paired *t* test is appropriate because the same subjects are tested on both occasions and whenever a parametric test is indicated. If the rigid mathematical assumptions cannot be met for parametric statistical testing, a nonparametric test should be selected, for example, the Wilcoxon matched–pairs signed–ranks test.[1]

Two–Group Pretest–Posttest Designs

Pretest–Posttest Control Group Design:.

$$O \quad X \quad O$$
$$O \qquad\ \ O$$

This design corrects for the deficiencies of the **ONE–GROUP PRETEST-POSTTEST DESIGN** by using a second group of subjects for control.[9] Subjects are selected and assigned randomly to the two separate groups. Pretest measurements are taken on each group. The experimental group is given some treatment or experimental procedure and, subsequently, post-test measurements are taken. Although pretest and posttest measurements are taken on the second or control group, no experimental treatment or procedure is administered to this group.[10]

The two–group design may be varied to include paired comparisons in which a number of pairs of subjects receiving different treatments are studied. Similarities (similar strength scores, blood pressures, ages, or weights) between two subjects are identified and the two subjects then constitute a pair. One member of the pair is randomly assigned to a designated treatment group; the other member is assigned to the other designated treatment group. This variation on the two–group design provides comparisons of two treatments free of systematic error, sources of internal invalidity; however, it is threatened by interaction of testing and treatment invalidity.

Pretest–Posttest Control–Group Design with Matching. Matching attempts to reduce differences between the experimental and control groups on the dependent variable at pretest. The researcher assigns subjects to the experimental and control groups so that they are matched (closely comparable) on pretest scores. This design is a variation of Two–Group Pretest–Posttest designs but is similar to the Pretest–Posttest Control–Group design. It is useful in studies where large mean differences between the groups are unlikely to occur and where the sample sizes are likely to be small. For example, in studies concerned with strength augmentation by electrical stimulation and the combination of isometric exercise and neuromuscular electrical stimulation, matching of pretest strength scores is appropriate so that subjects begin training with parity of muscular strength. This is particularly suitable if the subjects are active physically and will train only for a short period of time.

The suggested matching procedure is to rank all subjects on the basis of their pretest scores on the dependent variable. The first two subjects are randomly assigned to either the experimental or control group. This procedure is continued taking the next two ranked subjects, until all subjects have been assigned to groups.

The best approach to analyze data of these designs is to use analysis of covariance, in which the posttest means are compared using the pretest means as the covariate. If analysis of covariance assumptions cannot be met, analysis of variance of the posttest scores is appropriate.[1]

Posttest–Only Control Group Design. Occasionally an appropriate pretest cannot be located or the pretest has an effect on the experimental treatment. This design handles that situation by not administering pretests to the experimental and control groups. It permits the researcher to rule out any possible interaction between the two groups of subjects. This design,

$$X \quad O$$
$$O$$

has the disadvantages that: (1) pretest scores are not available on the dependent variable and, accordingly, cannot be used to control for any differences existing between groups on pretest; (2) the researcher cannot determine whether the experimental treatment has a different effect on subjects at various levels by forming subgroups; and (3) the design contains the threat of attrition to its internal validity.[1]

The independent t test is an appropriate statistical method to compare posttest scores of the two groups. The Wilcoxon matched–pairs signed-ranks test is a nonparametric method to use if the obtained scores depart radically from the normal curve.

Solomon Four–Group Design. This design enables the researcher to combine aspects of the Pretest–Posttest Control Group and Posttest–Only Control Group designs to study the pretest effect on the experimental group. The random assignment of four groups, two experimental and two control, is involved in this design:

$$
\begin{array}{ccc}
O & X & O \\
O & & O \\
& X & O \\
& & O
\end{array}
$$

One group receives the pretest and the experimental treatment; a second group is given a pretest and a posttest, but no experimental treatment; the third group is not given a pretest but receives the experimental treatment and a posttest; the fourth group receives only the posttest. This design permits testing of the difference between experimental and control groups in addition to the interaction of pretest scores and the experimental treatment. Although this is a powerful experimental design, it requires a large number of subjects and a lot of researcher effort.

Statistical analysis of the data generated by this design is complex and requires the services of a computer and a statistician. A form of analysis of covariance is used to analyze data.[1]

Cross–Over Designs

If different treatments are applied to the same subject in random order at different times, the design is a cross–over design, also called change–over and shift designs. It is used only when the administration of treatments applied during one period of time does not extend to or affect subsequent treatments applied during another period of time.[9] Suppose that the administration of some form of heat causes benefit (residual effect) for 30 minutes. If another form of treatment (heat or cold) is administered before the end of the residual effects of the first treatment, contamination results and the cross–over design is not being used appropriately.

This design maximizes subject performances and eliminates the influence of testing on a training process, such as that of studying effects of static and dynamic exercises.[19] The authors of this program studied two groups of subjects performing static exercise and two groups of subjects performing dynamic exercise. At the end of 29 days, one group performing static exercise shifted to dynamic exercise and one group performing dynamic exercise shifted to static exercise. The effects of given tasks on each group can be studied by using this design. By transferring tasks between two groups and retaining the other remaining groups as controls, the results support the concepts that load is not important in performing exercise as long as subjects perform to the point of fatigue, and that the best training technique for a particular type of exercise is that type of exercise itself.[19]

This two–group design is used appropriately with the independent *t* test (when scores of each group are independent of each other) or the paired *t* test (when scores of pretest and posttest are dependent, that is, taken from paired subjects). If more than two groups are involved in the analysis concomitantly, then the analyses of variance would be the appropriate statistical method (Chapter 10).

Sequential Trials

The method of sequential trials was introduced to medical research many years ago,[15] but its use has not been reported often in physical therapy literature.[16] The sequential method either groups patients in pairs, in which each member is randomly assigned to one of two treatments, or it permits comparisons of one patient on a series of trials. Comparisons made of a single patient on a series of trials are used when studying effects of chronic disease, whereas comparisons of paired patients are used when studying effects of acute diseases where time for study is limited.[15] In the situation in which responses of paired patients are compared, patients are added and compared until a conclusion is drawn about which treatment is better. A ''stopping rule'' based on the results obtained in the investigation defines the way in which the decision to stop is made. The plan for stopping the investigation is made in advance of the trials and may be determined by formulas for binomial distributions.[6,15,20,21]

The sequential trials method offers economy of subjects and time by setting a fixed upper limit to the number of subjects required in an investigation. The greatest reduction in sample size occurs when wide differences between the treatments are recorded. The method is useful when the researcher wants to select the better of two treatments, when it is convenient to pair subjects on two different treatments, or when a study should be stopped for ethical reasons as soon as a decision can be reached about which treatment is better.[22] The design offers the researcher the ability to estimate a characteristic of a population with a certain level of accuracy.[15] A sequential trials design is not suitable when the above situations cannot be met and when considerable time is necessary to follow up patient responses to treatment. This situation does not permit economy regarding subjects because the study might include pairs of patients whose responses could not be determined until after substantial follow–up periods. Readers are advised to study details of analysis of sequential trials by reading the cited references.[6,15,20,21]

Quasi–Experimental Designs

Quasi–experimental designs lack random assignment of subjects to experimental and control groups; therefore, they do not meet all the conditions of experimental design. Random assignment of subjects to experimental and control groups is not always possible. Although this group of designs contain a good level of internal and external validity, they do not possess complete experimental control. Interpretation of results when using quasi–experimental designs must be done with some reservation.

Nonequivalent Control Group Design. This design is similar to the Pretest–Posttest Control Group Design discussed previously; however, it differs in that subjects are not assigned randomly to the different groups.

$$O \quad X \quad O$$
$$O \qquad O$$

By systematically assigning one intact patient group to the experimental groups and another intact group to a control group, a lack of randomization takes place. This condition of systematically assigning intact subject groups permits some biases to occur in the groups, which causes the study to become invalid. The groups may differ in some characteristics that may confuse the interpretation of the results. Using a pretest compensates somewhat for the lack of randomization.

Earlier controls such as randomization, subjects-to-groups or groups-to-experimental-treatments, and use of analysis of covariance were discussed as possibilities for reducing initial (pretest) differences between experimental and control groups. These measures can compensate for the weakness of this design.[22]

The analysis of covariance is the statistical approach for handling data gathered with an experiment using this design. Occasionally the *t* test is appropriate for analyzing data of this design.

Time–Series Design. A single group of subjects is measured at pretreatment and posttreatment. Between the measurement intervals, treatment is administered to the group. The time–series design is a version of the pretest-posttest design and may be performed with or without a control group.[1]

The single–group time–series design involves the repeated measurement of a group of subjects prior to the administration of a treatment (independent variables) and following the treatment. The effect of the treatment, if any, is shown by a directional change in the line connecting the scores recorded before and after the administration of the treatment. The single-group time–series design does not include assigning subjects randomly to a group or the employment of a control group. History and instrumentation are the threats to validity in this design.[7]

A control group can be used with an experimental group in the time-series design; this is called the multiple time–series design. Use of a control group corrects for the threat of internal invalidity by history and instrumentation effects. Although the control group does not receive treatment, data on the dependent variable are collected over the same periods for both groups so that comparisons can be made between the two groups of subjects.

Time–series designs are easily analyzed by conventional statistical methods. The t test can be used to compare mean scores of the last pretreatment and first posttreatment scores of the two groups. Caution must be exercised, however, in interpreting significant t ratios. The patterns of the lines connecting all measured mean scores must be considered in the interpretation so that a significant t ratio is in isolation from the direction of other lines. Lines that vary considerably may not change because of the experimental treatment. Figure 9.1 offers an example. Pattern A shows that performance was increasing prior to treatment so no effect is indicated. Pattern C is variable and shows performance was increasing prior to treatment. Pattern B shows a treatment effect because the line changed after the treatment was administered.

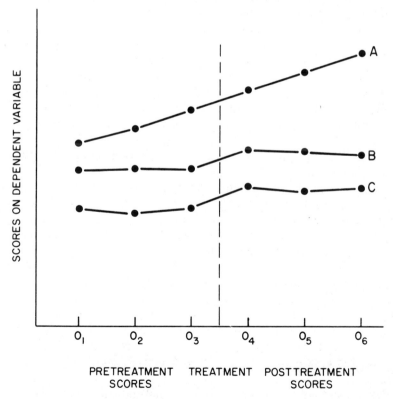

Figure 9.1 Possible patterns of a single-group time-series design. O_1 to O_3 indicates mean pretreatment scores and measurement intervals; the broken vertical line indicates the administration of treatment, and O_4 to O_6 shows the mean posttreatment values and intervals.

Single–Subject Designs

Single–subject designs involve measurements on one subject or patient receiving conventional or experimental treatment over a period of time. This design is similar to the time–series design but involves a single subject rather than a single group of subjects. It differs from the case report by using greater experimental control, whereas the case report is limited to impressionistic description.[1]

Single–subject designs are used to explore effects of independent variables on the behavior of a single subject.[23] They have been used to demonstrate treatment effects on a patient[24,25] and behavior modification of students in a classroom.[1] Three characteristics are common to single–subject designs: (1) the dependent variable (the subject's performance) is continuously and repeatedly measured across time; (2) the subject serves as his or her own control when comparing performances pretreatment and posttreatment; and (3) the multiple measurements provide some evidence of the treatment effectiveness. The designs enable the observer to examine changes in subject performance as they occur, and, with several data points, the observer later can predict subject performances.[23] I take the position that single–subject designs are useful in pilot work that may eventually lead to experiments using group designs and are good documentation sources of patient management. They are, therefore, of considerable value as a progress measure. Single–subject designs require measurements of quantitative data which are good physical therapy documentations. As mentioned earlier, a single subject is not always representative of a population or does not provide a firm basis for scientific prediction and inference. Caution must be exercised in generalizing about patterns of single–subject designs.

When data points are joined by lines, patterns in data are established which provide the essential information for interpretation. Patterns are interpreted visually, by the primary method, or statistically. Visually, the observer or researcher notes the degree of variability, trend, and level of the pattern produced by multiple measurements across time. The variability effect consists of the dissimilarity of scores recorded for a particular experimental condition. The direction that the pattern takes is the trend; the level of the pattern is reflected in the amount of change in the values of the data.[23] Variability of scores is important in single–subject designs. It can be examined within a specific measurement period (e.g., pretreatment) and across measurement periods (e.g., treatment–posttreatment). The plotted data points help depict variability, trend, and level patterns (Fig. 9.2).

Patterns are not evaluated by conventional statistical methods and may be controversial. The t test can, however, be used to compare mean scores between pretreatment and posttreatment measurements. If many measurements are available, analysis of variance can be used.[23]

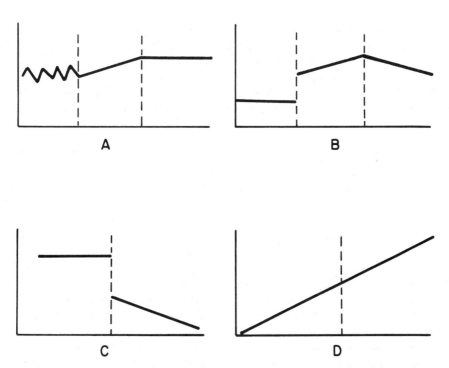

Figure 9.2   Some possible patterns across experimental conditions: Graph A shows changes in variability and trend, Graph B shows change in level but no change in treatment, Graph C shows changes in level and trend, and Graph D shows no change. The dotted lines represent treatment period.

Single–subject designs can be considered A–B–A designs with the non-treatment condition or period of time symbolized as A and the treatment condition or period of time symbolized as B.

The A–B design. In this variation of single–subject designs, the therapist determines the dependent variable to be measured and measures it repeatedly during the pretreatment or baseline period.

$$O \quad O \quad O \quad X \quad O \quad X \quad O \quad X \quad O$$
$$A \qquad\qquad\qquad . \qquad\qquad\qquad\qquad B$$
$$.$$

This condition of pretreatment measurements can pose a problem for clinicians who are obligated to treat patients immediately after initial assessment. For patients having chronic problems (e.g., neurological), a delay of treatment until several measurements can be taken may not pose a problem. Measurements are continuously taken during the experimental treatment period. Approximately the same length of time and number of measurements should be observed for each phase (nontreatment and treatment) of a single–subject study.

This design does not provide information about the behavior of the subject (as to what might have happened if the particular treatment had not been administered). Any change in behavior during the course of treatment may have occurred regardless of the particular treatment. Another flaw of this A–B design is that it does not provide a full experimental analysis of the treatment effects. This design does nonetheless establish the baseline for the single–subject designs; because of its weaknesses, however, stronger designs are preferred.

The A–B–A design. This design is an extension of the simpler A–B design in which a posttreatment phase is measured following the treatment; otherwise the same steps as the A–B design are followed.

```
O  O  O  X  O  X  O  X  O  O  O  O
   A     .  B           .     A
         .                 .
```

Although this design has good internal validity, the observed treatment effect is dependent on the particular baseline conditions imposed in this study. That is, the therapist can conclude only that the treatment effect occurs consistently for that particular baseline.[1]

The A–B–A–B design. The design introduces two within–subject replications of treatment to satisfy the ethical question of reduced treatment time to accommodate the pretreatment time.

```
O  O  O  X  O  X  O  X  O  O  O  O  X  O  X  O  X  O
   A     .        B     .     A     .        B
         .                 .           .
```

Ending the study with a treatment phase strengthens the interpretation of treatment effects.[7]

Analysis of Covariance

The analysis of covariance is a statistical procedure used to control for initial differences between groups. If pretest scores indicate that the dependent variable is different between groups, then analysis of covariance can adjust scores on the dependent variable for the initial differences on some other variable (the covariate). Usually the posttest scores are adjusted for initial pretest differences.

The analysis of covariance is similar to matching groups for increased control on a variable. With this technique, groups are placed on parity with the control variable and are then compared.[26] The effect of an extraneous variable is controlled by removing it prior to the testing for group differences.

The analysis of covariance is a complex and lengthy statistical procedure difficult to compute by hand. It is recommended that a statistician and a computer program be used for analysis.

Designs for Analyses of Variance

In experimental research the investigator is often interested in comparing more than two treatments or variables in a single experiment. The randomized, randomized blocks, factorial, and repeated measures designs are discussed briefly for the purpose of introducing terms and concepts that appear frequently in research literature. No attempt is made in this book to fit these particular designs to the proper statistical calculations. These mixed designs are for analysis of variance. Summary tables that coincide with these designs are also presented.

The randomized design is the proper scheme to use with the one–way analysis of variance presented in Chapter 10. "One–way" implies that a single response measure is involved with the analysis of variance design. The remaining designs (factorial, randomized blocks, and repeated measures) are presented only to acquaint the student with terms used in the research literature, especially since the researcher studies more than one variable in most investigations. The appropriate procedures of analyses for these designs are covered in most books of intermediate level statistics.

Randomized Design. This design permits the means of two or more independent random groups of subjects receiving variations of a single response measure to be compared for difference. A single response measure is a variable common to all treatments; the treatments, however, may be varied. In the example of Table 10.5 the intramuscular temperatures (dependent variable) of the gastrocnemius were measured before and after application of heat by hot packs, infrared, short wave diathermy, and ultrasound. The temperatures were measured by a thermistor and the fictitious data in the table represent the difference between before and after values. Twenty–eight subjects were assigned randomly to four different treatment groups so that seven subjects are treated in each of the treatment groups. The general design for the random samples used in the example of Table 10.5 was

	1		
A	B	C	D
S_1	S_2	S_3	S_4

where 1 represents the one independent variable (heating agent); **A, B, C,** and **D** represent (each) level heating agent of hot packs, infrared, short wave diathermy, and ultrasound, respectively; and *S1, S2, S3, S4* are the samples, each containing seven randomly assigned subjects. Since subjects are assigned randomly to one of the groups and receive a particular treatment without being influenced by another form of treatment, the groups constitute independent random samples of subjects and a randomized design. This design may also be called a one–way analysis of variance because only one independent variable (heating agent) is used. An unlimited number of levels (heating agents) can be used as long as the same dependent variable (intramuscular temperature) is measured from subjects in the sample of each level. In the example cited four heating agents were used to cause elevation of heat; a fifth level could have been a control group or some other heating agent.

In reading the research literature, many tables representing the various methods of **ANOVA** will be encountered. In the randomized design (one-way **ANOVA**) used for collecting and analyzing data contained in Table 10.6 the investigator might report the analysis as shown in Table 9.2

If the results from the study described above are to be meaningful, controlled variables must be sex, mass, and ages of patients; type, severity, and location of the injury; and duration of the injury. If these variables are not similar in characteristics, then the effects from the treatments will give ambiguous results to any of the variables outlined. For example, if sexes and ages are not similar, the researcher cannot determine whether the most favorable effects are attributable to the type of heat, the healing power of younger subjects, or the sex characteristics of the subjects. Uncontrolled variables in a simple randomized design can interact with treatment or other effects to influence or contaminate (confound) the outcome. Control of variables is critical in this design.[27] The one–way analysis of variance is the proper statistical method for this design. The analysis of variance enables the measured scores to be broken down into the proportion resulting from the treatment or experimental effects (X_1) and into a proportion attributable to error or chance variation (X_E). The randomized design for two or more groups compared on a single response measure can thus determine the components of the measured score, $X = X_T + X_E$.

Factorial Designs. The researcher is limited in ability to test complex problems if only the randomized design is available for studying different treatment effects of a single independent variable. Factorial designs enable

Table 9.2
Summary of One-Way Analysis of Variance with Equal Sized Samples (Example for Table 10.5)

Source of Variation	Sum of Squares	Degrees of Freedom	Mean Square	F
Between (heating methods)	0.370	3	0.123	1.051*
Within (error)	2.810	24	0.117	
Total	3.180	27		

* Not significant at .05 level.

the researcher to compare concomitantly two or more treatment (independent) variables within the same experiment. These designs enable the researcher to use the same subjects for estimating the effects from the two or more variables; this results in economy of subjects and time. Two or more variables are permitted to affect the outcome of the results and, therefore, each variable (main effects and independent) can influence another variable (main effects and independent) to cause interaction (crossing of levels of experimental effects to confound effects). That is, one or more independent (main) variables can affect the dependent variable, but two or more independent (main effects) variables can also have a joint effect (interaction) on the dependent variable.

In biofeedback training of patients having tension headaches, acceptable practice includes the use of audio and visual modes of feedback. Some physical therapists prefer autogenic (self–suggestion) to progressive relaxation (muscular contraction) techniques with electromyographic biofeedback. An experiment can be designed to contrast groups of patients using audio or visual modes with patients receiving autogenic and progressive relaxation techniques. If two independent variables (modes and techniques) are compared and each variable has two different levels (modes: audio and visual; techniques: autogenic and progressive relaxation), the design is a 2×2 factorial design. The patients are chosen and assigned randomly and independently for each level of the design. This 2×2 factorial design can be depicted as

$$
\begin{array}{ccc}
 & \multicolumn{2}{c}{1} \\
 & A & B \\
A & S_{111} & S_{121} \\
2 \quad B & S_{211} & S_{221}
\end{array}
$$

where 1 is one independent variable (modes) with two levels, **A** (audio) and **B** (visual); 2 is the second independent variable (techniques) with levels **A** (autogenic) and **B** (progressive relaxation). A total of four samples (cells) must be obtained with an equal number of subjects in each sample or cell. If eight patients in the above example are assigned to each cell, then a total of 32 patients are required. The first subscript number of the cell (S) designates the row, the second subscript number designates the column, and the third subscript number designates the subject to be identified. For example, S_{215} is the fifth subject of the audio–progressive relaxation sample.

The summary of the analysis for the 2×2 factorial design is shown in Table 9.3.

In designs that are more complex than the randomized design, treatment variables which might influence each other in the variance are partitioned out into interaction. Sometimes the interaction of variables is the most

Table 9.3
Analysis of Variance Summary for a 2 × 2 Factorial Design

Source	SS	DF	MS	F
Columns (main effect-modes)	SS_1	1	$SS_1/1$	MS_1/MS_w
Rows (main effect-techniques)	SS_2	1	$SS_2/1$	MS_2/MS_w
Interaction (modes-techniques)	$SS_{1\times2}$	1	$SS_{1\times2}/1$	$MS_{1\times2}/MS_w$
Within (error)	SS_w	$4(n-1)$	$SS_w/4(n-1)$	
Total	SS_T	$4(N-1)$		

valuable portion of an analysis. Each factor (main effect) is also partitioned out into individual components for examination of influences. Many combinations of factors can be analyzed in a factorial design, but the example here is basic to the design class.[28]

In addition, the error proportion can be determined. The factorial design offers flexibility to the researcher for studying as many variables and levels of variables as desired. The complexities and number of subject groups in the design increase as the numbers of variables to be studied increase. A 3 × 2 × 4 × 5 factorial design which restricts the data from one subject to one data cell requires 120 groups, and with 20 subjects assigned randomly to each one of the groups, a total of 2400 subjects is required in the experiment. This particular design is very complex and unlikely to be used often but could technically be computed.

Randomized Blocks Design. A randomized blocks design is a basic factorial design to which one or more block factors have been added.[27] A block is a classification variable in which subjects are placed into subgroups or blocks. Subjects in each block are assigned at random to any number of manipulated treatments with the constraint that each treatment occurs only once in each block.[29] Classifying subjects is similar to adding another variable to the design for study. Sex is often a significant factor whenever men and women are used in an experiment and the researcher wants to know what differences occur on the other variables being investigated between subjects of different sexes. By blocking or subgrouping subjects according to sex, the experiment becomes relatively homogeneous. The blocking technique reduces the error component. The equation to represent the concept is $X = X_T + X_E$ where X_T is broken into components of treatment factors, interaction between treatment factors and blocks, and blocks. The 2 × 2 factorial design discussed previously is compared with the randomized blocks design in which patients have been blocked into levels of symptoms, mild and severe (Table 9.4).

The summary table for randomized blocks design will differ from the 2 × 2 factorial design by blocks replacing rows and interaction replacing

Table 9.4
Variation in a 2 × 2 Factorial Design and a Randomized Blocks Design

	2 × 2 Factorial Design				Randomized Blocks Design	
	1				1	
	A	B			A	B
A	S_{11}	S_{12}		1	S_{11}	S_{12}
2				Blocks		
B	S_{21}	S_{22}		2	S_{21}	S_{22}

interaction and error, respectively. In the randomized blocks design, the interaction factor serves as the error factor, eliminating the component of interaction by main effects.

Repeated Measures Design. Repeated measures implies that each subject involved with the experiment is measured for each response measure (variable) investigated. In four angles of knee extension with and without a wedge under the knee during maximum isometric contraction of the knee extensors, each subject is measured for each of the six levels. In the randomized blocks and factorial designs, separate groups of subjects were used for each factor measured. Repeated measures design can be built into the randomized blocks and factorial designs.[27]

Since each subject is exposed and measured on each response measure, much of the variability that exists between different subjects is automatically limited. The sensitivity of the experiment is increased. The subject serves as his own control.[30] Pairing or matching of subjects improves the homogeneity of groups of subjects and was already discussed in the two–group and randomized blocks designs. In the repeated measures design, the ideal pair for a given experimental subject is achieved by having each subject be his or her own match.[27]

The design in Table 9.5 is conservative for subjects. Each subject serves as his or her own control, making this design useful for sophisticated analyses. All main effects or treatments can be given to each subject or measurements can be made on any designated factor.[27]

The notation of the numbering sequence (e.g., X_{321}) for this design is first subscript number = level of first factor ($X_{3..}$), second subscript number = level of second factor ($X_{.2.}$), and third subscript number = subject ($X_{..1}$). Summary of data broken down by a $4 \times 2 \times 25$ factorial design of analysis of variance with repeated measurements on each factor, knee angles and wedge–on–wedge[31] is shown in Table 9.6.

The reader may see tables similar to Table 9.6 in the research literature but should not be perplexed; the abbreviations are known as sum of squares (*SS*), degrees of freedom (*DF*), mean square (*MS*), and the *F* ratio, respectively. The significance of the *F* ratio is given in the table or at the bottom of the table and indicates the outcome of the analysis for quick and easy interpretation of the findings.

Table 9.5
A 4 × 2 Factorial Design with Repeated Measure on Each Factor

		Subjects	A	1	B
	A	1	111		121
		.	.		.
		.	.		.
		.	.		.
		n	$11n$		$12n$
	B	1	211		221
		.	.		.
		.	.		.
2		.	.		.
		n	$21n$		$22n$
	C	1	311		321
		.	.		.
		.	.		.
		n	$31n$		$32n$
	D	1	411		421
		.	.		.
		.	.		.
		.	.		.
		n	$41n$		$42n$

These designs enable the researcher to make comparisons involving highly homogeneous material, thus increasing the power of the test, to conserve on the number of subjects required for any given investigation, because each subject is used more than once, and to reduce any history or maturation effects, because subjects are repeatedly measured over time.[27]

One problem with the use of repeated measures design is the carry–over effects caused by repeated physical performances in which each subject

Table 9.6
Summary of Analysis of Variance of Maximal Isometric Force of Knee Extensors with and without a Wedge

Source	SS	DF	MS	F
A (wedge)	64.98	1	64.98	1.43*
AS (Error)	1,088.02	24	45.33	—
B (angles)	25,278.52	3	8,426.17	16.23†
BS (error)	37,372.98	72	519.06	—
AB (interaction)	696.18	3	232.06	1.01*
ABS (error)	16,441.14	72	228.34	—
S (subjects)	61,082.18	24	2,545.09	—
Total	106,965.68	199		

* Not significant at .05 level.
† Significant at .01 level.

must engage to complete all measurements of the variables being studied. In strength measurements, the researcher must avoid causing muscular fatigue because of the number of repeated performances needed over all measures for collecting data through repeated measurements. Subjects tested on too many measures over a long period of time generally yield data confounded by unwanted variables.[32]

The **ANOVA** is extremely versatile and can be adapted to most of the designs presented. There are methods available that can handle data for samples of unequal size.[27,30] The reader is advised that the "designs" presented in this chapter are not mutually exclusive (one variable cannot be used with another variable), but are used in various combinations. For example, a study might be prospective and longitudinal with subjects selected by a stratified sampling technique and the independent variable administered by means of a double–blind design.

SUMMARY

The established objectives and nature of the experiment determine the appropriate design chosen. Several sources of internal and external validity are discussed briefly to acquaint the reader with the need for establishing suitable control in experimental research. Various designs are presented that can be selected by the researcher depending on the variables to be controlled in his or her study. Selection of the appropriate experimental design is important, so that any change in the posttest can be assigned only to the treatment that was manipulated by the researcher. For greater detail about the designs included in this chapter as well as additional designs, the reader is advised to consult such authors as Borg,[1] Gay,[7] Campbell and Stanley,[8] Dayton,[27] Winer,[30] and Keppel.[33] Table 9.7 provides a summary of the research process presented thus far.

Table 9.7
Cumulative Summary of the Research Processes Presented

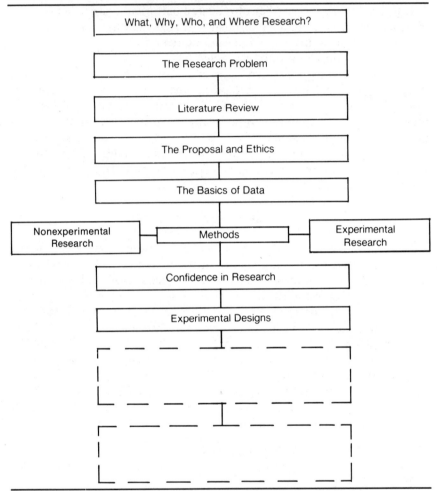

REFERENCES

1. Borg WR, Gall MD: Educational Research: An Introduction, ed 3. New York, Longman, 1979
2. Curwen MP: The clinical trial: An exercise in logic. Physiotherapy 56: 482–486, 1970
3. Slater SB: Let's reduce the understanding gap. 2. The design of clinical research. Phys Ther 46: 265–273, 1966
4. Gonnella C: Let's reduce the understanding gap. 2. The method: What and Why? Phys Ther 50: 382–385, 1970
5. Kelimbet ZA: Review of research methods as they apply to physiotherapy, with emphasis on the clinical trial. Physiother Canada 28: 35–37, 1976

6. Cox DR: Planning of Experiments. New York, John Wiley & Sons, Inc, 1958

7. Gay LR: Educational Research: Competencies for Analysis & Application, ed 2. Columbus, OH, Charles E Merrill Pub Co, 1981

8. Campbell DT, Stanley JC: Experimental and Quasi Experimental Designs for Research. Chicago, Rand–McNally & Co, 1967

9. Lehmkuhl D: Let's reduce the understanding gap. Part III. The experimental design: What and Why? Phys Ther 50: 1716–1720, 1970

10. Ethridge DA, McSweeney M: Research in occupational therapy. Part III: Research design. Am J Occup Ther 25: 24–28, 1971

11. Schenck, JM, Forward EM: Quantitative strength changes with test repetitions. Phys Ther 45: 562–569, 1970

12. Makrides L, Richman J: Research methodology and applied statistics, Part 5: Experimental design. Physiother Canada 33: 6–14, 1981

13. Bracht GH, Glass GV: The external validity of experiments. Am Educ Res J 5: 437–474, 1968

14. Meyers LS, Grossen NE: Behavioral Research Theory, Procedure, and Design. San Francisco, WH Freeman and Co, 1974

15. Armitage P: Sequential Medical Trials. Springfield, IL, 1960

16. Gonnella C: Designs for clinical research. Phys Ther 53: 1276–1283, 1973

17. Cox KR: Planning Clinical Experiments. Springfield, IL, Charles C Thomas Publishers, 1968

18. Silverman FH: Research Design in Speech Pathology and Audiology: Asking and Answering Questions, Englewood Cliffs, NJ, Prentice–Hall, Inc, 1977

19. DeLateur B, Lehmann J, Stonebridge J, et al: Isotonic versus isometric exercise: a double-shift transfer–of–training study. Arch Phys Med Rehabil 53: 212–216, 1972

20. Rao CR: Linear Statistical Inference and Its Applications, ed 2. New York, John Wiley & Sons, Inc, 1973

21. Armitage P: Statistical Methods in Medical Research. New York, John Wiley & Sons, Inc, 1971

22. Burdette WJ, Gehan EA: Planning and Analysis of Clinical Studies. Springfield, IL, Charles C Thomas Publishers, 1970

23. Wolery M, Harris SR: Interpreting results of single–subject research designs. Phys Ther 62: 445–452, 1982

24. Ostendorf CG, Wolf SL: Effect of forced use of the upper extremity of a hemiplegic patient on changes in function. Phys Ther 61: 1022–1028, 1981

25. Martin JE, Epstein LH: Evaluating treatment effectiveness in cerebral palsy: single–subject designs. Phys Ther 56: 285–294, 1976

26. Currier DP, Mann R: Muscular strength development by electrical stimulation in normal individuals. Phys Ther 63: 915–921, 1983

27. Dayton CM: The Design of Educational Experiments. New York, McGraw–Hill Book Co, 1970

28. Cain RB: Elementary Statistical Concepts. Philadelphia, WB Saunders CO, 1972

29. Ferguson GA: Statistical Analyses in Psychology and Education, ed 5. New York, McGraw–Hill Book Co, 1981

30. Winer BJ: Statistical Principles in Experimental Design, ed 2. New York, McGraw–Hill Book Co, 1971

31. Currier DP: Evaluation of the use of a wedge in quadricepts strengthening. Phys Ther 55: 870–874, 1975

32. Singer RN: Experimental Research. In Hubbard AW (ed): Research Methods in Health, Physical Education, and Recreation, ed 3. Washington, Am Assoc Health Phys Educ Rec, 1973

33. Keppel G: Design and Analysis: A Researcher's Handbook. Englewood Cliffs, NJ, Prentice–Hall, 1973

Part Three

HYPOTHESIS TESTING

10

Parametric Tests

The great tragedy of science—the slaying of a
beautiful hypothesis by an ugly fact.
T.H. Huxley

Research is performed to answer specific questions relevant to physical therapy; that is, to contribute to the body of knowledge. A researcher conducts studies only after having knowledge about the problem; the researcher operates within some frame of reference and the study is directly related to a problem within that reference. Raw data represent recorded observations which, on examination, imply certain conclusions or trends intuitively. Although this approach can sometimes yield information for making important inferences, failures in interpretations often occur because the meaning of the data is not always obvious. Chance variations can mask information suggesting conclusions other than what mere visual examination of the data might reveal. Chance variations can sometimes produce regularities as well as irregularities. If the researcher is deceived by what the data are showing, an erroneous conclusion can be disseminated and adopted. The science of statistics has been developed to help the researcher make fewer errors when inferring from collected data.

Research is performed to uncover information not obvious by other methods. The researcher performs experimental and nonexperimental research to compare results from two or more different groups or techniques. The researcher performs research to test hypotheses. What are hypotheses? How are they tested? How does the researcher know whether a hypothesis is right or wrong? This chapter attempts to answer these questions and offer some methods for analyzing experimental data. Expressions using the word "experiment" pertain not only to experimental but to nonexperimental research. Nonexperimental research becomes experimental whenever two different methods are compared. For example, two types of admission interviews may be compared or three forms of a written test administered to the same group of students.

HYPOTHESES AND HYPOTHESIS TESTING

Hypotheses

The term hypothesis has been defined in many ways. A hypothesis is an idea based on some plausible or factual knowledge about a problem. A hypothesis is a conjecture or an idea about the relation between two or more variables. Wilson[1] has defined a hypothesis as a trial, idea or a tentative suggestion about the nature of things. Kerlinger[2] defined a hypothesis as a conjectural statement, a tentative proposition, about the relation between two or more observed phenomena or variables. A statistical hypothesis is an assumption about a parameter of a population.[3] Hypothesis testing is using data from a sample to support or refute a statement about the population.[4]

In Chapter 2 the concept of a problem was discussed and was defined as an answerable question, an interrogative sentence. A problem asks, a hypothesis states. Problems and hypotheses express relations between two variables. An hypothesis is always in declarative form and carries clear implications for testing the relation between variables.[2] The problem asks, but cannot be tested in question form. To answer the research question, the researcher must make a declarative statement about what the specific relation is. For example, an hypothesis might be: "Dynamic exercises are better than isometric exercises for increasing strength throughout the entire range of joint motion," "An ergometer causes less energy expenditure than a treadmill for a given load," or "Ice packs and hot packs are equally effective for treating patients having chronic low back strains." These statements are in declarative form; they are statements that can be tested. They are hypotheses.

Examination of the above three hypotheses reveals that they differ in more ways than the content area to be tested. They differ in the way that the statements are directed. The first hypothesis states that dynamic exercises are better than isometric exercises under a specific condition. The word "better" implies that the mean of dynamic exercise data must be larger than the mean of isometric data if the hypothesis is true. The second hypothesis states that the ergometer requires less energy than a treadmill in performing a particular amount of work. This hypothesis is opposite that of the first, because the mean value of the ergometric data is believed to be less than that calculated for treadmill data. If the calculated mean values were actually reversed in the first two examples, the hypotheses would be false. These two hypotheses indicate direction, with each hypothesis indicating a specific but opposite direction that is tested to determine whether these are true statements (hypotheses). The third example is somewhat different from the first and second. The third hypothesis represents a special case in hypothesis testing and is referred to as the "null" hypothesis.

Null means without value or without significance.[5] In hypothesis testing, the null hypothesis implies that the difference between the means of the different variables is equal to zero, that there is no difference between the means, or that the effect of each variable is the same. The null hypothesis is used commonly in experimental research because of its simplicity.

A researcher usually does not know the exact scores of a population; he or she does not know the mean or standard deviation of the population. In fact, the researcher seldom, if ever, knows details about the population, so hypotheses are formed about the population's parameters. The hypothesis is a convenient statement about parameters and it can be tested. Hypothesis testing enables the researcher to compare theoretical results with those obtained by experimentation. The null form serves as a simple starting point by stating that no difference exists between two variables, that is, the two variables are related. Since the null form states that no difference exists between variables, an alternate hypothesis must be developed which states that a difference does exist between variables. Thus, two outcomes are possible for a research investigation. Gathering and analyzing data are ways of determining whether theoretical and experimental results are in agreement or whether the difference in results warrants rejection of the theory. The null form of hypothesis testing offers the researcher a simple, convenient, and versatile way of testing the probability of agreement between theory and observation. The null hypothesis is a clear and unambiguous statement.

Further examination of the three stated hypotheses discloses that none of these hypotheses offers the researcher an alternative decision. If the null hypothesis states that the means of the various variables are equal, what about when the means are not equal? If the mean differences are tested statistically and are found to be different, all the researcher can say is that the hypothesis is false if two groups are involved. What about the situation where three of five means are equal (or nearly equal) but two means are different? In hypothesis testing, the researcher must have two hypotheses, an original and an alternate hypothesis. The null hypothesis is used most commonly as the original hypothesis and can be written symbolically as H_0 (read as H sub-zero). The null hypothesis, "Ice packs and hot packs are equally effective for treating patients having chronic low back strain," can be expressed as an equation. Suppose data collected from using ice packs are designated as sample A, and sample B represents data from using hot packs. Since testing hypotheses is really testing the differences between means of two variables, and since statistics are unbiased estimates of parameters, then the equation expressing the null hypothesis can use symbols for parameters. The exemplary null hypothesis can be written as $\mu_A = \mu_B$ or as $\mu_A - \mu_B = 0$ (μ represents the mean of the population). The alternative hypothesis can also be expressed as an equation, H_1: $\mu_A \neq \mu_B$ or $\mu_A - \mu_B \neq 0$. In narrative form, the alternate hypothesis can be stated as "Ice packs and hot packs do not have the same effect on patients having chronic low back strains." These two hypotheses now offer the researcher choices in decision making. If the statistical analysis indicates that the mean differences are the same, the researcher then concludes that the null hypothesis is true and rejects the alternative hypothesis as false. In practice, the researcher, because of background knowledge or frame of reference, usually hopes that the data will support the alternative hypothesis. If collected data support the null hypothesis then the different treatments (ice and hot packs) have the same effect; but if the data support the alternative hypothesis by indicating that a significant difference occurs between means, then the inference can be made that treatment A is better or worse than treatment B. In the situation where a significant difference between means occurs, the larger or largest mean is then inferred as being superior to the variable or variables having the smaller or smallest mean.

Hypotheses can be expressed as directional hypotheses also. If a researcher has some evidence (personal observations or literature reports showing trend) to believe that one method is better than another, then a directional hypothesis can be stated. For example, a directional hypothesis is that dynamic exercises (A) are better than isometric exercises (B) for increasing muscular strength throughout the entire range of joint motion. The equation for this directional hypothesis (original) can be written: $\mu_A > \mu_B$. The alternate hypothesis then would be expressed symbolically as: $\mu_A \lesssim \mu_B$. Note that in statistics the symbol > refers to greater than, < refers to less than, and − refers to equal when used with a symbol of direction. The equation, $\mu_A \lesssim \mu_B$ can be read as the mean for ice pack effect (μ_A) is less than or equal to the mean for hot pack effect (μ_B). In this situation, the researcher hopes for support of the original hypothesis if hot packs are believed to be better than ice packs. The alternate hypothesis offers a choice of another outcome. If the researcher hopes that the data supports the ice packs, then the equation for the original hypothesis would be $\mu_A > \mu_B$.

In experimental studies in which statistical analyses are made, the rule is that the researcher must devise two hypotheses. The hypotheses are formed (stated) before data are collected; the hypotheses can be stated in the protocol (Chapter 4). Data are collected for confirming or refuting the hypotheses (hypothesis testing). The procedure in decision making is to choose one hypothesis as true and reject the other as false. The decision of nonrejection or rejection of the null hypothesis is based on the outcome of the data analyses (difference between means).

Criteria for Rejection and Use of Hypotheses

Hypotheses are essential in the scientific approach; without them there is no way to explain the collected data, dependent variables, or phenomena. Hypotheses must be written simply in language easy to comprehend. Hypotheses should suggest investigations and arguments which, if they do not answer the specific question, will at least bring the researcher closer to the solution. Hypotheses are used to contrast, compare, or verify the relation of two or more variables at some more or less remote point in time.[6]

Hypotheses provide direction to data and the method in which the data is gathered. The methods for organizing and analyzing the data are decided by hypotheses; the decisions and the inferences to be made are suggested by hypotheses. Failure to pose the proper hypothesis relative to the research problem can cause decreased proficiency of the investigation. The basis of experimentation rests on the ability of the researcher to devise productive hypotheses and design proper experiments to test them.

At this point, the introduction of some new concepts and review of some concepts presented previously should help in synthesizing the idea of hypothesis testing and direction, as well as how to determine whether a hypothesis is right or wrong.

INFERENCES FROM DATA

Descriptive Statistics

Sampling is the procedure of collecting data from a few subjects, events, or characteristics so that the researcher can learn something about a population. Sampling procedures make the theory of probability practical in research by enabling the researcher to use inductive reasoning to say something about universal characteristics; for example, ice packs are superior to hot packs in the treatment of chronic low back strains. A statistic calculated from a sample is the best estimate of a parameter of the population. The best estimate of central tendency is the mean which describes the central most characteristic of a sample, or, if inferred to the population, the mean of the population. The mean is used in testing hypotheses because it is the average score of the data and is the best estimate of the average score of a population.

Hypothesis testing asks the question of whether the means of two groups differ or not. In theory, the question is whether the difference between means reflects sampling from two different populations.[7] The question is whether the difference between the means of two or more samples will be small enough to be attributed to sampling variability. If the difference between the means is small (no significant difference), the researcher concludes that no true difference exists between the means of the populations (ice packs and hot packs are equally effective). On the other hand, if the difference between the sample means is large enough to be attributed to the effects of the experimental manipulation (significant difference), the researcher concludes that a true difference exists between the two methods of treatment (effects of ice $>$ or $\geqq$ hot packs).

Because of chance variations, means of samples can vary within the population. Suppose a sample of patients having rheumatoid arthritis is selected and the mean wrist extensor strength is found to be 10 kg. Another sample of patients having rheumatoid arthritis is selected in which many variables are controlled (sex, age, severity of disease, similar motion, and motion measured with the same instrument under similar conditions), and the mean wrist extensor strength is subsequently found to be 13.5 kg. Sampling and measuring can continue indefinitely by drawing subjects independently and randomly. Each mean strength value calculated is not exactly the same as that calculated for any other sample, but when analyzed statistically, no significant difference is found. That is, all means may have ranges from 10 kg to 14 kg, but the data support the null hypothesis (no difference exists between wrist extensor strength of patients having rheumatoid arthritis given specific controlled conditions). Another way of interpreting the null hypothesis when the means range within certain values that are not statistically different is to say that the means do not differ from zero. The researcher can state that the mean differences result from chance variations and that the samples were drawn from the same parent population. If all possible samples are drawn from a parent population and the mean of each sample is calculated and then placed into a single sample, the single sample will be a distribution of sample means rather than a single sample of raw scores or values. The standard deviation of the sample of means (standard error of the mean, $S_{\bar{x}}$) can be calculated to represent the variability of the sample of means. If the standard error of the mean is squared, the variance of the sample is formed (Chapter 5). When dealing with experimental and control groups of subjects in a research study, which can be conceptualized from Figure 10.1, the variance can be visualized as occurring from two sources.

The method of determining the standard error of the mean in Figure 10.1 is not practical; we must determine its value by drawing all possible samples of a parent population. This situation is similar to taking measurements directly from the population, something that is physically and economically impossible for a researcher. Fortunately, an estimate of the standard error of the mean can be calculated from raw data collected from any one of the samples; for example, Sample 1 of the figure. Since the variability of the means of all possible random samples depends on the number of scores in a sample and the standard deviation of the data of that sample, the formula used for determining the standard error of the mean ($S_{\bar{x}} = s/\sqrt{n}$) can be used for a single random sample.

Within–groups variance is the variability that occurs within a particular sample: for example, variance occurring within Sample 1 in Figure 10.1. Just as the means can be different for every sample so can the variances of each sample be different. Within–groups variance refers to the difference between scores of subjects within the same sample and can be caused

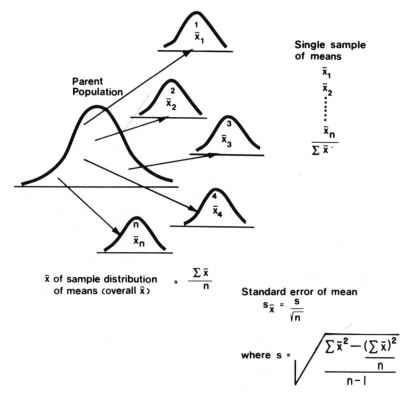

Figure 10.1.   Samples are drawn from a parent population.

by the instruments, the researcher, measured strength differences of subjects, fatigue, or even amounts of enthusiasm.

The second source of variance is referred to as between–groups variance. If one group of patients is given ice packs and another group is given
hot packs and the dependent variable is the total number of treatments, the
difference in the mean number of treatments between the two groups is
partially reflected by the between–groups variance. Returning to Figure
10.1, the between–groups variance is represented as the variance occurring between group two and group four. Between–groups variance is the
difference of group means from the overall mean and is represented symbolically as: s^2 total $= s^2$ within–groups $+ s^2$ between–groups. Note: Use
of variance here is not quite correct. In partitioning the variability which
occurs in methods of hypothesis testing (viz, analysis of variance), the sum
of squares is the correct term (Chapter 5). Sum of squares is, in effect, only
a proportion of the variance computation presented for determining variance. For reasons of convenience in approaching the topic of significance,
variance is used.

Degrees of Freedom

In calculating the variance and standard deviations (Chapter 5), the symbol, $n - 1$, appeared in the formula

$$s = \sqrt{\frac{\Sigma X^2 - \frac{(\Sigma X)^2}{n}}{n - 1}}$$

Degrees of freedom is a concept which enables the statistic, in this case the standard deviation, to be an unbiased estimate of the population's standard deviation. Degrees of freedom (df) is the number of scores in an array that are free to vary when such constraints as the mean and the number of scores must remain fixed. For example, in a sample with a mean of 50 and $n = 20$, 19 ($n - 1$) scores are free to vary (19 df). In other words, if you have 20 scores which provide a mean of 50 in which the mean and number of scores must remain the same (fixed), 19 of the scores can be altered to any other 19 scores chosen arbitrarily without changing the mean value of the data or the total number of data. In the equation $s_{total}^2 = s_{within}^2 + s_{between}^2$ the degrees of freedom for s_{total}^2 is calculated by $n - 1$, the degrees of freedom for $s_{between}^2$ is calculated by subtracting 1 from the number of groups (K samples) or $K - 1$, and the degrees of freedom for s_{within}^2 is found by subtracting the df for between-groups variance from the df for variance total, $df\ s_{within}^2 = df\ s_{total}^2 - df\ s_{between}^2$.

Significant Difference

Researchers can determine whether the difference between the means of two or more variables is consistently different by similar amounts. The researcher really wants to know whether the difference between two means is truly different and how reliable the difference is. Two methods are available to the researcher to solve the dilemma. A study can be repeated many times and if the differences between means remain similar, then the researcher can conclude that the differences are true and consistent. This approach is analogous to measuring the entire population to determine the true or real situation. Both approaches (repeated studies and measuring a population) are the best approaches in absolute terms. As discussed previously, in practice these approaches are costly and time-consuming and are not used routinely. The alternate approach to this dilemma is to apply statistical methods to the data to determine whether differences between the means of samples are statistically different. Earlier, the standard deviation calculated from a sampling distribution of means was called the standard error of the mean and expressed by the symbols $s_{\bar{x}}$ or **SEM**, and the equation $s_{\bar{x}} = s/\sqrt{n}$ or ($s_{\bar{x}}^2 = s^2/n$). The standard error of the mean (**SEM**) of a sample of means has the same effect in practice as repeating a study many times for determining the reliability of the differences between means. In effect, this statistic, when used in computing the t ratio (t test), is similar to within–groups variance, which is actually computed in the analysis of variance. In the concept of significant difference, a ratio is formed of the between–groups variance and the within–groups variance. The ratio is calculated and formed from the data collected from two (t test) or more variables (analysis of variance, **ANOVA**), and is referred to as the obtained value (t or F ratios). Once the statistic representing the obtained value between two or more variables is computed, the researcher must determine whether the value of the computed statistic (t or F ratio) could be attributed to chance or attributed to the effects of the experimental treatments. At this point, the theory of probability is applied to test the hypotheses. If the difference between means more probably results from chance, then the conclusion is that the original hypothesis is true. On the other hand, if the difference between means more probably results from the effects of the treatments, then the original hypothesis is rejected and the alternative hypothesis is accepted as true.

Levels of Significance

In hypothesis testing, the obtained ratio which is calculated by subjecting the collected data of the sample or samples to statistical procedures is compared with a calculated probability of the statistic. That is, the obtained value (ratio) is compared to a baseline value appropriate to the statistical test used in analyzing the data for the particular design chosen for the study (e.g., t test or **ANOVA**). The appropriate baseline (that which fits the design) is, in effect, the level of significance (**LOS**), which is an arbitrarily designated level of confidence or probability that the researcher sets for rejecting the null hypothesis. The **LOS** is associated with the researcher's probability or risk of committing an error when failing to reject the null hypothesis. The concept provides a way of comparing a calculated statistic (ratio of differences between means and their standard error) with a norm for the purpose of committing fewer errors in the decision-making process. Note that the researcher must specify the **LOS** in advance of the collection of any data. The appropriate time and place to state the arbitrarily chosen level of significance is when writing the proposal (protocol). The hypotheses and levels of significance are never contrived after the data have been collected. Researchers must maintain a degree of ethics in the conduct of a study, and the **LOS** is stated in advance to indicate what risk the researcher is willing to take in making the conclusion or inference. For most purposes in physical therapy, the 5% (0.05) or 1% (0.01) level of significance is satisfactory. The nature of the study assists the researcher in determining the level of significance. In Chapter 7, the concept of error was discussed and, because research deals with prediction, estimation, and probability, the true outcome or score is never really known (unless every member of the population is measured). Error is always present and for this reason the researcher takes a risk when making a conclusion or inference from an experiment. How much risk is the researcher willing to take? The level of significance serves to answer the question. If the 5% level is selected, then the researcher is stating that he is willing to be wrong five times out of a 100 chances. Another way of stating this is to say that if the study is repeated 100 times, the outcome would vary from the true course five times. Thinking positively, the researcher may say that the outcome of his study will be correct 95 times out of 100 trials. This is a practical use of the theory of probability. Suppose the researcher is unwilling to risk being incorrect five times out of 100 and, therefore, chooses the 1% **LOS**. By doing this, the researcher has decreased the risk to being wrong to only one time in 100; in decreasing risk, however, he has subjected the data to more rigorous scrutiny.

In Chapter 5, the concept of the normal curve was presented. The time is now appropriate to repeat the discussion of the normal curve. The normal curve has a mean of zero and a standard deviation of ± 1.0. Also, the normal curve can be sectioned into areas by the standard deviation, and the areas can be used as probabilities.

Look at Figure 10.2. If you add the percentages of area on both sides of the mean, about 95% of the area is represented between ±2 standard deviations (**SD**) and about 99% of the area is represented between ±3 **SD**. When the researcher selects the 5% **LOS**, he really is setting the limits for rejecting the original hypothesis at ±2 **SD** from the mean.

Suppose the researcher collects appropriate data for ice packs and hot packs in the treatment of patients having chronic low back strains and the unit of measure is total number of treatments (**TNT**). The appropriate test is selected for testing the data (*t* test), the appropriate calculations are made, and the researcher arrives at an appropriately obtained value to the

Figure 10.2. Normal curve showing areas between ordinals at different standard deviations.

t ratio. The obtained value is now compared with the value appropriate to the selected **LOS**. The value appropriate to a particular **LOS** is found in a table of norms and is called the critical value. In essence, the obtained value is compared with the critical value. If the calculated probability of the statistic is higher than the **LOS** established for the study, the original hypothesis will be true, and there is no difference between means. If the obtained value (*t* ratio) is smaller than the critical value of the table for the appropriate **LOS**, the original hypothesis is true. This situation is illustrated in Figure 10.3; when the 5% **LOS** has been selected, the null hypothesis is supported if the obtained value falls between the hatched areas.

If the obtained value (*X*) is less than the critical value (*Y*), then the original hypothesis is supported, because the 5% **LOS** sets the limits at ±2 **SD** and any obtained value falling within the area *X* (noncritical) between ±2 **SD** is less than the critical value which established the limits at ±2 **SD** and −2 standard deviations. This situation also indicates that the calculated probability of the obtained value from the collected data (statistic) is higher than the **LOS** established for the study; therefore, the original hypothesis is supported. The use of ±2 **SD** is used as an example; in the normal curve, 2.5% of the area of the curve actually falls to the right of +1.96 **SD** above the mean and 2.5% falls to the left of −1.96 **SD** below the mean at the 0.05 **LOS**.

Conversely, the original hypothesis is false if the calculated probability of the statistic (obtained value) is equal to or less than the **LOS** established. The obtained value will be larger than the critical value (tabular value) established for the specific **LOS** when the original hypothesis is less tenable than the alternate hypothesis.

In the situation in which the obtained value (calculated ratio) exceeds the critical value (tabular ratio), the original hypothesis is false because the obtained value *X* falls outside the limits of the noncritical area established by *X* at the 0.05 level (Figure 10.4). The researcher can conclude that the two samples were not drawn from the same population, that the obtained value was not the result of chance variation, but that, presumably, the obtained value resulted from the effects of the treatment intervention (experimental method). If ice and hot packs were compared (ice packs having

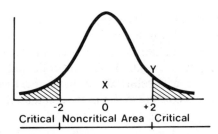

Figure 10.3. Critical and noncritical areas under the normal curve; *LOS* = 0.05.

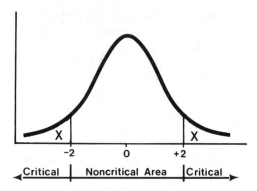

Figure 10.4. Critical and noncritical areas under the normal curve; $LOS = 0.5$.

the smaller mean **TNT**) and if the obtained value exceeded the critical value at the 0.05 **LOS**, the researcher could designate the original hypothesis as false, choose the alternate hypothesis as true, and conclude that ice packs are superior to hot packs in the treatment of chronic low back strains. The inductive reasoning (inferring from the specific or experimental results to the general or population) is based on the results of the samples and inferred to the population. Remember, if the 0.05 **LOS** was selected and only one experimental study was conducted, the researcher has no guarantee that the data and conclusion are not erroneous. The conclusion could have been based on data obtained from among those five times out of 100 occurrences (this will be discussed later).

The probability level (**LOS**) established by the researcher is also referred to as alpha (α). If the calculated probability of the statistic is greater than ($>$) α, then the original hypothesis is supported and is stated as being nonsignificant, or true. If the calculated probability of the statistic is equal to or less than ($\leqq$) α, the original hypothesis is false and the results of the calculated data are statistically significant or significantly different from zero.

Tails

Another new concept must be introduced at this point. When the researcher specifies the level of significance (α), the limits of critical and noncritical areas under the normal curve are established. On the basis of the established limits (0.05 or 0.01 **LOS**), the collected data already calculated are compared to a baseline or norm in the form of a ratio. The baseline value varies according to the **LOS** selected. Earlier the statement was made that the researcher decreases the risk of error when going from the 0.05 level to the 0.01 level of significance. In doing so, the areas under the curve increase, because, instead of using ± 2 **SD**, the researcher now uses ±3 **SD** at the 0.01 **LOS**. Note that as the levels change from 0.05 to 0.01, the area increases, the tail limits shift peripherally, and the probability increases. As the researcher decreases his risk of drawing wrong conclusions from the data, the restrictions for reaching significance are increased. The critical values increase in size at the 0.01 **LOS** and the obtained values are larger for the 0.01 level than for the 0.05 level. The researcher must pay the price of decreasing risk by increasing the magnitude of the obtained ratio to exceed the critical value to accept the true hypothesis. This means that the effects of the experimental treatment or method must be greater at the 0.01 **LOS** than at the 0.05 **LOS** to become significant.

At the time the researcher selected the appropriate design, test, and level of significance for the experimental study, the number of tails must be selected. Returning to Figure 10.3, you see hatched areas at either end of the normal curve. These hatched areas are referred to as tails and, in this particular illustration, two tails are shown. Ordinarily, two tails are used to test hypotheses when no direction is indicated. The null hypothesis is such a case where no direction is indicated by the wording or equation, $\mu_A = \mu_B$. The researcher cares what direction the data take when forming the null hypothesis but cannot bias the data or outcome. In practice, the researcher hopes to accept the alternate hypothesis and conclude that a particular treatment is statistically significant or better than another. If one views hypothesis testing with this situation in mind, then the alternate hypothesis is really more important. Since the alternate hypothesis, when accompanied by the null hypothesis, also does not indicate direction, $\mu_A \neq \mu_B$, but merely indicates that a difference occurs, then the obtained value from the data falls outside the established limits (level of significance arbitrarily selected) either in a positive or negative direction. If the obtained value exceeds the critical value, the researcher can designate the null hypothesis as false and choose the alternate hypothesis. Then that difference occurs outside the mean and limits to the right of the normal curve (positive tail) or to the left of the normal curve (negative tail). Two tails are working for hypothesis testing when no direction is indicated in the original hypothesis.

Going back to the hypothesis that ice packs are better than hot packs for the treatment of chronic low back strain, you will note that direction is indicated by the word "better," which implies that the researcher possesses some prior knowledge (personal observations or review of literature) that one method of treatment is better than another, but that the two methods have not been tested to determine which is better under specific conditions. Hypotheses of $\mu_A > \mu_B \gtrless \mu_B$ indicate direction and require one tail in testing because the researcher has indicated prior to data collection that one method is more (positive direction, above mean) or less effective (negative direction, below mean) than another (Figure 10.5).

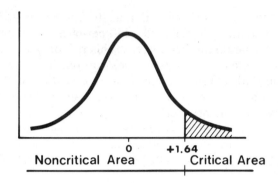

Figure 10.5. Noncritical and critical areas for one–tailed test; $\alpha = 0.05$.

The one–tailed test requires a smaller critical value (1.64 at the 0.05 **LOS**) for significance than the two–tailed test; however, the restriction for a one–tailed test is rigid because it requires prior knowledge about the variables being compared. The two–tailed test is more commonly used in hypothesis testing than the one–tailed test. Tailed–testing applies to the *t* test, but in the **ANOVA**, the *F* ratio is mostly presented as a one–tailed test, so the researcher need be concerned about tails mostly when using the *t* test. (Procedures for *t* and **ANOVA** tests are discussed later in this chapter.)

Errors

Errors are always present in measurement and testing theory. The risks involved in selecting the level of significance were discussed briefly. Even though the researcher selected the **LOS** arbitrarily and, in doing so, indicates the risk he is willing to take in making conclusions and inferences, errors exist regarding the decision to reject the original hypothesis or not. The errors associated with selecting hypotheses are called Type I and Type II. A Type I error is made when the original hypothesis is really correct but is ignored by the researcher in favor of the alternate hypothesis, which is incorrect. A Type II error is made when the original hypothesis is incorrect and is considered true by the researcher rather than the alternate hypothesis, which is really correct. Type I and II errors are easier to conceptualize if summarized in tabular form (Table 10.1).

Table 10.1
Conditions in Rejecting Hypotheses

	True Hypothesis	False Hypothesis
Do not reject the hypothesis	Decision is correct	Type II error
Reject the hypothesis	Type I error	Decision is correct

The ability of a test to expose a false original hypothesis is related to its power. A statistical test has high power when a false original hypothesis is exposed at a high level of probability.[3] The **LOS** relates to the power of the test, but generally the 0.05 and 0.01 levels of significance are sufficient for most studies in physical therapy. If the experimental treatment contains considerable risks or hazards for patients, then higher levels of significance are essential. For example, in pharmacological experiments where a particular drug may cause secondary complications or even death, a very high significance level must be used before accepting a potent drug for marketing; perhaps 0.0001 **LOS**. For situations like this, animals (rats) are used experimentally before the drugs are tested for human reactions. The theoretical idea is to avoid Type I errors whenever possible by selecting proper designs, tests, and levels of significance. Many researchers consult statisticians and seek assistance for experimental designs and tests when planning a study. This view has merit and is certainly recommended for the beginning researcher. Statistics and research design are a science and must be learned before their models can be applied to an investigation.

Type I and Type II errors and power of a test are discussed in many textbooks on statistics; the interested student is referred to statistics books.

ANALYSIS OF DATA

The *t* Test

The *t* test, sometimes called Student *t* test, is used only for experiments involving the two–groups design. The two–groups design refers to the variable measured on each of two independent groups. Designs are discussed in Chapter 9. The *t* test is not appropriate for comparing more than two groups, because chance of error in interpreting significance is increased greatly when used for multiple comparisons. The *t* test is often misused in the literature. A good discussion is given by Michels.[8] Note that the "*t*" is always a lower case letter and should be written properly. The *t* test is appropriate for studying the effect of a particular ultrasonic dosage (e.g., 1.5 watts/cm^2/unit time) on peripheral nerve conduction. The conduction is measured in advance of the ultrasound (pre), ultrasound is administered (treatment), and then the conduction is measured 3 minutes following ultrasound (post). Determination of any difference between mean difference (difference between pretreatment and posttreatment means) of nerve conduction from ultrasound on peripheral nerve to the mean difference of conduction obtained from a sample not subjected to any treatment (control). The two groups of data then are analyzed for determining statistical significance.

The t test is a rugged and flexible test. The test can be adapted to different situations. Three situations where the t test is appropriate are presented with the appropriate calculations.

t **Test (Independent Samples, Equal Size).** This variation of the t test examines the significance of a difference between the means of two samples or samples that have been drawn from the same or different populations.[3] Assumptions made when using this test are that two samples (X and Y) are independent and randomly distributed, are of equal size, and are drawn from normally distributed populations having equal variances.[3,4] The formula for determining the ratio of t is:

$$t = \frac{\overline{X} - \overline{Y}}{S_{\overline{x}-\overline{y}}}$$

where $S_{\overline{x}-\overline{y}}$ is the standard error $= \sqrt{s_{\overline{x}}^2 + s_{\overline{y}}^2}$ and $df = n_x + n_y - 2$.

Suppose we are interested in testing whether a hip angle of 70° causes a difference in quadriceps femoris muscle force different from that of a hip angle of 80° when subjects are performing knee strengthening exercises. The null hypothesis, H_0: $\mu_x = \mu_y$, will be tested against the alternative hypothesis H_1: $\mu_x \neq \mu_y$, at the 0.05 level of significance. A sample of subjects (volunteers) is collected and tested for maximum isometric muscular force (knee positioned 60° from full extension) with hips angled at 70° (X). Another sample of equal size is measured under exactly the same controlled conditions but the hips are angled at 80° (Y) by a back support.[9] Since we do not know whether quadriceps femoris muscle force will be increased, maintained, or decreased by changing the hip angle from 70° to 80°, no direction is indicated in the hypothesis (2–tailed). The samples contain eight measures for illustrative purposes only. Calculations are shown in Table 10.2.

The data obtained from the computation of the exemplary data yield a t ratio of 2.150. This value is compared with a baseline value (critical value) found in Appendix, Table C. Table C gives the probabilities with which various values of t will be equaled or exceeded in random sampling from a normal curve. The appropriate degrees of freedom for the example ($n_x + n_y - 2$ or $8 + 8 - 2 = 14$ df) is determined, and then the row of the table (left–hand column) containing 14 degrees of freedom is entered. Because the test is two–tailed, read down from the top of the table for 0.05 **LOS** until the row for 14 df is met. The critical value "2.145" is located. Since the obtained value $t = 2.150$ exceeds the critical value $t_{c(0.05,\ 14df)} = 2.145$, our decision is to accept the alternative hypothesis.

$$t_{\text{obtained}} > t_{\text{critical}} \therefore H_0 : \mu_x = \mu_x \text{ is false}$$

The results of this example can be interpreted to mean that a hip angle of 70° is superior to a hip angle of 80° for enhancing quadriceps femoris mus-

Table 10.2
Computation of the Independent t Test with Equal Sample Sizes: Effects of Hip Angles on Quadriceps Femoris Muscle during Knee Strengthening Exercise

X (kg 70°)	Y (kg 80°)
42	30
48	41
55	52
50	42
48	35
62	55
55	43
40	32

$$\sum X = 400 \qquad\qquad \sum Y = 330$$
$$(\sum X)^2 = 160{,}000 \qquad\qquad (\sum Y)^2 = 108{,}900$$
$$\sum X^2 = 20{,}366 \qquad\qquad \sum Y^2 = 14{,}172$$
$$\bar{X} = 50.00 \qquad\qquad \bar{Y} = 41.25$$
$$s_x^2 = 52.29 \qquad\qquad s_y^2 = 79.93$$
$$s_{\bar{x}}^2 = \frac{s_x^2}{n} = 6.54 \qquad\qquad s_{\bar{y}}^2 = \frac{s_y^2}{n} = 9.99$$

$$S_{\bar{x}-\bar{y}} = \sqrt{s_{\bar{x}}^2 + s_{\bar{y}}^2} = \sqrt{6.54 + 9.99} = \sqrt{16.53} = 4.07$$

$$t = \frac{50.00 - 41.25}{4.07} = 2.150 \qquad t_c = 2.145_{(0.05, 14df)}$$

cle force of subjects performing knee strengthening exercises isometrically.

t **Test (Independent Samples, Unequal Sizes).** Occasionally during the process of conducting a two–groups experiment, subjects fail to report for testing, or, for other reasons, subjects cannot be obtained for two groups of equal size. In the previous example, the standard error of the means common to both samples was found by the formula,

$$S_{\bar{x} - \bar{y}} = \sqrt{s_{\bar{x}}^2 + s_{\bar{y}}^2}.$$

When samples are unequal in size, the scores of the smaller sample will contribute more to the variance estimate than the scores of the larger-sized sample. This situation creates an advantage for one sample that cannot be accepted if a comparison between two samples is to be made without bias. The mathematical procedure to prevent bias between samples having unequal sizes is to weight the variances rather than average the variances, as was done in the previous example. The weighted procedure used to prevent bias between variances of two unequally sized samples is called pooling variances.[3] The pooling is performed during the computation of the sample variances, and therefore, the formula is somewhat different from that used previously for obtaining the variance.

$$s^2_{pooled} = \frac{\left[\sum X^2 - \frac{(\sum X)^2}{n_x}\right] + \left[\sum Y^2 - \frac{(\sum Y)^2}{n_y}\right]}{df_x + df_y}$$

The degrees of freedom (e.g., df_x) are equal to $n - 1$ in each case.

The unequal sized samples, in addition to pooling variances, cause a change in the formula for determining the standard error of means ($s_{\bar{x}-\bar{y}}$) and is expressed by the formula

$$s_{\bar{x}-\bar{y}} = \sqrt{s^2_{pooled} \frac{(n_x + n_y)}{n_x n_y}} \quad \text{or}$$

$$s^2_{\bar{x}-\bar{y}} = s^2_{pooled} \frac{(n_x + n_y)}{n_x n_y}$$

The computation of an exemplary problem will serve to illustrate the procedure of the t test for two unequally sized, independent samples. Suppose we are interested in testing whether the use of a biofeedback method (X) is effective in reducing spasm. A sample of patients having whiplash injuries to the cervical region accompanied by secondary spasm of the trapezius is measured for electrical activity of the trapezius, treated by biofeedback therapy for 1 week, and then measured for electrical activity of the trapezius (X). Another sample of patients having similar injuries is not treated for 1 week, is measured and remeasured for electrical activity of the trapezius, and serves as a control (placebo) group (Y). Since we are interested in testing whether the use of biofeedback method (X) is effective in reducing spasm, a directional hypothesis is indicated, because "reducing" implies direction (1–tailed t test). Hypotheses are formed as H_0: $\mu_x \geq \mu_y$ and H_1: $\mu_x < \mu_y$ at the 0.05 level. Table 10.3 shows the computation for the exemplary t test of independent samples of unequal sizes. The scores represent differences between premeasurements and postmeasurements of microvolts. The obtained value from the computation of the exemplary data yields a t ratio of -2.603. This value is compared with the critical value found in the Appendix, Table C, for a one–tailed t test (read down from the top of the table for 0.05 **LOS** and 10 df to locate the number "1.812."). Because the obtained value exceeded the critical value (left side of normal curve), the decision is to accept the alternative hypothesis, that a difference between the means exists.

$$t_{obtained} > t_{critical} \therefore H_0: \mu_X = \mu_Y \text{ is false}$$

The object of biofeedback therapy is to get relaxation of the contracted muscle; in this case, decreased microvoltage in sample X (biofeedback)

Table 10.3
Computation of the Independent t test with Unequal Sample Sizes: Comparison of Biofeedback Method and Control Group (Artificial Data)

X (BF, μV)	Y (Control, μV)
30	44
25	45
15	33
5	16
12	32
10	
28	

$$\sum X = 125 \qquad \sum Y = 170$$
$$(\sum X)^2 = 15,025 \qquad (\sum Y)^2 = 28,900$$
$$\sum X^2 = 2,803 \qquad \sum Y^2 = 6,330$$
$$\bar{X} = 17.86 \qquad \bar{Y} = 34.00$$
$$n_x = 7 \qquad n_y = 5$$

$$s^2_{pooled} = \frac{\left[2,803 - \dfrac{15,625}{7}\right] + \left[6,330 - \dfrac{28,900}{5}\right]}{6 + 4} = 112.09$$

$$s_{\bar{x}-\bar{y}} = \sqrt{\frac{112.09\,(7 + 5)}{7 \times 5}} = \sqrt{38.43} = 6.2$$

$$t = \frac{17.86 - 34.00}{6.2} = -2.603 \qquad t_{c(.05, 10df)} = 1.812$$

indicates a reduction in spasm, which is a favorable effect. No significant difference was found between sample means before the experiment began; therefore, the researcher can conclude that the significant difference obtained between means can be attributed to the experimental treatment, biofeedback. Biofeedback therapy appears effective among the sample of patients having spasm of the trapezius musculature. The independent distributions of this example were biofeedback therapy and control (placebo), whereas the dependent variable was the measured electrical activity (microvolts). The samples were independent of size n_1 and n_2 from two normally distributed populations with unequal variances.

Paired t Test. Matching or pairing members of one sample with members of another sample is a method of reducing variability and thus increasing the power of a test. The paired or dependent t test is appropriate for experimental designs contrived to reduce variability between groups. The paired t test is appropriate in the one–group design in which pretest results are compared with the posttest results among the same members of a sample. The cross–matching design is appropriately used with the paired t test. Matching members according to similarity of scores obtained during pilot work is a suitable way of assigning subjects to the paired t test.[3] The assumptions for this test are that random samples of paired differences are from a normally distributed population of differences.[4]

Consider a sample of subjects whose right and left superficial radial nerve (sensory) latencies from the distal third of the forearm are measured after receiving an application of ultrasound and ultrasound–electrical stimulation over the location of the nerve branch. Measurements of the latencies from the right arm are designated X ; those recorded from the left arm are assigned Y. The null hypothesis is stated as H_0: $\mu_X = \mu_Y$ and the alternative hypothesis as H_1: $\mu_X \neq \mu_Y$ at the 0.01 **LOS**, two–tailed. The test deals with the differences between each pair of scores rather than the difference between means of the samples. Formulas for each step in reaching the t ratio are somewhat different from those used in the independent t tests and will be presented in Table 10.4 with the computations. The t ratio is expressed by the formula

$$t = \frac{\overline{D}}{S_{\overline{D}}}$$

where $\overline{D}$ is the mean, $\overline{D} = \Sigma D/n$, and $S_{\overline{D}}$ is the standard error of the mean, $S_{\overline{D}} = \sqrt{(d^2/n - 1)/n}$.

Note the change in degrees of freedom compared with that calculated for independent t tests. In independent t tests, the degrees of freedom was

Table 10.4
Computation of the Pair t Test: Radial Nerve Latencies after Two Methods of Ultrasound

X (Ultrasound, msec)	Y (Ultrasound-electrical stimulation, msec)	$X - Y$ D	$D - \overline{D}$ d	$(D - \overline{D})^2$ d^2
2.3	2.7	−0.4	−0.32	0.1024
2.5	2.2	0.3	0.38	0.1444
2.4	2.6	−0.2	−0.12	0.0144
2.0	2.5	−0.5	−0.42	0.1764
2.6	2.5	0.1	0.18	0.0324
2.5	2.4	0.1	0.18	0.0324
2.6	2.5	0.1	0.18	0.0324
2.4	2.6	−0.2	−0.12	0.0144
2.5	2.3	0.2	0.28	0.0784
2.4	2.7	−0.3	−0.22	0.0484
		−0.8		0.6760

$\overline{D} = \dfrac{\Sigma D}{n} = \dfrac{-0.8}{10} = -0.08$

$S_D^2 = \dfrac{\Sigma d^2}{n - 1} = \dfrac{0.6760}{9} = 0.0751$

$S_{\overline{D}}^2 = \dfrac{S_D^2}{n} = \dfrac{0.0751}{10} = 0.0075$

$S_{\overline{D}} = \sqrt{S_{\overline{D}}^2} = \sqrt{0.0075} = 0.0867$

$t = \dfrac{-0.08}{0.0867} = -0.923$ $t_c(0.01,\ 9\ df) = 3.25$

calculated as $n_x + n_y - 2$, but in paired t tests, the pairs are considered as one group and the degrees of freedom is calculated as $n_{xy} - 1$. Pairing or matching scores in the two groups reduces variability, which in turn decreases the size of the standard error.[3] If the data were treated as independent samples, the df would have been 18 rather than 9. The critical value for the 0.01 level and 18 df is 2.878, whereas the critical value for this paired t test example with 9 df is 3.25 (2–tailed, Table C, page 332). Since the critical t values for the paired t test are greater than those required by the independent t test of similar sized groups, the former requires a greater obtained value for rejecting the null hypothesis. The researcher using the paired t test thus can place more confidence in his decision about the null hypothesis.

In the example, the obtained t value of -0.923 was less than the critical value $t_c(0.01, 9\ df) = 3.25$, so that the null hypothesis $H_0: \mu_x = \mu_y$ is true. The rate of nerve conduction is effected similarly by ultrasound and ultrasound-electrical stimulation.

Interpretation of the t Tests. One of the objectives in a course of research methods is to improve the student's ability to read the research literature. Reports of research studies in which t tests were used are not always informative about type of test (independent or paired), the number of tails (1 or 2), and levels of significance. Authors of research studies owe the readers this particular information. Also, the t tests are sometimes used improperly for multiple comparisons, but the test is really only effective in comparing two distributions. Two unrelated variables should not be tested with the t test; for example, effects of isokinetic exercise (force) and effects of manual therapy (range of joint motion) on elbow extension. If isokinetic exercise and manual therapy effects are treated as two methods effecting the variable motion (range of) of the elbow joint, then the t test for independent groups can be used.

The ability of a test to assist in supporting an original hypothesis when it is true and in rejecting the hypothesis when it is false is very important to the researcher. Three conditions improve the power of t tests. The first condition is to decrease the magnitude of the variance; the second is to increase the difference between means; and the third is to increase the size of the sample. Increasing the numbers of scores in samples reduces the size of the standard error of the differences which has the effect of enlarging the t ratio.

Some assumptions about the t tests already have been mentioned. Morehouse and Stull[3] have provided a clear discussion about the basic assumptions of the independent t tests. Conclusions drawn from the independent t tests are suspect if the variables are not distributed normally. If for some reason scores are skewed (clustered into a certain region of the curve) or if the researcher has some doubt about the distribution of data, then nonparametric tests should be considered. For example, if strength (force) measurements are being converted into + or − symbols or into descriptive terms (fair or poor) as in the manual muscle test, nonparametric tests (Chapter 11) should be used to analyze the data. One assumption is that the scores of one group do not influence the scores of the other group (independence). When scores are matched or paired, the use of the independent t test is violated and the paired or correlated t test would be more appropriate.[3] Tests are available for verifying the homogeneity of variances of the different groups. If the variances are markedly different, such tests should be used to determine homogeneity. The student is referred to Cochran and Cox[10] for this topic. Wide divergence of sample sizes or extremely small samples are not recommended for use with t tests. The t test tables go as low as 1 df, so that values are available for very small samples; however, small amounts of information are not always representative of the population characteristic and therefore should be avoided. Actually, only drastic violations of the basic assumptions will have serious consequences.[11] The use of large sample sizes in experiments using hypothesis testing is the best preventive for nonviolation of basic statistical assumptions.[12]

The t tests are parametric tests that estimate the parameter of the populations being tested.

ANALYSIS OF VARIANCE

In the discussion about sum of squares earlier in this chapter, between– and within–groups variability was mentioned as a component of the total sum of squares. The t tests are a special case in which the between–groups sum of squares cannot technically be partitioned out of the total sum of squares. In effect, the mean difference serves as between–groups variability but is a weak and limited version of the concept of partitioning total sum of squares into within– and between–groups variability. This does not flaw the t tests because they are excellent for the job for which they were mathematically designed. Remember that t tests only handle the comparison between two groups, and between–groups sum of squares cannot be partitioned out; it must be relegated to the means of the different groups. The t ratio can be formulated as

$$t = \frac{\text{difference between two means}}{\text{within–groups sum of squares}}$$

Analysis of variance (**ANOVA**) is a statistical method that divides the sum of squares $\Sigma (X - \overline{X})^2$ into additive parts with each part assigned to a known source, cause, or factor.[12] The sum of squares of groups is a large proportion of the total sum of squares and generally is explained in terms of variance, and the F ratio (F) can be expressed as

$$\frac{\text{Mean square}_{between}}{\text{Mean square}_{within}}$$

ANOVA is an extension of the t tests because, in its simplest terms, it can be used to test the significance of the difference between the means of two or more populations.[12]

The null hypothesis for **ANOVA** is used similarly to the way hypotheses were used in the t tests. In the t tests, the ratio involves the difference between two means (H_0: $\mu_1 = \mu_2$), whereas in **ANOVA** the ratio includes differences between more than two means. The null hypothesis in **ANOVA** might be H_0: $\mu_A = \mu_B = \mu_C \ldots -\mu_n$. An alternative hypothesis is also used and is usually given in the narrative form, H_1: at least two means differ. Methods of accepting the hypotheses are the same for t tests and **ANOVA**. If variations between means are due to sampling variabilities, then the null hypothesis is accepted; but if the variations are not attributed to sampling fluctuations, the null hypothesis is considered false. Unlike the t tests, a significant F ratio tells the researcher that a significant difference exists between the smallest and largest means only. Other differences of significance must be determined by special post hoc (after–the–fact or retrospective) analysis. Methods of post hoc analyses will be discussed later.

Since the F ratio is formed by sums of squares in the numerator and denominator, two different degrees of freedom are needed to compare the obtained F value to the baseline, critical F value. This condition influences the shape of the F distribution by causing it to be skewed positively.

The ratio (Fig. 10.6) deals with squared values and, therefore, no negative values are formed for the F distribution; this results in the zero point being at the extreme left and the median being 1.0. Most F tables present critical values for one–tailed tests because most computed F ratios fall to the right of 1.0 in the F distribution.

Theory of Analysis of Variance

ANOVA, like the t tests, determines whether the difference between means of different samples is drawn from the same population. Unlike the t tests, the **ANOVA** is appropriate for testing the differences between more than two means and offers more design options to the researcher than the t

Figure 10.6. Hypothetical F distribution.

tests. The differences between more than two means can be tested simultaneously and the pooled within–groups variance can serve as an estimate of error variance, which is important to the researcher.

ANOVA is an arithmetic scheme and is accomplished by partitioning the sum of squares [$\Sigma (X - \overline{X})^2$ or $\Sigma X^2 - (\Sigma X)^2/n$] into additive parts so that each additive part can be assigned to a known source, cause, or factor. These additive parts of known sources, causes, and factors are used to estimate the variance of the population.[12] The simplest model on which **ANOVA** is based is the randomized model; the concept of randomness is the foundation of statistical probability. The partitioning of the total sum of squares (SS) can be expressed as $SS_{total} = SS_{between} + SS_{within}$. Different authors use different terminology for expressing the components of the total sum of squares; for example, between–groups SS are sometimes called treatment and within–groups SS are sometimes called error SS. The total sum of squares is the sum of squares of the deviations from the overall mean for all scores, $\Sigma (X - \overline{X})^2$. Most books on statistics use a form of summation notation in **ANOVA** to differentiate sample and total values, and the student pursuing courses in statistics will become familiar with these. For illustrative purposes a very simple method of using upper case letters for total values and lower case letters for sample values is used here. That is, x = sample values and X = total values.

The between sum of squares is the sum of the products for all samples of all scores in a given sample multiplied by the square of the deviations of a given sample mean from the overall mean:[3]

$$SS_{between} = \Sigma\, n_{all}\, (\overline{x} - \overline{X})^2$$

The sum of squares within is the sum of the squared deviations of all scores from their respective sample means:[3]

$$SS_{within} = \underset{\text{samples scores}}{\Sigma \quad \Sigma}\, (X - \overline{x})^2$$

The population variance can be estimated once the above calculations are completed by finding the mean squares (MS) of the partitioned parts:

$$MS_{between} = \frac{SS_{between}}{df_{between}}$$

where df is $K - 1$ (K = number of samples) being tested.

$$MS_{within} = \frac{SS_{within}}{df_{within}}$$

where df is $(N - 1) - (K - 1)$, N = total number of scores. The mean square for within is an extension of $(s_{\bar{x}}^2)$ and is a pooling of the sum of squared deviations from the means within all groups. Once the sum of squares and mean squares are calculated, the F ratio can be found by dividing $MS_{between}$ by MS_{within}.

$$F = \frac{MS_{between}}{MS_{within}}$$

Theoretically, if only sampling fluctuations have occurred between samples, the $MS_{between}$ will equal the MS_{within} and a ratio of 1.0 is formed. On most occasions using **ANOVA**, the $MS_{between}$ will be larger than MS_{within} to provide an F ratio larger than 1.0. If experimental effects are at work in the study, the results will be evident in the F ratio when the $MS_{between}$ is many times larger than the MS_{within} value. Special F tables are available for comparing the obtained value from the computations to the critical value of the table (Appendix, Table D). If one thinks of df for $MS_{between}$ being at the top of the F table, then little difficulty will be encountered when obtaining the critical value. Tables often have rows of values associated with the df_{within} rows and these represent different levels of significance. The appropriate row and column for level of significance must be found when locating the critical F value.

Example of One–Way Analysis of Variance

Computation of a hypothetical situation involving four methods of applying heat to the body is illustrated in Table 10.5. Because the one–way **ANOVA** is a randomized model, each sample contains different subjects who were assigned randomly to the different methods (samples). One–way refers to the one independent variable common to all samples. The independent variable in the present example is methods of heating. The null hypothesis is H_0: $\mu_A = \mu_B = \mu_C = \mu_D$, and the alternative hypothesis (H_1) is that at least two means will differ. The 0.05 **LOS** is used, the methods of applying heat are hot packs, infrared, short wave diathermy, and ultrasound. The intramuscular temperatures (dependent variable) of the gastrocnemius are measured for each application of heat by a thermistor.

In Table 10.5, the degrees of freedom for $MS_{between}$ is found by $K - 1$ samples $(4 - 1 = 3)$, and for MS_{within} by $(N - 1) - (K - 1)$ or $[(28 - 1) - (4 - 1) = 27 - 3 = 24]$. The F ratio obtained $< F_{critical}$ ∴ H_0: $\mu_A = \mu_B = \mu_C = \mu_D$ is true.

The F ratio is less than the critical value of Table D in the Appendix; the conclusion can be made that the null hypothesis is true; the difference between the means is not significantly different from zero. If the hypothesis is true, then no difference in heating muscle is obtained by the different methods. The obtained F ratio must exceed 3.01 to be significant (i.e., accept the alternate hypothesis).

Table 10.5
Computation for One-Way Analysis of Variance with Equal Sample Sizes: Temperature Differences of Various Forms of Heat (Fictitious Data in Degrees)

Hot Packs	Infrared	SW Diathermy	Ultrasound	
2.0	1.6	2.3	2.3	
1.5	2.6	2.1	2.3	
1.8	2.5	2.3	2.1	
3.1	1.9	2.2	2.3	
2.2	2.2	2.1	2.5	
2.3	2.0	2.3	2.4	
2.4	1.8	2.4	2.9	TOTALS
$\sum x = 15.30$	14.60	15.70	16.80	62.40
$\sum x^2 = 34.99$	31.26	35.29	40.70	142.24
$\bar{x} = 2.19$	2.09	2.24	2.40	

$$SS_{total} = \sum X^2 - \frac{(\sum X)^2}{N} = 142.24 - \frac{62.4^2}{28} = 3.18$$

$$SS_{between} = \sum samples \frac{(\sum x)^2}{n} - \frac{(\sum X)^2}{N}$$

$$= \frac{15.3^2 + 14.6^2 + 15.7^2 + 16.8^2}{7} - \frac{62.4^2}{28} = 0.37$$

$$SS_{within} = SS_{total} - SS_{between} = 3.18 - 0.37 = 2.81$$

$$MS_{between} = \frac{0.37}{3} = 0.123 \qquad F = \frac{0.123}{0.117} = 1.05$$

$$MS_{within} = \frac{2.81}{24} = 0.117 \qquad F_{c(.05,\ 3\ \&\ 24\ df)} = 3.01$$

Example of One–Way Repeated Measures Analysis of Variance[13]

The precision of an experiment can be improved by matching or pairing different subjects or groups of subjects who receive different treatments. Using the same group of subjects, all receiving different treatments, provides the highest degree of comparability. Experiments using this approach of matching subjects on all treatments are called repeated measures designs (Chapter 9). The repeated measures may be used in any basic design and analysis of variance.

Repeated measures designs have advantages over randomized designs. Using the same subject over all treatments improves the power of the design by involving comparisons of homogeneous subjects. The repeated measures designs are efficient because they reduce the number of subjects needed in other designs (viz, randomized designs). Repeated measures designs control the time factor when treatments are given over time (that is, each subject is treated under the same time condition, which reduces invalidity caused by growth and development factors).

Repeated measures designs do not permit different treatments to be applied simultaneously. In the situation where little time passes between different treatments (insufficient wash–out time), carry–over effects can accumulate or influence subsequent treatment outcomes. Despite these drawbacks, the repeated measures designs are considered applicable for experimental research. The simplest form is presented here. It is used for two or more treatment combinations.

Computation of a hypothetical situation involving three methods of exercise is illustrated in Table 10.6. The null hypothesis is $H_0 : \mu_A = \mu_B = \mu_C$, and the alternate hypothesis (H_1) is that at least two means will differ. A 0.05 LOS is used; the methods of exercise are isometric, electrical stimulation, and the combination of isometric and electrical-stimulation exercise. The torque is calculated in Newton meters. In Table 10.6, the degree of freedom for $MS_{treatment}$ is found by K − 1 samples (3 − 1 = 2); $MS_{subject}$ is $n - 1$ subjects in a sample (6 − 1 = 5); and $MS_{interaction}$ is $(K - 1)$ samples $\times (n - 1)$ subjects $(2 \times 5 = 10)$. The F ratio obtained > F critical, $\therefore$ H_1 is true (at least two means differ; for example, 4.33 and 9.33).

Table 10.6
Computation for One–Way Repeated Measures Analysis of Variance: Torque Differences of Various Forms of Exercise (Fictitious Data in Newton Meters)

Subject	1	2	3	Totals
		Treatments		
1	3	5	6	14
2	5	9	10	24
3	2	5	9	16
4	6	11	12	29
5	7	12	8	27
6	3	8	11	22
$\Sigma X =$	26	50	56	132
$\Sigma(X)^2 =$	676	2500	3136	
$\Sigma X^2 =$	132	460	546	1138
$\overline{X} =$	4.3	8.3	9.3	

SS_{total}
$$= \Sigma X^2 - \frac{(\Sigma X)^2}{N} = 3^2 + 5^2 + \ldots 8^2 + \ldots 11^2 - \frac{(132)^2}{18}$$
$$= 1138 - \frac{(132)^2}{18} = 1138 - 968 = 170$$

$SS_{treatment}$
$$= \Sigma \text{ samples } \frac{(\Sigma X)^2}{n} - \frac{(\Sigma X)^2}{N} = \frac{26^2 + 50^2 + 56^2}{6} - \frac{(132)^2}{18}$$
$$= 1052 - 968 = 84$$

$SS_{subject}$
$$= \Sigma \text{ subjects } \frac{(\Sigma X)^2}{n} - \frac{(\Sigma X)^2}{N} = \frac{14^2 + 24^2 + \ldots 22^2}{3} - \frac{(132)^2}{18}$$
$$= 1027.33 - 968 = 59.33$$

$SS_{interaction}$
$$= SS_{total} - SS_{treatment} - SS_{subject} = 170 - 84 - 59.33$$
$$= 26.67$$

$MS_{treatment}$
$$= \frac{84}{2} = 42 \qquad MS_{subject} = \frac{59.33}{5} = 11.87$$

$MS_{interaction}$
$$= \frac{26.67}{10} = 2.67 \qquad F_c(.05, 2 \ \& \ 10 \ df) = 4.10$$

The obtained F ratio is greater than the critical value of Table D in the Appendix. The conclusion is that two or more means differ and a post hoc analysis of means must be performed to determine which means differ from each other.

The **ANOVA** is extremely versatile and can be adapted to most of the designs presented in Chapter 9 (random, factorial, and repeated measures). Certain methods can be used to handle samples of unequal size, but are not discussed in this book.

Post Hoc Analysis of Means

When the F ratio is tested for significance by comparing the obtained F value to a tabular value (critical value) and is found to exceed the critical value, the decision is to accept the alternative hypothesis. The alternative hypothesis is that at least two means are different. This alternate hypothesis is all that can be interpreted from a significant F value at this point. The interpretation is only that the mean having the smallest value is significantly different from the mean having the largest value when all means of the samples are rank ordered. What about the other means? If the F value is significant, the question is answered only by performing further analyses. Analysis of the significant means is called post hoc, postmortem, or a posteriori analysis. Several tests are available and are named after the men who developed them. These tests perform pairwise contrasts and are based on the avoidance of committing a Type I error. Because of their bases, each test incorporates varying degrees of conservatism and special tables are available for each procedure, although some procedures use similar tables. The procedures are presented according to their conservatism of the risk of the Type I error.

If the calculated F ratio in the above example is not significant (less than the critical value), no further analyses (post hoc) for the ANOVA is necessary. The null hypothesis would not be rejected.

Duncan Procedure. The Duncan Procedure was designed for samples of equal size, but sample means of unequal sizes can be compared by using the harmonic mean ($\overline{X}_h = n/(1/\Sigma X)$).[4] The standard error of a mean, $S_m = \sqrt{MS_{within}/n}$, is multiplied with an appropriate "multiple-range" value to provide an estimate of the standard error of the difference between ranked pairs of means. The level of significance is greater for pairwise contrasts for means separated by large numbers than for the small numbers of ranked positions.[13]

Newman–Keuls Procedure. Newman–Keuls procedure, sometimes referred to as Student–Newman–Keuls procedure, tests all pairwise contrasts at the same level of alpha so that the "studentized range" (special table) accounts for the magnitude or rank separation of the pair of means entering into a contrast. The studentized range protects the alpha levels

(LOS), which vary according to the rank separation of pairs or means. The procedure is similar to Duncan's except for the protected levels of alpha. The two procedures are considered middle–of–the–road post hoc analyses.[13]

Tukey Procedure. This procedure uses a fixed–range test to compute one critical value for all comparisons of means regardless of the number of steps separating the means. Tukey's procedure of "honestly significant difference" yields fewer significant differences than the previous two procedures. The procedure is easy to use, can be used for equal- and unequal-sized samples, and uses the "studentized range" table of Newman–Keuls.[3]

Scheffé Procedure. Scheffé's test involves the calculation of t ratios for each comparison, followed by comparisons with a special critical t'. This procedure is the most conservative and will yield the fewest significant differences among the post hoc tests presented. The probability of committing a Type I error is never higher than the established alpha level in this test.[3]

Researchers must decide the risk they are willing to take when selecting post hoc tests (0.05 or 0.01 LOS). Review of the literature seems to favor the middle–of–the–road tests. Authors should report the type of post hoc analyses used in determining significance of the means in analysis of variance. The reporting of post hoc tests is usually found in the results section of the narrative report.

CORRELATION

Correlation is a method of determining the degree of association (correspondence, agreement, relation) between two variables. The method of computing a correlation coefficient is appropriate for those research projects in which an attempt is made to determine relations. The relation must be logical, as determined by the researcher prior to calculating a correlation coefficient. For example, determining the relation between the severity of cancer among patients and the number of pickles they eat each week might be ridiculous if it led to the interpretation that pickles cause cancer. Correlation is concerned with a bivariate distribution in which scores have been recorded for two variables or two sets of scores from a single variable. An example of the latter is when you are interested in having patients perform some motor skill with the left and right hands and then try to determine the degree of association existing between the two performances (dexterity determinations). Karl Pearson, a behavioral scientist, devised a method known now as the Pearson product moment correlation method;[14] the coefficient is designated by the symbol "r". This symbol r when standing alone denotes Pearson product moment correlation and can be found in tables or narratives of reported research studies. Pearson product moment correlation should not be confused with other types of correlation, such as rank order correlation to be presented later in Chapter 11. The Pearson product moment correlation method is the most frequently used method of determining the agreement between two variables.

When two variables are correlated, the variables tend to vary together: (1) one variable systematically becomes larger, while the other variable systematically becomes larger; and (2) one variable systematically becomes larger, while the other variable systematically becomes smaller. In the first situation, the variables are correlated positively if both variables tend to vary in the same direction, larger or smaller. A person's height is usually correlated positively with body weight; both variables have a tendency to vary together in an upward (positive) direction. Coins vary in size with their values, the smaller the coin, the less the value (the one- and ten-cent pieces are exceptions, but the general trend holds true, although imperfectly). The second situation occurs when one variable becomes larger and is paired with a variable that becomes smaller; the variables in this situation are said to be correlated negatively. When a person becomes older (positive trend in age), muscular strength tends to lessen (negative trend). In mathematics, the negative sign masks the positive sign so that the correlation is a negative relation (trends in different directions). Another example of negative correlation is the correlation of items on a semantic differential scale, where the descriptive terms are polar opposites. For example, in the assessment of **PAIN**:

Hurt   0   Pleasant

The researcher hopes, however, that the results obtained from the instrument correlate positively with some specific attitude.

The correlation coefficient not only detects the degree of variation between two variables but also detects the direction of variation. The coefficient is an index of relation (correspondence, agreement, association) between two variables and is expressed as a single numerical value. The value can range from a perfect positive correlation of $+1.00$ to a perfect negative correlation of -1.00. The midpoint bisects the range and is designated as zero. A zero correlation indicates that no relation exists between the two variables. The relation between two variables can take on any value (decimal number) ranging between $+1.00$ and -1.00; the coefficient is a continuous variable with set limits.

Scatter Diagrams

The examples of correlation cited can be graphed in a vivid fashion. A scattergram is a graphic illustration showing the manner in which scores of two variables vary concomitantly. As a rule, the scores of the X variable are graphed on the horizontal axis of the graph, and scores of the Y variable are graphed on the vertical axis of the graph (in graphing correlation both variables are given equal standing, so that either variable can be plotted on the X and Y axes). For purposes of illustrating different relations between two variables, fictitious data will be used for the figures.

The scattergrams depicted are different because the points of the X and Y variables either follow a straight line (Figs. 10.7 and 10.11) or else depart from a straight line by varying amounts. A basic assumption of the Pearson product moment correlation method is that the association between the variables is linear, that the relationship between the variables follows a straight line. The magnitude of the correlation coefficient is reflected by the departure of the measures from the straight line. In Figures 10.7 and 10.11, all the points fall on a straight line (if the points are joined) and the relations are perfect. In Figure 10.7, the scores of the X variable tend to increase, while scores on the Y variable tend to increase by equal amounts—a perfect positive correlation. The direction of the perfect correlation depicted in Figure 10.8 is negative because, as scores of the X

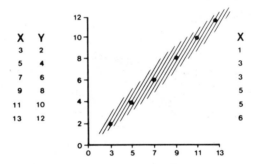

Figure 10.7. Perfect positive correlation. Note: In Figures 2 to 6, the shading around the points of the graphs is used to emphasize the relation.

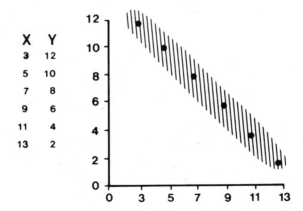

Figure 10.8. Perfect negative correlation.

variable increase, the scores of the *Y* variable decrease by equal amounts. The relations shown in Figures 10.9 to 10.11 vary in direction and magnitude.

Computation of Correlation

Several forms of the formula are available for computing the correlation coefficient, but, in keeping with the theme of the variance in statistical

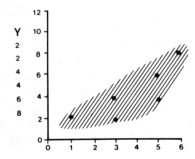

Figure 10.9. High positive correlation.

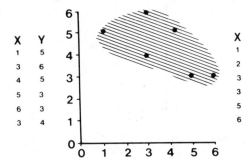

Figure 10.10. Low negative correlation.

Figure 10.11. Low positive correlation.

calculations, most formulas used in this book have commonalities (variance). The basic formula for r is:

$$r = \frac{\Sigma XY - \frac{(\Sigma X)(\Sigma Y)}{n}}{\sqrt{\left[\Sigma X^2 - \frac{(\Sigma X)^2}{n}\right]\left[\Sigma Y^2 - \frac{(\Sigma Y)^2}{n}\right]}}$$

where

r = correlation coefficient
ΣXY = sum of the cross–product of X multiplied by Y
ΣX^2 = sum of squared scores (also for Y)
ΣY^2 = sum of scores squared (also for Y)
n = number of paired scores

The formula caused three operations of division by the positions of n; therefore, a more convenient form of the formula, which represents a savings in efficiency, is:[3]

$$r = \frac{n\Sigma XY - (\Sigma X)(\Sigma Y)}{\sqrt{[n\Sigma X^2 - (\Sigma X)^2][n\Sigma Y^2 - (\Sigma Y)^2]}}$$

An example of testing for reliability of an instrument using some data should help to explain the formula (Table 10.7). The reliability determined by the test–retest method in Table 10.7 is $r = 0.96$, which is highly correlated. The repeated measurements are dependent on the instrument (volume cylinder).

Interpretation of the Correlation Coefficient

The coefficient is an index of convenience developed in theory and modeled by mathematical formulas for practical use. Because limits of $+1.0$ to -1.0 were chosen arbitrarily, the reader can only interpret the obtained index values in relative terms.[14] The coefficient is not a proportion or a percentage. An r of 0.96 has the same value as an r of -0.96, but the concomitant variation of the two variables tends to vary in different directions. The numerical size of the coefficient does not permit any interpretation about the magnitude of the variables.

The coefficient value does not imply a cause-and-effect relation between the two variables. The reader cannot determine the cause of the relation other than by the way the scores actually vary with each other. Suppose separate groups of young adult women and men are tested for strength by measuring maximum isometric muscular contractions of the quadriceps femoris muscle. The bivariate distribution of scores yields a value of $r =$

Table 10.7
**Results and Computation of Test–Retest Reliability of Measurements Recorded from a
Volume Cylinder Using Hands of Various Sizes**

Test (mm of water displaced)	Retest (mm of water displaced)
36.0	36.0
18.0	17.0
22.0	22.0
17.0	16.0
24.0	24.0
20.0	23.0
20.0	18.0
8.0	10.4
12.0	16.6
14.0	15.6
13.0	12.8
22.0	24.0
16.5	15.0
17.2	16.4
10.4	10.0
22.8	19.6
15.0	16.0
10.4	10.4
9.8	10.0

$\Sigma X = 328.10$
$\Sigma X^2 = 6{,}451.29$ $\Sigma XY = 6{,}475.82$
$(\Sigma X)^2 = 107{,}649.61$

$\Sigma Y = 332.80$
$\Sigma Y^2 = 6{,}563.20$
$(\Sigma Y)^2 = 110{,}755.84$

$$r = \frac{n\Sigma XY - (\Sigma X)(\Sigma Y)}{\sqrt{[n\Sigma X^2 - (\Sigma X)^2][n\Sigma Y^2 - (\Sigma Y)^2]}}$$

$$= \frac{19 \times 6{,}475.82 - 328.10 \times 332.80}{\sqrt{[19 \times 6{,}451.29 - 328.10^2]\,[19 \times 6{,}563.20 - 332.80^2]}}$$

$$= \frac{13848.90}{\sqrt{14924.90 \times 13944.96}} = \frac{13848.90}{14426.61} = 0.95995 = 0.96$$

0.98; the researcher should not conclude, however, that the quadriceps
femoris muscle strength of women and men are equal. In all probability,
the women were athletic and endomorphic, whereas the men were sedentary and ectomorphic. Previous studies have indicated that women have
about 70% of the strength of men.[9,15]

To avoid some problems of interpretation, the coefficient is squared.
The coefficient of determination is the name given to the squared correlation coefficient, r^2. The r^2 value is the ratio of the explained sum of
squares of variable Y divided by the total sum of squares of variable Y. If
the coefficient of determination is used, then the value is a proportion of
the retest variance, which is associated with the preexisting variance. The
coefficient of determination ranges between zero and $+1.00$ (squaring con-
verts a negative score into a positive score). The r^2 value is a better

indicator or predictor of the relative importance of the different magnitudes of r than the correlation coefficient alone.[16]

Correlation can be used in experimental research as well as nonexperimental research for determining relation between two variables and hypothesis testing.

REGRESSION ANALYSIS

We have seen how the relation of two variables can be projected through an index. Sometimes a single score of one variable can be predicted when the corresponding score of the other variable is known.[17] Regression analysis is the method used to determine the linear relation between two variables when predicted values of one variable are desired. When a relation exists between two variables, we can attempt to predict a score of one variable within the limits of the scores on which the correlation coefficient is based.[3] Correlation and prediction form close relations and one method can be projected to the other. Unlike correlation in which each variable is given equal standing, regression analysis calls the X variable from which prediction is based the independent variable, and the dependent variable, which is being predicted, is Y. This rule holds true when setting the results of regression analyses in graph form.

With the scattergram we were able to form a vivid image of the relation between the two variables, and with the correlation coefficient, a numerical value can be assigned to provide a relative index of that idea. Now an equation can be introduced to express the relation between two variables.

Computation of Regression Analysis

Like the method of Pearson product moment correlation, regression analysis also assumes that two variables are related in a linear fashion. If a scattergram is plotted and the geometric form does not resemble a straight line, but rather a curved line (curvilinear), the regression analysis discussed here is not appropriate. The technique provided for regression analysis is valid only for the situation in which the two variables resemble a straight line (linear relation). The linear regression line is sometimes referred to as the line of best fit.[18] The equation for a straight line is:

$$Y' = a + bX$$

where

Y' = the predicted Y value
a = intercept of Y
b = slope of the line
X = X variable on which prediction is based

This equation of a straight line represents the relation among a series of points formed by their coordinates. According to the above equation, the dependent variable, Y, will equal a when the independent variable equals zero. The point where the line of best fit and Y meet is the Y intercept, or the distance on Y between zero and the point of intersection; b is the tangent of the angle formed by X and Y.[16] In Figure 10.12, the mean electrical activity in microvolts root mean square of the left anterior deltoid is 5.2 when X (time in seconds) is zero, or the noise level of the electromyographic unit when the muscle is not contracting.

The regression line is computed by using the scores of a bivariate distribution and locating coordinate points for the average of the scores containing a minimum of error.[18] The symbols a and b in the equation are statistics computed from gathered data. The equation, $Y' = a + bX$, can be found by first solving for b and then for a.

$$b = \frac{\Sigma XY - \frac{(\Sigma X)(\Sigma Y)}{n}}{\Sigma X^2 - \frac{(\Sigma X)^2}{n}}$$

$$a = (\bar{Y} - b\bar{X})$$

Using data supplied in Table 10.8, a regression line can be formed from the scores for predicting future outcomes of the dependent variable. If the

Figure 10.12.   Voltage of contracting muscle as a function of time. (Reprinted with permission from Currier DP: Measurement of muscle fatigue. Phys Ther 49: 724–730, 1969).

Table 10.8
Prediction of Electrical Activity of Muscle from Contraction Time

X Time (seconds)	Y Electrical Activity (RMS)
10	5.96
20	5.98
30	6.02
40	6.06
50	6.27
60	6.58
70	6.91
80	7.20
90	7.52
100	8.03

$$\Sigma X = 550 \qquad\qquad\qquad \Sigma Y = 66.53$$
$$(\Sigma X)^2 = 302,500 \qquad\qquad (\Sigma Y)^2 = 4,426.24$$
$$\Sigma X^2 = 38,500 \qquad\qquad \Sigma Y^2 = 447.47$$
$$\Sigma XY = 3,850$$

$$\bar{X} = 55.0 \qquad\qquad \bar{Y} = 6.65 \qquad r = .95$$

$$b = \frac{\Sigma XY - \dfrac{(\Sigma X)(\Sigma Y)}{n}}{\Sigma X^2 - \dfrac{(\Sigma X)^2}{n}} = \frac{3,850 - \dfrac{(550)(66.53)}{10}}{38,500 - \dfrac{302,500}{10}}$$

$$= \frac{3,850 - 3,659.15}{38,500 - 30,250} = \frac{190.85}{8,250} = 0.023$$

$$a = (\bar{Y} - b\bar{X}) = 6.65 - (0.023)55 = 6.65 - 1.27$$
$$= 5.38$$
$$Y' = 5.380 + .023X$$

value of 45 seconds is recorded for X, the predicted Y' value becomes $Y' = 5.380 + 0.023 \times 45 = 6.420$ RMS (root mean square). If for some reason you were interested in predicting the electrical activity of the contracting muscle, wanted to establish a particular amount of time (X), and solve for Y' in the equation, the Y' would be an estimate of the corresponding score on the other variable (electrical activity). Suppose we take an X value recorded in the time column of Table 10.8 and solve for Y', let us say 40 seconds; the predicted Y' value would be 6.30 RMS. The predicted value of 6.30 is not the same as that of 6.06, which was obtained (Table 10.8) by actually measuring the electrical activity. The difference of 0.24 RMS between the two scores is not exact. The predicted score can, however, be considered our best estimate of muscular activity without actually measuring the electrical activity of muscle contracting for 40 seconds. The larger the number of data examined and used in the computation of the equation, the better our estimate becomes. One thousand data are better than 10 or 100 data. According to error theory, the predictor equation will never be perfect.

Determination of the correlation coefficient before the regression analysis assists the researcher in decision-making, that is, whether or not to compute a line of best fit. Unless the correlation coefficient is very high, the equation will not be a good predictor. Caution must be exercised in using linear regression for predicting. The relation must be appropriate for what is being predicted. A high correlation can be demonstrated for quantitative electromyographic activity of muscle and muscular force during contraction. The association between the two variables is linear, so that as force increases so does the electrical activity of muscle. After cursory observation, one might be inclined to simulate this association into clinical practice for measuring the strength of a patient's involved muscle group. The difficulty arises when making intercomparisons with different subjects, different muscles of different subjects, and different muscles of the same subject because of several factors (age, sex, strength, fitness, impedance, and mass differences); the comparisons are very erratic. Sampling the electrical activity of one muscle cannot predict the outcome of another. The idea is appealing, but one must be cautioned about the appropriateness of predictor equations if the variables are not related physiologically or conceptually. The correlation coefficients can be very high between the two variables, but the coefficients are not necessarily indicative of cause and effect.

TEST OF SIGNIFICANCE OF CORRELATION

Often one reads in research reports that the calculated correlation coefficient r was significant. This reporting of a significant r is enough to warrant attention in improving the student's ability to read and interpret the literature. The use of the word "significance" or "significant" in testing correlation coefficients does not carry the same importance as it did with the t tests or analyses of variance. The interpretation of a significant r only means that that particular coefficient value is not expected if the hypothesis stating that there is no relation between variables is true.[3] The distribution of r does not satisfy any distributions (normal, t or F) so far presented. The correlation coefficient, however, can be transformed into a t distribution where t is represented by the equation

$$t = \frac{r\sqrt{n-2}}{\sqrt{1-r^2}}$$

Hypotheses can be formed as a null hypothesis, H_0: $\rho = 0$, and as an alternative, H_1: $\rho \neq 0$. The letter "ρ" (rho) is the parameter for the statistic "r". When the null hypothesis is false, the interpretation is that the calculated r is statistically significant from zero. Another interpretation is that the value of the correlation coefficient obtained is unlikely to have resulted by chance variations if ρ was indeed equal to zero.[3] One must realize that the r value required to reach significance is dependent on the sample sizes, and if a very large number of scores is included in the samples (e.g., $\ge$ 1,000), the significant r value will be close to zero. Table C of the Appendix used for the critical values of the t distribution is also used for the transformed r values for determining significance. The levels of significance, again, are determined arbitrarily by the researcher. Hypothesis testing is similar to that used for the t tests and the F ratio. Ferguson has suggested that little importance should be given to this formula when small samples sizes (n = <20) are used unless the coefficients are large.[12]

After observation, the difference between the obtained r value and zero is obvious and using the above test would thus be fruitless. If some value other than zero is used to compare significance of the obtained r value, then a method of transforming the r value to a ''Z_r'' value is possible with a special transformation table. This method results in the comparison between Z and r having some importance. Ironically, authors seldom report the method of transformation used in determining significance of r in their studies. A conservative view assumes that the t transformation is used more commonly in the literature, especially since the method is frequently presented in many statistics textbooks. The Z_r transformation uses natural logarithms in the conversion for improving parity with r and Z values. The significance of the difference between correlation coefficients can be performed through the Z_r–transformation methods for hypotheses testing. Again, a special table is available in many statistics books for the convenience of the researcher who does not need to make the log transformations.[3]

SUMMARY

An hypothesis is a conjectural statement about the relation between two or more variables. If the hypothesis is clearly and specifically stated, it can be tested. The null hypothesis is a special form in hypothesis testing and implies that the difference between the means of the different variables is equal to zero. The null hypothesis is used commonly in experimental research because of its simplicity.

Hypothesis testing enables the researcher to make inferences based on collected data with a relative degree of reliability. Hypothesis testing is based on the theory of probability.

This chapter answers what hypotheses are, how they are tested, and how risks in hypothesis testing are determined. Appropriate statistical tests are presented for testing hypotheses. Table 10.9 provides a summary of the research processes presented thus far.

Table 10.9
Cumulative Summary of the Research Processes Presented

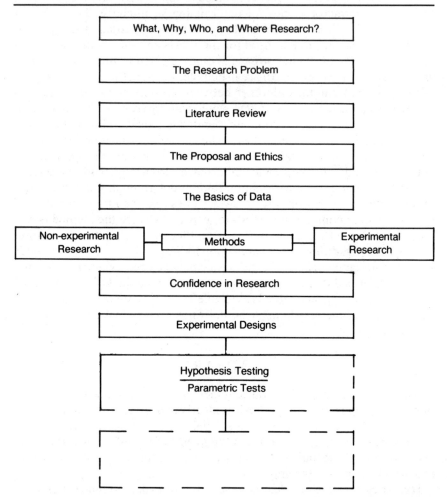

REFERENCES

1. Wilson BE: An Introduction to Scientific Research. New York, McGraw–Hill Book Co, Inc, 1952
2. Kerlinger FN: Foundations of Behavioral Research, ed 2. New York, Holt, Rinehart & Winston, Inc, 1973
3. Morehouse CA, Stull GA: Statistical Principles and Procedures with Applications for Physical Education. Philadelphia, Lea & Febiger, 1975
4. Remington RD, Schork MA: Statistics with Applications to the Biological and Health Sciences. Englewood Cliffs, NJ, Prentice–Hall, Inc, 1970
5. Random House Dictionary of the English Language, Unabridged ed. New York, Random House, 1967

6. Cajal SR: Precepts and Counsels on Scientific Investigation: Stimulants of the Spirit. Mountain View, CA, Pacific Press Publishing Assoc, 1951

7. Meyers LS, Grossen NE: Behavioral Research Theory, Procedure, and Design, ed 2. San Francisco, WH Freeman and Co, 1978

8. Michels E: Letters to the editor: Use of the t-test. Phys Ther 50: 102–104, 1970

9. Currier DP: Positioning for knee strengthening exercise. Phys Ther 57: 148–152, 1977

10. Cochran WC, Cox GM: Experimental Designs, ed 2. New York, John Wiley & Sons, Inc, 1957

11. Boneau CA: The effects of violations of assumptions underlying the t-test. Psych Bull 57: 49–64, 1960

12. Ferguson GA: Statistical Analyses in Psychology & Education, ed 5. New York, McGraw–Hill Book Co, 1981

13. Dayton CM: The Design of Educational Experiments. New York, McGraw–Hill Book Co, 1970

14. Roscoe JT: Fundamental Research Statistics for the Behavioral Sciences, ed 2. New York, Holt, Rinehart and Winston, Inc, 1975

15. Williams M, Stutzman L: Strength variation through the range of joint motion. Phys Ther Rev 39: 145–152, 1959

16. Sokal RR, Rohlf FJ: Introduction to Biostatistics. San Francisco, WH Freeman and Co, 1973

17. Daniel WW, Coogler CE: Statistical applications in physical medicine: Part II. Am J Phys Med 54: 25–47, 1975

18. Alder HL, Roessler EB: Introduction to Probability and Statistics, ed 6. San Francisco, WH Freeman and Co, 1977

11

Nonparametric Tests

It is better to be satisfied with probabilities
than to demand impossibilities and starve.
F. C. S. Schiller

Statistical procedures are divided into parametric and nonparametric statistics. Chapter 10 included tests of significance (t, analysis of variance) on which inferences can be made about the parent population. This group of statistics is called parametric. "Metric" refers to measurement procedures, and "para" refers to the assumptions about the population from which data are obtained.[1] Assumptions for parametric statistics are (1) that the samples are random, (2) that scores are independent of each other, (3) that experiments are repeatable with constancy of measurements from experiment to experiment, (4) that data are normally distributed, and (5) that samples have similar variances.[2] The parametric group of statistics then requires certain methods with desirable characteristics that yield unbiased, consistent, efficient, and sufficient estimates of the population.[3] Calculations are sometimes demanding in that they require long mathematical procedures, and results are sometimes difficult to interpret or understand by persons not well-versed in mathematics.

All statistical tests have assumptions; however, nonparametric statistics refers to a class of statistics that does not require assumptions as rigid as those of the parametric class. "Nonpara" implies this. Because this group of statistics does not require assumptions signifying a certain form of distribution or does not make statements about parameters or equality of variances, nonparametric statistics sometimes is referred to as distribution–free method.[4] In statistics, robustness is the degree to which a test can stray from the assumptions before changing the probability too much. The nonparametric class trades the power (large sample sizes) of the parametric tests for robustness, (generality).[2,5] The assumptions are that the samples are randomly and independently chosen and that the experiments are repeatable. No assumptions about the shape of the distribution have to be met as with the parametric class; nonparametric tests can test the null hypothesis, but the hypothesis is not stated in terms of parameters of

270

parent populations. Nonparametric statistics does not estimate parameters but rather tests the null hypothesis in a general form with samples that come from populations having the same distribution. The alternative hypothesis then tests samples that come from populations with different distributions. Methods requiring few and weak assumptions about the populations being sampled are less efficient than the corresponding parametric methods. Chances of committing Type II errors are increased with nonparametric statistics.[6] Table 11.1 groups statistics and statistical tests according to their classification and appropriate use by design.

USES

Nonparametric tests are used in the behavioral sciences when there is no basis for assuming certain types of distributions. Siegel[5] advocates that nonparametric tests be used for nominal and ordinal levels of measurements, whereas parametric tests are appropriate for analyzing interval and ratio data. In practice, levels of measurement are sometimes "downgraded" from ratio and interval to ordinal or nominal scales for the convenience of a measuring instrument or interpretation. For example, muscular strength or force (force = mass × acceleration) is a variable which yields ratio data because a true zero point exists in the level of measurement.[5,7] Muscular strength is absent with paralysis (true zero point). The manual muscle tests convert the ratio characteristics of force (mass and acceleration) into an ordinal scale by assigning grades of relative position (N, G, F, P, T, O or 5, 4, 3, 2, 1, 0). Williamsen[8] has countered that statistical tests are selected to meet certain goals or to answer specific questions rather than to match levels of measurements with parametric or nonparametric procedures. Gaito[9] has also offered a good argument against contaminating measurement theory with statistical theory. Levels

Table 11.1
Summary of Statistics and Statistical Tests Presented in Book

Classification	One–group	Design Two–group	Multi–group

Nonparametric	mode
	median
	chi–square
	percentile
		chi–square
		median test
		Turkey quick test
		Rank correlation
		Wilcoxon matched-
		  paired signed–ranks
		  test
		Mann–Whitney U test
			Kruskal–Wallis one-
			way *ANOVA*

Parametric	mean
	coefficient of variation
	standard deviation
	correlation (r, R)
		t tests (independent
		  and paired)
		regression analysis
		  (linear)
			Analysis of variance
			(*ANOVA*)

of measurement are not used in the application of nonparametric statistical procedures in this chapter.

Calculations of nonparametric tests are generally easy to perform[10,11] and to apply[10] and have considerable intuitive appeal as shortcut techniques.[6] Caution must be exercised because of their ease and convenience in calculation. Nonparametric tests are used when the assumptions of parametric tests cannot be met, when very small numbers of data are used, and when there is no basis for assuming certain types or shapes of distributions.[8] Nonparametric tests are never substituted for parametric tests when the parametric tests are more appropriate. Parametric tests are more powerful than nonparametric statistics and deal with continuous variables, whereas nonparametric tests often deal with discrete variables. Caution must also be exercised in using results from analyses of nonparametric tests for making inferences, because small numbers of data are used and no assumptions about parent populations are made.

Nonparametric tests are used if data can only be classified, counted, or ordered, for example, rating staff on performance or comparing results from manual muscle tests. These tests should not be used in determining precision or accuracy of instruments because the tests are lacking in both areas.

ADVANTAGES

The techniques of nonparametric tests are generally simpler to calculate mathematically than the parametric tests they replace.[6,11] These tests may be performed quickly and easily without automated instruments (computers and calculators).[11] Nonparametric tests are easier to understand and explain. The tests are easy to calculate and reduce concern for assumptions; they are designed for small numbers of data including counts, classifications, and renumerations. These tests are robust and can be used effectively in behavioral research.

DISADVANTAGES

Nonparametric tests are not as powerful as parametric tests and, therefore, are somewhat limited for experimental research. The ease of calculation and reduced concern for assumptions have been referred to as quick and dirty statistical procedures.[12]

Nonparametric tests are available for determining relations and significance. Conditions for using parametric tests were discussed in Chapter 10; the conditions necessary for nonparametric tests follow.

RANK CORRELATION

Earlier, the Pearson product moment correlation (r) for computing the association or relation between two variables was discussed. This method is used for testing validity and reliability of instruments and for correlational investigations. Spearman's rank correlation (ρ) is a nonparametric method of computing correlation from ranks. The method is similar to Pearson's, with the computed value ρ providing an index of the relation between two groups of ranks. If the original scores are ranks, the computed index will be similar in value to that computed by the product moment method. The difference between the two methods is that the product moment method assigns weight to the magnitude of each score, whereas the rank method is concerned with the ordinal position of each score.[8]

The coefficient of rank correlation (ρ, rho) ranges from $+1$ when paired ranks are changing in the same order to -1 when ranks are changing in reverse order. Zero is an indication that paired ranks are occurring at random. The formula for rank correlation is

$$\rho = 1 - \frac{6 \sum d^2}{n(n^2 - 1)}$$

where $\sum d^2$ is the sum of squared differences between ranks, 6 is a constant, and n is the number of paired scores.

Suppose 10 student physical therapists are drawn at random from a large class; each student has been rated on a 10–point scale for a recent clinical experience, and each student has a grade–point average (GPA). The coefficient of ranks will be computed to determine the extent of agreement between the two sets of scores (clinical experience rating and GPA). In the rank correlation method, the procedure is to replace the raw scores by assigning an appropriate rank to each score of each set. Ranks for each set correspond to the total number of scores in that set.

If the relation is a true one (real data), it is interpreted as a fair relation between clinical experience ratings and grade–point averages. The example illustrates what happens when obtained scores are similar (tied ranks). When tied ranks occur (e.g., column Y of Table 11.2), each score is assigned the average rank which the tied scores occupy. The GPA of 3.2, for example, had two scores occupying ranks 3 and 4, since ranks 1 and 2 were occupied by scores of 3.6 and 3.5, respectively. The average rank for the score 3.2 is obtained by adding ranks ($3 + 4$) and dividing by the number of ranks occupied (e.g., $3 + 4 \div 2 = 3.5$ ranking).

Since ρ is equivalent to r of the product moment method, the assumption is made that ranks are the first integers or raw scores, as in the product moment procedure. When many tied ranks appear in the computation, in the above example, the sum of squares of ranks departs from the sum of

Table 11.2
Computation of Coefficient of Rank Correlation: Clinical Rating and Grade-Point Average
(GPA) of 10 Student Physical Therapists (Artificial Data)

X (Clinical Rating)	Rank	Y (GPA)	Rank	(X − Y)	d^2
9.0	4	3.0	6.5	−2.5	6.25
8.0	6	2.9	8.0	−2.0	4.00
10.0	1	3.5	2.0	−1.0	1.00
6.0	9	3.0	6.5	2.5	6.25
8.3	5	3.1	5.0	0	0
7.0	8	2.7	9.0	−1.0	1.00
9.2	3	3.6	1.0	2.0	4.00
5.0	10	2.5	10.0	0	0
7.2	7	3.2	3.5	3.5	12.25
9.3	2	3.2	3.5	−1.5	2.25
					37.00

$$\rho = 1 - \frac{6\,(37.00)}{10\,(100-1)} = 1 - \frac{220.00}{990.00} = 1 - .22 = .78$$

squares of the first integers as in r.[3] This departure affects the ρ value.
When there are substantial tied ranks, the researcher is advised to use
Pearson's product moment correlation method.

TESTS FOR SIGNIFICANCE

There are nonparametric tests available to replace the three parametric
tests presented in Chapter 10 (correlation, t, and analysis of variance).
Representative nonparametric tests are discussed in this section.

Rank Correlation

Rank correlation can be used for hypothesis testing. The hypothesis H_0:
$\rho = 0$ and H_1: $\rho \neq 0$ can be tested for significance. For 20 paired scores or
more, the formula $t = \rho \sqrt{(n-2)/(1-\rho^2)}$ approximates a t distribution
with $n - 2$ degrees of freedom.[3,7,13] The $n - 2$ degrees of freedom is
peculiar to testing the significance of r from zero and the slope of a line
from zero.[3] The table for the parametric t distribution can be used as a
baseline (critical values) for comparing obtained t for rank correlation and
the critical t value (Appendix, Table C).

If the ρ value from 22 pairs of data was 0.78, the values are then substituted in the formula for t, the t value of 5.58 is then obtained

$$t = 0.78\,\sqrt{\frac{22-2}{1-0.78^2}} = 0.78\,\sqrt{\frac{20}{0.39}} = 0.78 \times \sqrt{51.28} = 5.59$$

and, locating the critical value for the 0.05 level of significance for 20 df, we find a t value of 2.21 for a two–tailed test:

$$t_{\text{obtained}} > t_{\text{critical}} \therefore \text{accept } H_1 : \rho \neq 0$$

The results can be interpreted to state that the coefficient of $\rho = 0.78$ is significantly different from zero. The hypotheses having direction (one–tailed) can also be tested for significance by using the one–tailed levels of significance in the table for t distribution.

One–Group Test

Chi–Square. Occasionally one sample chi–square is used when the apportionment of subcategories (K) of a sample into mutually exclusive and exhaustive sets is compared with expected theoretical frequencies. The chi–square (χ^2) test is based on the difference between an observed frequency for some category (K) and that expected from a known probability. The assumptions are that the subcategories $(K_z\text{'s})$ are standard scores, have normal distributions, and are independent.[8] The null hypothesis can be written to show the probability of observed frequencies differing from expected frequencies, $H_0 : D = O - E$ and an alternative hypothesis of $H_1 : D \neq O - E$, where D is the difference, O is the observed frequency, and E is the expected or theoretical frequency. The formula for chi–square is

$$\chi^2 = \Sigma\left[\frac{(O - E)^2}{E}\right]$$

The categories (K) are classes of a quantitative variable or components of a discrete or continuous variable. The χ^2 distribution is used to test significance in a way similar to that in which the t or F distributions are used. The null hypothesis states that no difference exists between the observed and expected frequencies; if the obtained chi–square value is less than the critical chi–square value, the indication is good that observation agrees with expectation. On the other hand, an accepted alternate hypothesis means that a significant difference exists and cannot be explained by sampling variations. Tables are available for indicating the values required to select hypotheses. The degrees of freedom are $K - 1$ in the single sample chi–square, and the 0.05 and 0.01 levels of significance are generally used to determine significance.[3]

An example of the chi–square sample using fictitious data is illustrated in Table 11.3. Suppose the directors of a physical therapy department wanted to know which of four brands of transcutaneous electric nerve stimulators (TENS) was preferred by patients.

Table 11.3
Computation of Chi-Square for Single Group: Preferred Use of Transcutaneous Electric
Nerve Stimulators (Fictitious Data)

TENS	O	E	$O - E$	$(O - E)^2$	$(O - E)^2/E$
A	10	22.5	−12.5	156.25	6.94
B	15	22.5	− 7.5	56.25	2.50
C	30	22.5	7.5	56.25	2.50
D	35	22.5	12.5	156.25	6.94
					$\Sigma = 18.88$

As shown in Table 11.3, χ^2 obtained $= 18.88$, χ^2 critical $= 7.82$ (0.05, 3 df) $\therefore$ select H_1: $D \neq 0 - E$.

The hypothesis tested is whether the observed frequencies are equal to the expected frequencies (22.5). The value of 22.5 is derived from the probability of preferring any one TENS based on the opinions of 90 patients selected to use all four TENS units at various times. Since four TENS units are being observed and 90 patients are using them, 90 divided by 4 is 22.5, or the theoretical expected frequency of preference. The values entered in the observed frequency column (O) are the frequencies of preference indicated by the 90 patients who underwent a trial period with each instrument. The obtained χ^2 value exceeds the critical value of χ^2. The hypothesis selected favors the alternative hypothesis that the observed frequencies are not equal to the expected frequencies. The director wants to eliminate one or two units of TENS based on the probability of them ever being preferred by patients as frequently as expected.

Appendix, Table E, can be consulted for the appropriate critical values at the desired levels of significance.

Two–Group Tests

Chi–Square. The 2×2, or four–fold contingency table of the chi–square test is used to determine the significance of differences between two independent samples. The hypothesis is whether the two samples differ on some variable with a frequency with which sample observations can be classified.[5] In this use of chi–square, the number of degrees of freedom is $(2 - 1)(2 - 1) = 1$.[3] An example serves to describe the test. Suppose a physical therapist studies the relation of skill acquisition of a new activity among subjects having left- and right-arm dominance. The null hypothesis, H_0, states that there is no difference between skill acquisition of left-handed and right-handed subjects. The alternate hypothesis, H_1, states that right–handed subjects do better than left–handed subjects in skill acquisition. The task for the seated–subjects is to succeed in four successive trials of putting a ball into a distant basket.[14] Each subject (10 left-handed and 10 right-handed) was given 50 trials; the numbers of successes and failures were counted. The hypotheses were tested at the 0.05 level. The 2 × 2 contingency table shows the results of the experimental procedure (data are fictitious):

	Left	Right	
Success	A_{20}	B_{18}	38 $(A + B)$
Failure	C_{30}	D_{32}	62 $(C + D)$
	50 $(A + C)$	50 $(B + D)$	

The formula for calculating chi–square is

$$\chi^2 = \frac{N(AD - BC)^2}{(A + B)(C + D)(A + C)(B + D)}$$

where N = the total number of trials and the letters correspond to specific blocks of the 2 × 2 contingency table.[3] The calculation of χ^2 from the above data is then:

$$\chi^2 = \frac{100(20 \times 32 - 18 \times 30)^2}{(38)(62)(50)(50)} = \frac{1,000,000}{5,890,000} = 0.17.$$

Appendix E is consulted for χ^2, $df = 1$, 0.05 level and the critical value, 3.84, is found. For $df = 1$, a $\chi^2 = 0.17$ indicates that no difference occurs between left–handed and right–handed subjects in skill acquisition of a new task. The null hypothesis, H_0, is supported.

The Median Test. Discrete and continuous variables are used with the median test. Note that continuous variables are treated as discrete in this statistical design. The median is determined for the two samples combined; scores above, equal to, and below the median are counted. This information is placed onto a table showing categories of scores and their totals. A chi–square statistic with 1 degree of freedom (2 samples) is calculated to test the hypothesis. The null hypothesis, H_0: $Md_A = Md_B$ is tested against an alternative hypothesis stating that the two populations do not have the same medians, H_1: $Md_A \neq Md_B$.[5] The median test is used to determine whether two independent samples of nominal level measures come from populations with the same median.[15]

The table for showing categories of scores and their totals can be displayed as

A	B	$A + B$
C	D	$C + B$
$A + C$	$B + D$	N

and the chi–square formula for the 2 × 2 tabular information can be calculated by the formula

$$\chi^2 = \frac{N(AD - BC)^2}{(A + B)(C + D)(A + C)(B + D)}$$

where N = total number of scores involved in all samples; A and C are values above the median of each sample, and B and D are scores equal to or below the median of each sample.

Consider a situation where the physical therapist wants to know the number of hours in which the patient is free from pain following two different methods of treating "tennis elbow." The hypotheses would be H_0: $Md_a = Md_b$ and H_1: $Md_a \neq Md_b$ and tested for the 0.05 level of significance, χ^2 obtained = $0.20 \geq \chi^2$ critical $(0.05, 1\ df) = 3.84$; ∴ the null hypothesis H_0: $Md_a = Md_b$ is true.

In the example (Table 11.4), two groups with equal numbers (10) of patients having "tennis elbow" are treated with different methods (a and b). All scores are placed in a single distribution and are rank ordered. The median (7) is determined. Scores in each column (A and C) larger than the median (7) are counted ($A = 4$, $C = 5$) and placed in the appropriate blocks of the table. Next, scores in each column (B and D) equal to or smaller than the median are counted ($B = 6$, $D = 5$) and placed in the proper squares of the table. The values entered in the labeled squares of the table are placed into the formula and solved for χ^2 (Table 11.4).

Since the obtained χ^2 value is less than the critical χ^2 value, the researcher has no reason to reject the null hypothesis and concludes that no difference exists between the relief times provided by the two methods.

Table 11.4
Computation of the Median Test: Two Methods of Treating "Tennis Elbow"

Method a (hours of relief)	Method b (hours of relief)					
1	2					
4	1					
6	8		$>$	$\geq$		
10	6					
8	12	a	4^A	6^B	10	
7	5					
6	9	b	5^C	5^D	10	
7	10					
17	15		9	11	20	
13	5					

median for combined groups = 7

$$\chi^2 = \frac{20\,(20-30)^2}{(10)\,(10)\,(9)\,(11)} = \frac{2000}{9900} = .202$$

Tukey's Quick Test. Suppose a group of patients ($N = 10$) having recent strokes are given a form of facilitatory training to reeducate a certain group of muscles assessed to be nonfunctional. Each nonfunctional muscle group is tested for tone before therapy begins and again at the termination of their biofeedback programs. A group of normal subjects is also measured before and after the experimental period, but they do not receive any therapy (control group). The myotonometer is an instrument that measures the resting tone of muscle by determining the amount of tissue depression possible under controlled conditions. The unit measured is an "MTM" and is an arbitrary unit.[16] Table 11.5 shows the amount of change in muscular tone for each subject during the experimental period.

The results are analyzed by Tukey's quick test. The MTM is a numerical unit that lacks great precision, and, therefore, produces data better suited to nonparametric testing, as with Tukey's test, than to a t test. From Table 11.5, the largest value in each group is located. The experimental group (facilitatory training) has the largest value (21 MTMs) and the control group's largest value is 6 MTMs. The number of values in the experimental group larger than the largest value recorded for the control group (6 MTMs) is counted. Eight values in the experimental group are larger than the largest value in the control group. Next, the number of values in the control group smaller than the smallest value in the experimental group (3 MTMs) is counted. Five values in the control group are smaller than the smallest value (3 MTMs) of the experimental group. The two counts are added ($8 + 5 = 13$) and, if the sum of the two counts is equal to or greater than seven, the conclusion is that the effects of the two treatments (facilitatory training and placebo in example) are different. The number seven is fixed and is the criterion value used in the comparative phase of Tukey's quick test. If the sum of the two counts is less than seven, the effects of the

Table 11.5
Increase in Muscular Tone Following Biofeedback and Placebo Program (Fictitious Data)

Experimental Group (MTM units)*	Control Group (MTM units)*
4	2
15	6
3	1
15	3
9	1
11	2
16	4
21	3
8	2
10	4

* Difference between before and after treatment measurements; MTM = myotonometer units.

two treatments are not different. In the example cited, the sum of the counts is 13; therefore, we conclude that the effects of facilitatory training are different from placebo effects.

In the event that both the largest value and the smallest value occur in the same group, the conclusion is that the two treatments do not have different effects.[11]

Wilcoxon Matched–Pairs–Ranks Test. This rank test is appropriate for two paired or related samples, and it considers the size and direction of the differences within pairs.[5] The difference (d) between each is found; if the paired numbers are equal, d is assigned zero. The difference (d) values can be negative or positive but are ranked by ignoring the sign. The smallest difference value is assigned the rank of 1 and so on. When tied ranks occur, each score is assigned the average rank which the tied scores occupy (similar to that used for rank correlation). After determining the ranks, the sign of the differences (ignored earlier) is now assigned to the particular rank. The original hypothesis that the sum of positive ranks will equal the sum of negative ranks is formed. A large difference between the sums provides support for rejecting the original hypothesis that the paired measurements are from the same population. The sum of the negative and positive ranks are compared. The smaller of the two sums is assigned T. The researcher then compares T with the number of paired scores having signs (ignore zeros) and the **LOS** selected. Appropriate tables for this test have been constructed by Ferguson[3] and Siegel[5].

Suppose two groups containing eight subjects are matched for sex, weight, and age and then rated by a perceived exertion rating scale (Chapter 6). One group rides a bicycle ergometer (X) and the other runs on a treadmill (Y) at a similarly fixed load and duration. The following are paired observations for X and Y:

X	15	19	16	14	17	18	16	17
Y	18	17	19	20	17	17	20	15
d	-3	2	-3	-6	0	1	-4	2
rank	-4.5	2.5	-4.5	-7	0	1	-6	2.5

The sum of the negative ranks is 22 and that of the positive ranks is 6. A Wilcoxon table indicates that for $n = 7$ (zero rank is ignored) at the point 0.05 **LOS** for a two–tailed test ($H_0: \mu_x = \mu_y$), the lower sum must be two or smaller to reject the null hypothesis. These data indicate that exertion from ergometer and treadmill activity of equal load and duration are perceived similarly by matched subjects.

When the number of ranks exceeds 25, the Wilcoxon table cannot be used; a table containing values of z in the normal distribution must be consulted. This latter table is found in standard statistical tests.[2-7] The negative and positive sums of ranks are found using the same approach for

N of less than 25. The letter T is assigned to the smaller number, placed in a formula where z (the normal deviate)[3] is calculated,

$$z = \frac{T - \dfrac{N(N + 1)}{4}}{\sqrt{\dfrac{N(N + 1)(2N + 1)}{24}}}$$

where N is the number of ranks and 4 and 24 are constants. Once z is found, its value is located in a table of the normal distribution and the probability for a two–tailed or one–tailed test is determined for a particular level of significance.

    Mann–Whitney U Test. This is a rank test for two independent samples and may be the best nonparametric alternative to the t test.[3] An example will explain this particular test.

    Suppose an experimental group of five rabbits receives laser treatment for their contrived wounds (X), and a control group of seven rabbits does not receive treatment for their contrived wounds (Y). The Mann–Whitney test is chosen because two independent samples containing small numbers of subjects and days to complete healing constitute the criteria. The null hypothesis is H_0: $\mu_x = \mu_y$, and the 0.05 significance level is selected. Consider the following scores and their ranks:

X	27	51	33	37	43		
rank	2	11	4	6	9		
Y	30	35	25	53	50	38	40
rank	3	5	1	12	10	7	8

    Each score is given a rank in ascending order of size: with a rank of 1 being the smallest value. Next, the ranks are ordered according to their identity.

rank	1	2	3	4	5	6	7	8	9	10	11	12
group	Y	X	Y	X	Y	X	Y	Y	X	Y	X	Y

The U is found by determining the number of X scores preceding each Y score. The U is: $1 + 2 + 3 + 3 + 4 + 5 = 18$ (rank $2X$ precedes $3Y = +1$, ranks $2X$ and $4X$ precede $5Y = +2$, ranks 2, 4 and $6X$ precede $7Y = +3$, and so on). Consulting a Mann–Whitney U test table for $n_y = 7$ (larger sample size), locate U value (18) on the left–hand margin and $n_x = 5$ at top of the table. The probability of occurrence under the stated null hypothesis is 0.562. The null hypothesis is true and the decision is that the data are nonsupportive for rejecting H_0.

The above procedure is appropriate only when the larger sample size is eight or smaller. Different procedures and tables are used for samples ranging between 9 and 20 and larger than 20, respectively. Procedures and tables for the Mann–Whitney test can be found in Siegel.[5]

Test for More Two Groups

Kruskal–Wallis One–Way Analysis of Variance by Ranks. The Kruskal–Wallis one–way analysis of variance by ranks functions like the conventional one–way analysis of variance. The null hypothesis posits whether the differences among samples show true population differences or whether they represent chance variations to be expected among several samples from the same population.[5] The Kruskal–Wallis technique also states that the ranks within each sample constitute a random sample from the set of numbers 1 through N.[13] The assumption, in using this test, is that the variable being tested has a continuous distribution.[5]

Scores in all samples are combined and arranged in order of magnitude so that ranks can be given to each score. The lowest score is assigned the rank of 1. The scores are then replaced in their respective samples with their appropriate ranks. The ranks for each sample are summed (ΣR). The assumption is that mean rank sums ($\overline{R}$) are equal for all samples and equal to the mean of the N ranks, $(N + 1)/2$, if the samples (K) are from the same population.[3]

Equal- and unequal-sized samples can be used in the Kruskal–Wallis test, because the sums of sample ranks (ΣR) are pooled in the formula. This pooling is similar to that of independent t tests of unequal sample sizes (Chapter 10).

The statistic "H" used in this test can be defined by the formula

$$H = \frac{12}{N(N + 1)} \left[\Sigma \frac{R^2}{n} \right] - 3 (N + 1)$$

where N is the number of scores in all samples combined; $\Sigma R^2/n$ is the sum of scores in a particular sample squared and divided by the number of scores in that particular sample; and n is the number of scores in a particular sample. The sum of scores, $\Sigma R^2/n$, is obtained by adding all of the group dividends together. The example shown in Table 11.6 is

$$\frac{68.5^2}{6} + \frac{46.0^2}{6} + \frac{56.5^2}{6} \text{ for}$$

$$\Sigma \frac{R_1^2}{n_1} + \Sigma \frac{R_2^2}{n_2} + \Sigma \frac{R_3^2}{n_3}.$$

The random sample distribution of H is approximated by a chi–square distribution of $K - 1$ degrees of freedom where K is the number of sam-

Table 11.6
Computation of the Kruskal-Wallis One-Way Analysis of Variance by Tied Ranks:
Methods of Teaching Pathokinesiology (Artificial Data)

Text and Lab (%)	Rank	Text (%)	Rank	Lab (%)	Rank
95	17	94	16	88	6.5
92	13.5	88	6.5	92	13.5
86	3.5	90	9.5	97	18
91	11.5	84	1	97	5
93	15	86	3.5	91	11.5
89	8	90	9.5	85	2
	$\Sigma = 68.5$		$\Sigma = 46.0$		$\Sigma = 56.5$

$T = t^3 - t$ ties	3.5	6.5	9.5	11.5	13.5
t (no. of ties)	2	2	2	2	2
$T(t^3 - t)$	6	6	6	6	6

$$H = \frac{\frac{12}{18(18+1)}\left[\frac{68.5^2}{6} + \frac{46.0^2}{6} + \frac{56.5^2}{6}\right] - 3(18+1)}{1 - \frac{30}{18^3 - 18}}$$

$$H = \frac{\frac{12}{342}[1666.75] - 57}{.995} = 1.34$$

ples. The chi–square probability of Appendix, Table E, can be used to determine the significance of H when each sample contains more than five scores. Special tables (not included in this book) have been prepared to use when there are only three samples with five or fewer scores in each.[5]

Tied ranks occur and are averaged in a way similar to that used in rank order correlation. However, a special denominator is used with the formula for computing H. The H value is usually smaller if computed without the special denominator. The special denominator corrects the deficiency caused by tied scores. H is computed by the above formula and divided by

$$1 - \frac{\Sigma T}{N^3 - N}$$

where $T = t^3 - t$. In this situation, t is the number of scores tied at a particular level of tied ranks. When no tied ranks are involved, the special denominator is not used. The formula for H when ranks are tied is

$$H = \frac{\frac{12}{N(N+1)}\left[\Sigma\frac{R^2}{n}\right] - 3(N+1)}{1 - \frac{\Sigma T}{N^3 - N}}$$

Table 11.6 provides an example of the computation for the Kruskal-Wallis one–way analysis of variance by ranks when ranks are tied. Suppose three sections of a class of physical therapy students are taught pathokinesiology by three different methods (using a text and laboratory exercises, using a text, or using laboratory exercises). The students are given a test at the end of the instruction. All recorded scores are rank ordered into a single (univariate) group. χ^2 obtained $= 1.34 < \chi^2_{critical}$ (0.05 **LOS**, 2 df) $= 5.99; \therefore H_0: R_1 = R_2 = R_3$.

The Kruskal–Wallis one–way analysis of variance by ranks is indicated when assumptions for the parametric **ANOVA** are not suitable for the data or when the level of data is less than interval measures.[5]

The obtained χ^2 value is less than the critical χ^2 value, so we conclude that the three methods of teaching pathokinesiology are equally effective.

A few nonparametric tests that appear occasionally in the research literature have been presented. This introduction enables the reader to understand some nonparametric statistics used in comparative research. Statistics presented in Chapters 10 and 11 are used with certain designs in controlled experiments. Some considerations for experimental design and control are presented in Chapter 9.

SUMMARY

Nonparametric tests refer to a class of statistics that does not require assumptions signifying a certain form of distribution or does not make statements about parameters or equality of variances. These tests are used for analyzing small-sized samples. Nonparametric tests are performed quickly and easily and are interpreted without difficulty. They are less powerful than parametric tests.

Tests of rank correlation and significance have been presented. Tests of significance include one–group, two–group, and multigroup designs. Table 11.7 provides a summary of the research processes presented thus far.

Table 11.7
Cumulative Summary of the Research Processes Presented

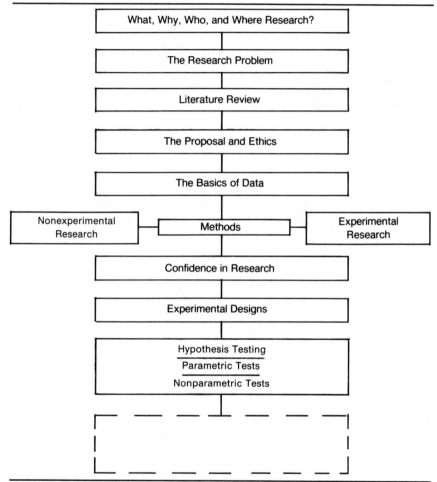

REFERENCES

1. Meyers LS, Grossen NE: Behavioral Research Theory, Procedure, and Design, ed 2. San Francisco, WH Freeman and Co, 1978
2. Schor S: Fundamentals of Biostatistics. New York, GP Putnam Sons, 1968
3. Ferguson GA: Statistical Analyses in Psychology and Education, ed 5. New York, McGraw-Hill Book Co, 1981
4. Remington RD, Schork MA: Statistics with Applications to the Biological and Health Sciences. Englewood Cliffs, NJ, Prentice-Hall, Inc, 1970
5. Siegel S: Nonparametric Statistics for the Behavioral Sciences. New York, McGraw-Hill Book Co, 1956
6. Freund JE: Modern Elementary Statistics, ed 5. Englewood Cliffs, NJ, Prentice-Hall, Inc, 1979

7. Morehouse CA, Stull GA: Statistical Principles and Procedures with Applications for Physical Education. Philadelphia, Lea & Febiger, 1975
8. Williamsen EW: Statistical Reasoning. San Francisco, WH Freeman and Co, 1974
9. Gaito J: Measurement scale and statistics: resurgence of an old misconception. Psych Bull 87: 564–567, 1980
10. Weinberg GH, Schumaker JA: Statistics: An Intuitive Approach, ed 4. Belmont, CA, Brooks/Cole Pub Co, 1980
11. Daniel WW, Coogler CE: Some quick and easy statistical tests for physical therapists. Phys Ther 54: 135–140, 1974
12. Tukey JW: Quick and dirty methods in statistics. 2. Simple analyses for standard designs. In Quality Control Conference Papers. New York, Am Soc Quality Control, 1951
13. McCollough C: Introduction to Statistical Analyses: A Semi–programmed Approach. New York, McGraw–Hill Book Co, 1974
14. Payton OD, Kelley DL: Electromyographic evidence of the acquisition of a motor skill. Phys Ther 52: 261–266, 1972
15. Cain RB: Elementary Statistical Concepts. Philadelphia, WB Saunders Co, 1972
16. Gordon AH: A method to measure muscle firmness or tone. Res Q J Am Assoc Health Phys Educ Rec 35: 482–490, 1964

Part Four

REVEALING RESEARCH

12

Reporting Research

Easy writing makes hard reading.
Samuel Putnam
Paris Was Our Mistress, 1947

The culmination of investigative efforts is the report. Research is never complete until the results have been reported. The report is the opportunity for the researcher to communicate with the scientific community by disseminating his findings orally at professional meetings or by publishing in a professional journal. The scientific community receives the report and responds. This response is formed through questions or correspondence, as well as any replication or extension of the reported research. Thus, communication is established between the researcher and the scientific community, and through the reporting process, the research is scrutinized by professional colleagues. Unless reported, the findings are lost forever and no one benefits from the researcher's time and efforts.

This section discusses reporting the research findings through written and oral presentations, with the major emphasis on publication.

PUBLICATION

The final step of the research process is publication of the results.[1] Publication in a reputable scientific journal is not, however, the ultimate goal; the true purpose of the investigative effort is to improve health.[2] Some therapists question the need to publish a study, particularly when the results might not support the investigator's original hypothesis.

Why Publish?

Publication is essential if physical therapy is to grow.[1] In 1960, Worthingham[3] stated that the realm of empiricism can be removed from physical therapy only through research presented and reported in the literature. She faulted physical therapists for their lack of contributions to the literature. Of 1800 National Foundation physical therapy scholarships,

14% of the recipients had undertaken graduate study, but only 6% of these had contributed to the professional literature.[3] An informal survey of the authorship of articles appearing in **PHYSICAL THERAPY** during the period between 1970 and 1974 provides evidence to indicate that some weaknesses from 1956 have been corrected. The percentage of authors with graduate degrees who contributed to the Journal during the 5-year period ranged from a low of 55% (1974) to a high of 71% (1971).[4] Despite increased contributions of physical therapists with graduate degrees, a proportionate increase of publishable papers has not kept pace with the increased Association membership.[5]

Michels[6] repeats A. C. Ivy[7] when he states that the most easily committed error in physical therapy is to believe that the treatment works if the patient improves following therapy. The same amount of improvement may have occurred without treatment.[6] We must produce evidence that what we do to patients is effective and, without it, patients would not have full recovery. Documentation of scientific evidence supporting the efficacy of techniques and procedures must be made through publication.[8] The results of research must be disseminated so that the information can be integrated into the world of science, which can only expand through the accumulation and interpretation of such knowledge.[9] The researcher must educate others who might want to replicate the study.[10] The published report provides a vehicle for igniting sparks (ideas) among interested investigators and serves to inform them about the completed study. Others can read the report, alter their own designs or methods, and perhaps improve on the reported investigation. A published study is valuable to the reader if a new twist has been given to an old idea, if literature has been reviewed critically, if an author's experiences are shared, or if illuminating situations are cited.[11]

The researcher is derelict in his responsibilities to colleagues and peers if the results of a study are not published. After all, why undertake a study and devote time and energy if the outcome is not shared? This question can be answered with several reasons. Writing is difficult and time consuming. Perhaps the investigator does not submit a manuscript for publication because of fear of rejection. Writing requires additional time and energies beyond those needed to conduct the study. Perhaps the researcher feels overwhelmed by the process associated with manuscript preparation. Or was the outcome of the study unexpected? The purpose of formulating a hypothesis is to test specific declarative statements, regardless of the outcome. The report makes a valuable contribution to the professional literature, regardless of whether the data supported the original or the alternative hypothesis. In either case, someone will be satisfied by the outcome and, therefore, the report is valuable. Perhaps a reader will make some minor revision of the design methods and subsequently resolve the problem by repeating the study.[1] Researchers must publish their results to contribute to the body of knowledge of physical therapy.

Format for Publishing Research

Published studies are expected to meet the same literary standards of organization and precision that apply to all forms of scientific or technical writing.[12] No exceptions can be made for physical therapists. I have heard many physical therapists claim that journal articles are too technical or do not have clinical application. Perhaps the therapist who makes such a statement is admitting that he does not understand research reports.

More than ever, we must write clearly and concisely to convey our thoughts in as few words as possible using vocabulary that everyone understands. Writing, to be effective, must be understood. The reader must understand the author's message without difficulty and the interpretation should be obvious.

The potential author selects a journal for submitting his manuscript and familiarizes himself with that journal's style. Each professional journal has a certain format to be followed for writing. Most journals have a section for "Instructions to Authors" which may differ according to the particular journal. Researchers who plan to submit their work for publication are strongly advised to consult the instructions of each particular journal. The information is intended to assist potential authors by stating the style and format in which submitted manuscripts are to be received. Specific formats are given for tables, illustrations, and references. Much of the information contained in this chapter will assist the researcher in submitting manuscripts to **PHYSICAL THERAPY**. I believe that physical therapists should submit most of their research reports to their own professional journals because: (1) Good research articles upgrade or maintain high quality levels of a journal. (2) More physical therapists read their own journals than those of other disciplines; the research results can be shared directly with those who will benefit the most from the information. (3) Publishing in the researcher's own professional journal is good for the profession because it contributes to the profession's growth and body of knowledge. Because physical therapists frequently pursue graduate study outside their own field (e.g., anatomy or physiology), they often publish in other journals to maintain an alliance with a particular discipline. Although this situation results in the loss of many good research reports to **PHYSICAL THERAPY**, it does broaden the exposure of the profession.

Components of Journal Research Reports

These components of a research report serve as guidelines when writing a report. Research appears generally as a journal manuscript, a thesis, or a formal document to a funding agency. The essential components are the same:

1. Title. The title of a manuscript is an important part of the paper because the reader often decides whether or not to read a paper on the basis of the title.[13] A brief title conveys the major ideas in the paper and should contain key words which represent the major aspects.[13-15] Because titles of reported studies are used for indexing purposes, the author should avoid the use of "A," "An," "Use of," or "Study of" in the beginning of the title.[14]

2. Abstract. The abstract, a brief summary presenting the major sections of the research report, can take the place of a summary section in the paper. Abstracts should include the reason for conducting the research, a description of the design and methods, and a summary of the results and conclusions. Most journals restrict the length of abstracts to 150 words, so a suggested strategy in writing the abstract is to construct a narrative containing key statements or thoughts from major sections of the paper.[13] The abstract should be written last, because it is a brief condensation of the entire study.

3. Introduction. This section is the beginning of the main report and sets the stage for the paper by presenting the framework on which the study was conceived. The word "introduction" is not used as a heading but is understood without labeling. The introduction contains the purpose, background for the study, the hypothesis, the research question, and a review of literature relevant to the topic of the paper. Information included in this section should be a synthesis of reports logically arranged in sequential or chronological order.

4. Review of Literature. If the literature review is extensive, this area may be optional and placed in a separate section from the introduction using the above heading. The literature review provides the background for work done by others; it cites discrepancies in previous attempts at resolving the identified problem; and it supports the reason for the study presented later in the discussion section. The literature review provides a valuable service to readers by giving them the opportunity to read about the topic in greater detail; it also saves the reader considerable time and effort in locating relevant information.

5. Method. This section describes, in sufficient detail to allow replication of the study, the subjects (number, type, height and weight, ages), the sampling method, materials, instrumentation, procedures, design, and statistical methods (e.g., tests, levels of significance or data analysis) used in the study.[13] The method section should include what the author did and the technical detail.[15] For clarity, the section may be divided into subsections according to subjects, apparatus, procedure, and design, but the wording should be succinct.

6. Results. The researcher must decide how best to describe the results so that all pertinent information is "squeezed" from the data. Findings and statistical analyses (e.g., significance and post hoc tests if appropriate) are presented in this section. No description of method or discussion takes place, only the reporting of the results. Descriptive statistics commonly presented include the mean, standard deviation, and correlational values, if appropriate. Tables or figures are suggested to reduce the length of the narrative report and to provide visual information for quick and easy interpretation. The same data should not be presented in both the narrative and in the table; only the highlights of tabular statistics are included in the narrative. Excessive statistical detail should not be reported because many readers do not understand statistics. Raw data are usually not presented because descriptive statistics provide representation of a group of numbers with a single value (a statistic) which enhances reader interpretation. Statistical findings in the narrative should be limited to the most pertinent; other details can be presented in tables, footnoted, or made available on request.[16] Organization of statistical reporting in the results section is important. A few sentences should identify the dependent variable and any highlights. Results should be reported from the general to the specific. Values of central tendency and variability are reported first to provide the background for the inferential statistics which usually are presented last.[16]

7. Discussion. The results are explained and interpreted in this section. Deductions are made from the data analyses. The literature review can be referred to to support the data, or the author can contradict reports cited in the literature. Inconsistencies borne out by the data or extensions of present theory suggested by data are discussed. Reasons for the outcome are given. The interpretation and discussion of the results must be consistent with the findings. If analyses indicate that the difference between means was not significant, then this should be stated; the author should not go beyond the limits of the research findings. If the null hypothesis is true, the author should not state that one mean is still higher than another or that the data still shows a trend despite the supported hypothesis. This approach misleads the reader and is erroneous. Statistical findings are usually reported in the results section and interpreted in the discussion section. If the statistics precede the interpretation in an organized fashion, interpretation and writing are simplified for the author and reading is easier for the audience. Occasionally the results and discussion sections are combined, but this requires more writing skill than if they are presented separately.[16] Implications for clinical practice and further research should be discussed to bridge the gap between research findings and application. The author also must acknowledge any weaknesses in the research design.

8. Summary and Conclusion. The summary of the study is already given in the abstract and need not be repeated at the end of the study. Research reports published a few years ago included a summary, but journals are now using abstracts instead. Since the abstract replaces the summary and precedes the main body of the manuscript, readers benefit from this shortcut to reading the literature. Conclusions based on the results are stated briefly and are in a separate section of the paper. If no abstract is given as a section of the report, then the conclusions are given as part of the summary and conclusions section. Conclusions summarize patterns from the findings, significance of the data, implications for practice, and suggested research needs (if this material does not already appear in the "Discussion section).

9. References. Journals usually specify the style in which references are to be cited in the text. Generally the reference list follows at the end of the paper, and references are cited chronologically in order of their appearance in the text or alphabetically, depending upon journal requirements. The potential author must consult the "Instructions to Authors" section of each journal when citing references. The recommended style is the one used by PHYSICAL THERAPY.[14]

Each reference cited in the paper is indicated by a superscript (of an Arabic numeral) at the end of the sentence or series of sentences pertaining to the work or author being cited. The same superscript is used whenever the reference is cited. If the reference is a journal article, the format is: author's last name followed by initials without internal punctuation; only three authors are listed, then "et al" is indicated and followed by a colon; title of the article with only the first letter of the first word capitalized; periods follow titles; name of the journal (abbreviated according to the form used by INDEX MEDICUS) with no punctuation; volume number of the journal followed by a colon; inclusive page numbers for the first and last page of the article followed by a comma; the year of publication with no punctuation. An example of a journal reference is:

Nelson RM: Facial nerve excitability: its reliability, objectivity and descriptive validity. Phys Ther 51: 387–390, 1971

A reference cited for a book is slightly different from that of a journal article. Superscripts are used for citing both references and are usually listed in chronological order. The sequence of a book reference is: author's last name followed by initials without internal punctuation and after three authors, the words "et al" preceding a colon; the title of the book with the first letter of each word capitalized with the exception of articles, conjunctions, and prepositions, followed by a period; if more than one edition of the book has been printed, then a comma replaces the period following the title, followed by "ed", the edition number and a period; the place of publication is given by the name of the city and state or country with internal punctuation, followed by a comma; the publisher's name is given with internal punctuation, followed by a comma; and the year of publication is placed at the end without any punctuation. Page numbers also should follow the date of publication when cited. An example is:

Hawker M: Geriatrics for Physiotherapists and the Allied Professions. Philadelphia, PA, JB Lippincott Co, 1976, p 61

If the book is one of a volume, the volume number follows the date of publication. Miscellaneous examples of references are:

No Author
Style Manual, ed 5. Washington, Am Phys Ther Assoc, 1986
Editor of Book[14]
Nelson RM, Currier DP (eds): Clinical Electrotherapy. Norwalk, CT, Appelton & Lange, 1987
Annual Reviews (yearbook)[17]
Am Physiol Assoc, Annual Review of Physiology, city, publisher, year
Encyclopedias[18]
Encyclopedia Britannica, year ed, s.v. "Physical Therapy"
Theses and Dissertations
Rooney JG: Effect of Variation in the Frequency and Carrier Frequency of High Intensity Electrical Stimulation on Muscle Fatigue and Pain Perception in Healthy Subjects. Doctoral Dissertation. Lexington, KY, University of Kentucky, 1988
Paper Read at a Meeting[14]
Name: Title. Read at the Annual Conference of the American Physical Therapy Association, Nashville, 1989

Format for other citations should be consulted in the style manual of the respective journal[14] or in books for writers.[17,18]

Before writing the research report, an outline of the report's contents is beneficial. The easiest approach is to follow the sequence of components of the research report just presented. Using the section headings and filling in the outlined requirements of each section will provide an "instant" guide. Each outline is modified and adapted to the purpose and nature of the report, but generally, the outline will follow the suggested outline shown in Table 12.1. More detail about writing the report is presented later in this chapter.

Some components of the written research report, the title, introduction, method and references are also parts of the proposal (Chapter 4). Fifty percent of the final written report is already prepared. After writing the proposal and collecting and analyzing data, only the results, discussion, conclusion, and abstract sections remain to be written.

Abstracts of Current Literature

Students are permitted to write abstracts of current research literature as partial fulfillment of course work, or these abstracts can be submitted for publication. The abstract is a summary of a recent article appearing in some health–related journal. PHYSICAL THERAPY requires the following format:

Heading. The heading includes the following information in sequential order: title of article with the first letters of words capitalized excepting

Table 12.1
Suggested Outline for the Written Report

Component	Suggested Comments
Title:	1. Concise description of study
	2. Place important words of the research in title (dependent variable, method, key words for indexing)
Introduction:	1. Nature of the problem, background, what led to study
	2. Purpose and scope, significance of outcome
	3. Literature review, synthesis of past studies
Method:	1. Describe subjects, instrumentation, procedures, design
	2. Provide sufficient detail for replication by readers
	3. Emphasize new or unique approaches
Results:	1. Describe general results, descriptive statistics
	2. Identify tables and figures
	3. Report analyses, significance and specifics
Discussion:	1. Discuss major cause-and-effect relations, present major conclusions that data supported
	2. Discuss the evidence provided by the data, refer to tables and illustrations
	3. Discuss and compare data with work of others from literature review, point out differences, recommendations
Conclusions:	1. Briefly emphasize conclusions discussed
Abstract:	1. Purpose
	2. Methods
	3. Results
	4. Conclusions

articles, prepositions, and conjunctions, followed by a period; last names and initials of the first three authors (additional names are cited as "et al"); enclosed in parentheses is the affiliation of the author(s), including city and state or country; abbreviation of the journal as listed in **LIST OF JOURNALS INDEXED IN INDEX MEDICUS;**[19] volume number followed by a colon; inclusive pages; and year of publication. An example is:

> Influence of Isometric Exercise and Passive Stretch on Hip Joint Motion. Mederros JM, Smidt GR, Brumeister LF, et al (University of Iowa, Iowa City, IA) Phys Ther 57: 518–523, 1977

Text. The body of the abstract includes the purpose of the research, the procedures, the results, and conclusion. The abstract, no longer than 250 words, is written in the past tense. No comments or judgments about the article are given because the abstract is a factual report describing the article.

Form. The abstract must be typed, double–spaced on standard sized paper; two copies should be submitted, an original and one duplicate. The first paragraph is not indented, but all other paragraphs have the first line indented. The abstractor's name, typed in uppercase letters, is flush with the right margin at the end of the review.[1,14]

Conference/Meeting Abstracts

A conference abstract is a brief summary (1 page) of a research project submitted to an organization for oral presentation at a meeting or conference. Specific instructions are established by the organization for the preparation and submission of the abstract. Readers are advised to obtain the instructions from the respective organization.

Caution must be exercised when citing and accepting information contained in conference abstracts published prior to the oral presentation. Oral or poster presentations given at conferences or meetings are submitted for peer review and acceptance is given months before the actual presentation. The researcher may have to submit an abstract of uncompleted research to meet a deadline for submitting conference abstracts. Published abstracts can therefore contain data based on an incompleted study or on a very small sample size in which the outcome may be altered substantially after completion. The reader must be aware of these discrepencies and not rely heavily on published abstracts for valid data.

Figures and Tables*

Readers of scientific publications frequently do not read each article entirely, but readers often look at the figures and tables which, if presented well, can entice the reader to read the article. Figures and tables are appealing and informative visual presentations of research results or text material. Because authors want to reach as many readers as possible, authors must be familiar with the general principles of constructing figures and tables. This section provides authors, or potential authors, with helpful information for the visual presentation of their results.

Figures. Figures are used to provide an overview of the results of the study and should be uncomplicated. Detailed information or results do not belong in figures. Figures can be drawings or photographs to illustrate text material, or graphs which show comparisons or trends.

Drawings and Photographs. A drawing or photograph clarifies text material so that the reader sees the subject clearly. Readers might have difficulty understanding what the author is trying to present unless a picture accompanies the text. The picture should be clear and as uncluttered as possible. The item should be photographed against a plain background and be in the forefront of the picture. In submitting photographs to a journal, authors must remember that photographs will usually be reduced to fit into one column or part of one column. If the photograph is cluttered with excessive material, the important points of the illustration will be lost completely in the reduction. Photographs accompanying articles should be

---

*This section on figures and tables has been reprinted from Physical Therapy 55: 768–772, 1975, by permission of the American Physical Therapy Association.

black and white glossy prints. Instantly produced pictures usually do not have as good a contrast as black and white prints.

Line drawings are more effective than a photograph. A line drawing effectively omits everything not essential to the understanding of the point the author wants to make.

Graphs

Graphs, like photographs, provide instant communication to the reader. By looking at a graph the reader can readily observe the trends or comparisons which, if presented in the text, might otherwise be obscure. Graphs should be self-explanatory and not require numbers within the body. A key identifying the different effects or methods can, however, be placed within the body of the graph (Fig. 12.1).

The author is responsible for the impression which a graph conveys; therefore, he must present the graph clearly. The spacing of units or divisions along the horizontal scale (abscissa) and vertical scale (ordinate) must be similarly proportioned. Disproportionate spacing of units along one scale can overemphasize one variable or characteristic and mislead the reader.

Bar graph. One of the simplest types of graphs for presenting discontinuous data is the bar graph, which appears in Figures 12.1 and 12.2. The bar graph presents frequencies of things or events through a series of bars or rectangles placed horizontally or vertically to the length or height of the bars proportional to the frequency of the things being measured. Usually

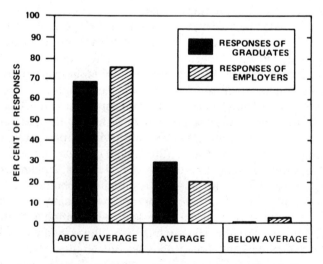

Figure 12.1. A simple bar graph. Note spacing between bars and key in the graph. (From Conine TA: A survey of the graduates of a professional physical therapy. Phys Ther 52: 855, 1972.)

Figure 12.2. A bar graph with horizontal rather than vertical bars. (From Conine TA: Teacher preparation based on functions and opinions of educators. Phys Ther 53: 876, 1973.)

each bar is separated by uniform spaces which are generally one-half the width of a bar and which enable the reader to make comparisons among data quickly and conveniently.

Histogram. A histogram is similar to a bar graph; however, it presents continous or grouped data and shows the frequency of things occurring within each group. The histogram is constructed by representing scores or observations grouped on the abscissa along with the frequency of scores or observations grouped on the ordinate. The bars of histograms are adjacent to each other so that the reader can readily discern the frequencies (Fig. 12.3).

Broken–line graph. A broken–line graph is useful for comparing changes in one characteristic with changes occurring simultaneously in another. The graph is constructed by plotting pairs of points of corresponding values of the two characteristics and then joining the consecutive points by a series of straight lines. The independent variable is plotted on the abscissa and the dependent variable is plotted on the ordinate. The graph is adapted conveniently to show different effects and methods which affect the two variables (Fig. 12.4).

Pie graph. The pie or circle graph is used to represent apportionment of a whole into its component parts. The component parts can be expressed as percentages, probabilities, or fractions of a whole. Labeling within the apportioned areas is permissible in the pie graph to prevent cluttering (Fig. 12.5).

Tables. Tables provide orderly and detailed arrangement of data. Tables provide clarity and increased meaning to data, which the narrative often

Figure 12.3. A histogram. Note that bars are adjacent to each other for ease in discerning the frequency of grouped data. (From Nelson R: Facial nerve excitation ability: its reliability, objectivity, and descriptive validity. Phys Ther 51: 387, 1971.)

Figure 12.4. A broken–line graph showing how the changes in one variable influence changes in a second variable. (From Bishop B: Vibratory stimulation: Part 1. Neurophysiology of motor response evoked by vibratory stimulation. Phys Ther 54: 1273, 1974.)

fails to accomplish. When data are presented in the tabular form of columns and rows according to logical and pertinent classifications of subject matter, the reader can interpret the results readily and conveniently.

Tables should clarify or emphasize certain aspects of the text but should not repeat the text. Often tables can present detailed material easily in less space than otherwise would be required in the text (Fig. 12.6).

In constructing tables, authors should limit them to as few points as possible. Complex tables will be passed over because they make tedious reading. In developing a table, authors should think of the size of a journal page. A table is usually limited to one column in the article and should be limited to no more than two columns unless it is presented sideways in the text, which, of course, makes it difficult to read. Only common abbreviations should be used in a table. The title of the table should indicate precisely what the table is about. Each column and row of numerical data

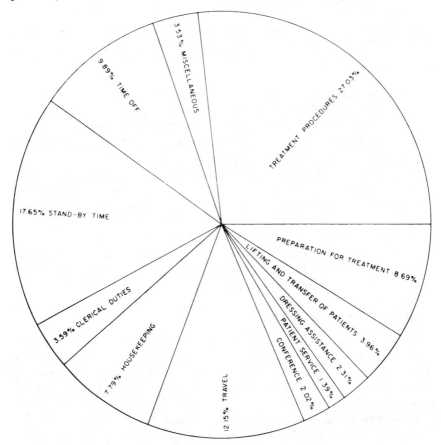

Figure 12.5. A pie graph is used to show values of parts in relation to a whole. (From Gray JM: Function of nonprofessional physical therapy personnel. Phys Ther 44: 103, 1964.)

TABLE 1. *Summary of Analysis of Variance for Muscle Tension During Test and Retest*

Source	SS	df	MS	F
Subjects		40		
Test	14653.51		366.34	
Retest	17820.20		445.51	
A (Elbow angles)		2		
Test	3629.89		1814.94	34.02[a]
Retest	5539.19		2769.59	60.90[a]
AS (interaction)		80		
Test	3023.51		37.79	
Retest	3638.34		45.48	
Total		122		
Test	21306.91			
Retest	26997.73			

[a] Significant at 0.01 level.

Figure 12.6. A table can be used to present statistical data with greater clarity than can be done in the text. (Modified from Currier DP: Maximal isometric tension of the elbow extensors at varied positions. Part 1. Assessment by cable tensiometer. Phys Ther 52: 1043, 1972.)

or variables must be labeled clearly with an identifiable unit. The same number of decimal places should be used when reporting data of the same characteristic. Zeros should be used in a table to indicate "none" if the rest of the data are numerical. If data are not available, a series of dots (. . .) should appear in the appropriate column.

Summary and Conclusions. Good figures and tables can enhance a written presentation by offering variety and convenience to the reader. Remember, figures present an overview and are kept simple and uncluttered; tables are reserved for presenting detail. Although the most commonly used figures and tables have been presented, the variations of ways in which data can be displayed really depend on the imagination of the author. In presenting pictorial information, however, the author must follow general rules and guidelines.

Common Faults in Writing

No infallible guide exists for good writing, nor is there any assurance that a person who thinks clearly will write clearly.[20] Although scientific journals have a certain required form for manuscript writing, the following section provides some of the aspects to be considered when writing the research report.

Punctuation. Clarity is achieved by good punctuation. The punctuation in the research report should follow the rules of current use. The writer should seek authoritative sources for proper punctuation.[14,20,21]

Brevity. When writing, the author should have something to say and be concise about it.[22] Effective scientific writing conveys the thought or idea to the reader directly, clearly, and succinctly.

Sanger[23] has offered some rules for writing: be simple, be specific, and be short. The best writing contains no unnecessary words and is presented in simple language. The vocabulary should be simple but appropriate. Good writing is interesting and alive and can be expressed with brevity.[23] Any time a five–word sentence is stated in 10 words, then the sentence is too long. Sentences can be reduced in length if the writer puts the manuscript away for a few days and then returns to it; freshness may prevail after a rest from writing. The author must review sentences critically to avoid misinterpretations.

Verb Tenses. Past tense is usually suggested since the research has taken place prior to the writing of the report.[13] The present tense is used in the presentation of the results, tables and illustrations;[21] for example, in "Table 2. Summary of Analyses of Variance on Effect of Varied Back Positioning on Force of Knee Extensor Muscles,"[24] both past and present tenses are used in the discussion of the results.[21]

Diction and Accuracy. The reader will have difficulty in interpreting what the author is saying or will be confused if words and phrases necessary to complete a thought are omitted, ambiguous statements are made, poor organization is present, points are raised but not discussed, or tables or figures are labeled inaccurately.

Phrases must relate to a specific word when used or the phrases become dangling words without meaning. Sometimes modifiers are misplaced in the sentence, and this destroys the emphasis. The normal order of subject and verb should not be reversed.[25]

Jargon is language peculiar to particular groups; jargon is unintelligible discourse for persons outside that particular group or profession. De Bakey[25] has called this imprecise language "gobbledygook." The writer must avoid words which may be understood by some but cannot be understood by most readers. Abbreviations such as **PRE** or **ROM** or the word "plinth" qualify as jargon. Flowery wording also is labeled jargon. Use of long unfamiliar words is often an attempt to confuse readers or to appear "learned," but the fact is, the learned writer uses simple, short words for effective writing.[22]

Other Concerns. The use of "It is," "There are," "This," and other indefinites causes the reader to search for the proper subject; complicated sentences result in misinterpretation and lack of smoothness in sentence transitions.[22]

The writer must be careful with compound constructions and modifiers. If a phrase, clause, or word is put into a sentence for additional information or explanation and it is not an essential part of the sentence, it must be set off by commas. Without the commas, the reader cannot tell a verb or noun from the modifiers.

The word "parameter" is frequently used to describe the characteristics of a trait or event. The word pertains to measures of a population in the science of statistics and is a mathematical term. If used in writing to express something other than a mathematical measure of the population, parameter is misused.

Numbers less than 10 are expressed in words, and numbers greater than 10 are expressed in numerals: for example, the active motion of the elbow was only five°, but the passive motion was 15°. Decimal and fractional amounts are usually written in Arabic numerals, 3.8 kilograms. In scientific writing, the metric system is used to express weights and measures. Temperatures are expressed in Celsius (centigrade). Abbreviations of the metric system are usually acceptable in the body of the text, for example, 15 cm.

Footnotes are used in the body of the paper to provide product information, such as the manufacturer's name and address, or to explain tables. Specific symbols are sequentially, in superscripts (*, †, ‡, §).[14]

Writing the Report

The research report is a statement and an interpretation of facts[21] and requires greater attention and higher standards than other kinds of writing.[25] Poor writing blocks efficiency, wastes the reader's time, and fails to communicate effectively.[25] Just as a plan is important for the composition and conduct of the research study, so must the written report be planned for effective communication. This section attempts to provide guidelines for writing the report.

Guidelines for Writing the Report

Keep the outline present (in view) when writing. Organize resource materials (reprints, notes, data sheets, tables, books) for ease of reference. Arrange the resource materials so that similar information is grouped together for logical order of reporting. Writing a topic sentence for each group helps to fill in the outline; no more than five main topic sentences should be used for effectiveness in any section. The last point to be presented will usually be the point the reader remembers, so the most important point(s) should be placed last.[25] Write a rough draft of the complete paper without stopping to regard detail or sentence structure. Write for flow of ideas in the organized plan.[21,26] Put the rough draft aside for 1 to 2 weeks and then return to the paper with a hypercritical approach for details, correct word use, and further development of ideas. Several rewrites will be necessary. Consider the reader: One of the most difficult tasks of writing is wording the paper to anticipate the reader's questions and presenting the paper in a way that enables the reader to grasp the meaning quickly and easily. Writing for the reader and revision of the paper are essential and cannot be overemphasized.[5]

Statements should be documented if they provide specific information or are open to question. Credit is given for the original work and ideas.[26]

When you think the report is in good form, give it to knowledgeable critics and to persons with little or no knowledge of the topic. Your best critic will be frank and offer the most constructive suggestions. If the reviewer with little or no knowledge understands the report, then the "average" journal reader will also understand. This "behind the scenes" review helps to produce a finished product of value. The most competent and prolific scientific writers go through the process of revision, rewrite, and preliminary critical reviews.

A young writer was once called before a faculty editorial committee, where a caustic critique of his or her poorly written paper was given. After the chairman's critique, the neophyte was ready to stop writing; the chairman, who was well known in the field, then produced a handful of letters and postcards representing rejections for manuscripts over which he had spent countless hours and effort. The conversation ended; the neophyte left the room without saying more than "Thank you." The moral of the story is that if you are going to do research and fulfill your obligation to communicate the results, be prepared to accept criticism from friendly and unfriendly reviewers, journal reviewers, and peer reviewers. Even with thorough planning, difficulties occur in publishing research reports. Professionals must accept the challenge and not be deterred by minor setbacks. Persistence and perseverance will help the therapist survive in the research arena. You may even find that research and publication make your professional life more stimulating and satisfying.

Copyright release statements are required by journals published in the United States. "Instructions to Authors" usually provides a sample of the statement that must accompany the manuscript. The statement must be signed by each author.

Journal Selection

Two kinds of journals exist among health professions: the refereed and the nonrefereed. The refereed journal is one in which manuscripts are reviewed by peers who judge each manuscript for its value to the profession, its accuracy and credibility, and then recommend its disposition. The manuscript accepted for publication reflects the judgment of the peer group and reflects its credibility in the profession. This review process is considered by health professionals to be more prestigious than publishing in a nonrefereed journal. A manuscript submitted to a nonrefereed journal is generally accepted by the journal's editor without peer review. **PHYS-ICAL THERAPY** is a refereed journal and is considered the standard of the profession.

Submission of the Research Report for Publication

Once the final draft is complete and submitted for publication, a time period elapses before a decision is reached about the manuscript. Time varies according to the workload of the volunteer reviewers, but ranges from 2 to 6 months. The course the paper follows after leaving your hands has been described for PHYSICAL THERAPY in "Whatever Happened to My Paper" by Davies.[27] After the journal receives the manuscript, an acknowledgement of receipt is sent and the manuscript goes to be reviewed by two or three reviewers. One of the consulting editors may be asked to review the manuscript also. The reviewers determine whether the paper should be accepted, rejected, or revised, along with suggestions for improvement. You are notified of their decision. Few manuscripts are accepted outright; about 60% to 65% are rejected because of poor writing. A few of the papers are rejected because the topic has been overexposed, or because the topic is not appropriate for the journal. A rejection does not mean that the manuscript will not be reconsidered; a rejection means reconsideration if a major revision is performed, as suggested. If the decision of the reviewers is for revision, then follow the suggestions and resubmit the revised paper.

The revised paper is treated like a new manuscript. To control bias, the manuscript is sent to other reviewers. The time for this review is usually shorter than that of the original submission, because the manuscript should be more readable. Once accepted, the paper is scheduled for future publication; the scheduling varies according to the topic and length of the paper. About 3 months before publication, the paper is edited by the journal editors and prepared for submission to the managing editor.[27]

The managing editor is responsible for preparing the paper for the printer. The type size is selected and the manuscript is marked. Next the paper goes to the printer where it is rearranged and marked for magnetic tape before actual printing. The tape is used to make galley proofs which is a proof printed from the tapes. Major revision cannot occur at the galley level. A copy of the galley proofs is mailed to the principal author to check for typographical errors and correction. The returned galley copy is rechecked by journal staff for accuracy. The managing editor lays out the format of the article as it will appear in the journal and returns the master galley to the printer. A series of correctional readings and transfer of copies takes place among the journal editorial staff, the printer, and printing plant personnel until the final form is authorized for placement on photosensitive aluminum plates. The image from the plates is printed on paper which is folded, collated, trimmed, and covered. The printing process requires 2½ months after the journal staff prepwork, which requires about 3 months.[27] A year or longer can transpire between submission of original manuscript and printed product.

Review by Editors

What do journal reviewers look at when reviewing a manuscript? The reviewers may have different reviewing styles, but similar criteria are used for judging the merits of the manuscript. The ultimate decision is based on whether the manuscript is worthy of publication and whether the principles for good writing were followed by the author(s). Reviews by manuscript reviewers are made independently; each reader reviews the manuscript for the appropriate title, organizational structure, and logical sequence, contents, writing style, and quality and quantity of illustrations and references.[28,29] Failure to state how the results of the study are important to physcial therapy may be cause for manuscript rejection.

Since the objective of publishing research reports is the dissemination of truth, the reviewers check each section of the manuscript for accuracy and technical details. An overview of the paper is judged for imagination, creativity, interest, and its contribution to physical therapy.[28]

Several factors are considered by reviewers when checking contents of a manuscript. Logical sequence and development of the topic must be apparent. The research must be relevant and sufficient. The assumptions must be valid and consistent with the purpose of the study. Detail must follow the sequence and proper information of components of the report, that is, method, results, discussion, and conclusion. The conclusion must be based on the experimental design of the study and method of analysis, and it must be supported by the findings.[29]

Revisions, Responsibility?

As DeBakey has said: "The editor of a scientific journal may be likened to a combined producer and director of a television series. Like a producer, he is responsible for selecting material that is interesting and important to his audience; like a director, he is also responsible for presenting it in an appealing and compelling way. Like both, he is subject to certain constraints that are imposed by his budget, his authors, his audience and his sponsors."[30]

The editor's task is to inform the author of the dilemma of major revisions of what may have been considered a masterpiece by the author and to educate the author through guidance to bring about improvement and revision without discouragement. If the editor prepares the revision, then the question of authorship is raised. The editor should give the author the chance to improve the manuscript according to suggestions without insisting too much on specific methods of expression. When accepted for publication, the editor has the additional task of facilitating the reader's comprehension by means of clarity, simplicity, and shortness without lowering standards of scientific writing.[30]

The author's task is to submit a paper written with clarity, simplicity, brevity, and accuracy. I believe that the manuscript is the author's responsibility and that the editors only guide and advise. After all, the principal author receives the credit for the article and also benefits from the assistance of the reviewers. The author should not be discouraged and disgruntled with the decision of revision or rejection. All is not lost! If the time and effort were worth performing the research and submitting the report in the first place, the additional time and effort required for rewriting are certainly worthwhile. Poor writing is not the fault of the editors. They are protecting the readers of the journal from poorly written, poor quality communication when they reject manuscripts.[30]

Manuscripts returned to the author(s) for revision may have detailed comments and suggestions attached for correction and improvement. Reviewers from different journals handle comments and suggestions with varying amounts of detail. Unfortunately, most journal reviewers are instructed to not edit but to offer general suggestions only. The author(s) must accept the review and correct identified flaws if publication remains as goal. When reviewers indicate that writing flaws are present, the author's responsibility is to rewrite the manuscript to improve credibility throughout, not merely to correct specific flaws and return the manuscript for another review. This latter approach not only delays publication by requiring additional revision(s), but can also lead to rejection of a revision. Rewriting a manuscript usually brings improvement in readability. Some authors rewrite manuscripts several times before submitting or resubmitting them. The reader benefits from the revisions and is protected against poor writing.

The reader has no guarantee that the study is accurate or that the information is factual when he reads a scientific article, because the outcome of a single, "one-shot,"[7] study is based on probability and a Type I error may have been committed without anyone's knowledge. The reader does, however, have some guarantee that the style, purpose, organization, and contents are consistent with the principles of good writing because of the numerous reviews. Errors can go undetected in the writing–publication process. Reviewers and editors do their best but occasionally miss an error in the data computations, or overlook a misprint or an incorrect reference. Although publication of scientific reports is the joint responsibility of the author and the editors, readers must learn to discriminate among speculation, hypothesis, inference, and fact.[7]

What the Reader Must Ask

Crocker[12] has given eight questions asked by journal referees in an attempt to increase the reader's ability to interpret and evaluate the research report. These questions and a brief discussion follow.

1. Is the research problem or purpose clearly defined? Although the problem and purpose of research are different, the author should provide information about the research problem, operationally define the variables, and give the purpose of the study. This information is usually found in the introduction to the article.

2. How does this research question relate to the current body of knowledge in the profession? The significance of the study is indicated in the literature review and conclusions.

3. How were data gathered? The author should state how data were gathered in the method section and provide the unit of measurement (found in method or results sections or in the tables). The data-gathering method is usually indicated by a description of the instrumentation, such as a questionnaire, interview, strain gauge, or graphic recorders. The author must convince the reader that the method was appropriate for the design and for solving the identified problem.

4. Is the size of the sample sufficient to answer the question? Journal referees (reviewers) are often impressed with large–sized samples, but a large–sized sample is not always essential. Experimental "overkill" is possible.[31] Crocker suggested that authors report the percentage of the population in the sample and the raw number so that readers can judge the appropriateness of sample size.

5. What is the sampling procedure? The author should state how subjects were obtained for the study. Sampling procedures are usually found in the method section. Subject attrition should also be mentioned in the paper in the discussion section.

6. Are the design procedures of the study described? Procedures are supposed to be described in sufficient detail so that any interested reader can replicate the study (necessary for determining reliability of the study). These procedures are discussed in the method section. The design is sometimes described in the method or results section, depending on how worded.

7. Are appropriate statistical procedures used? If correlational or comparative studies are presented, then the correct statistics must be used to describe and analyze the data. The level of statistical significance should be reported as well as any post hoc analyses if appropriate.

8. Is the article well organized? The suggested format of components of a research report must be followed unless the author is justified in deviating from the standard reporting procedure. The style of reporting must be looked at in a critical fashion to judge the research and the facts presented.

If ambiguous sentences are encountered, the reader must read and interpret with care.[12]

If these eight questions are followed by the author of a report, then publication chances are enhanced. Answering the questions is good exercise for the student to learn the principles of good writing, the essentials of a research report, and the methodical evaluation of the written report.

THE ORAL REPORT

The oral report, like the written report, is used to communicate the results of research. The speaker must organize the presentation for audience appeal. The report must be prepared with the audience in mind, keeping the report at the knowledge level of the audience. A report can be given to several groups, each group having a different level of knowledge about the subject; however, the essential features of the message still can be given to each group. The speaker must consider the composition of the audience, what they expect from the presentation, and what the most important information is to them. The speed of delivery for an oral presentation is slower than reading a written report; also less information can be given in an oral report. Reading aloud at a slow pace takes between 2 to 3 minutes per typed page. Voice aspects must also be considered along with audio and visual aids.

Since your voice is the principal vehicle of communication during your presentation, you must speak loudly enough to be heard by everyone in the room. You must enunciate clearly and distinctly. To put expression into your voice, use inflections. Use pauses and short periods of silence for effect. Movement and gestures, along with enthusiastic verbal delivery, will contribute greatly to animate and punctuate your presentation. Emphasize the talk with slides, repetition, review, and a pointer. Be authoritative and convincing by knowing your material and displaying confidence.

The oral report cannot replace the written report and vice versa. Each report is used to communicate the results of research, but the mode of each is different and, therefore, each requires different styles, format, and emphasis. Readers are urged not to submit for publication a report prepared for oral presentation without alteration and reamplification.

Format of the Oral Report

The oral presentation contains an introduction, a description of the procedure, and a discussion of the results. The introduction must catch the attention of the audience and provide the background for the study. Since the attention of the audiences rises and falls during most presentations, the beginning and end of the report are the most important parts.[32] Keeping this in mind, the presenter must make his most important points conspicuous during introductory and closing remarks. The introduction of the oral report is similar to that of the written report. The speaker can present the events that led up to the study, the problem that was derived from the events or review of the literature, and the purpose for conducting the study. Meeting or conference formats place limitations on the time allotted for the presentation of scientific papers. The time may vary between 10 to 60 minutes, but the usual time is 10 to 15 minutes per report. The introduction should be kept short, not to exceed 10% of the total time allotted.[33]

The study method is important. Because of time limitations, sampling and measuring procedures must be described clearly and concisely. Visual aids are valuable for emphasizing a point or reducing time for describing instrumentation. A picture can save many words, particularly if the procedure is complex and innovative. The speaker must decide before the presentation which aspects of the method are important and then set priorities or orders of presentation. Elaborate descriptions of subjects and designs can be reduced or eliminated. The time devoted to this portion of the oral report should be 17% to 25% of the total time allotted.

The results are reported, not discussed, at this point. Slides are valuable in presenting statistical data and results and will increase the audience's understanding of the explanations. Slides may include tables and graphs and may be repeated for emphasis. The pertinent features of the findings are presented as simply as possible. The research findings are one of the most important features of the presentation. The pace for presenting the findings should be slower than the pace for the introduction and method portions. Seventeen to twenty–one percent of the total presentation time should be allotted to permit audience understanding of pertinent points.

The discussion of the results follows and is the featured portion of the report. The speaker interprets the results and develops the theory for or against the findings. Pertinent literature is cited to support or contradict the data. Practical applications of the new knowledge can be discussed. Twenty–nine to fifty percent of the total time should be given to the discussion.[33]

The remaining 8% of time is devoted to a brief summary and conclusions. Conclusions presented separately serve to emphasize the discussion by repetition of important features. Usually, the rules governing oral reports allot additional time for a question and answer period.

To hold the attention of a difficult audience, Small and Krause[32] have suggested a provocative and unconventional pattern for oral presenters: Begin with conclusions, then justify the conclusions with the findings, and finish with a review of the literature. Table 12.2 provides guidelines for presenting research studies.

Table 12.2
Guidelines for Presenters and Discussants of Original Investigative Studies[a]

The session for Original Investigator Studies is to provide a mechanism of communication through which physical therapists may present the results of their investigations. These sessions follow the pattern of similar meetings of other organizations. A format of these sessions has been developed and considerations for presenters are offered:

Distribution of Time (20 minutes per paper)

1. The presenter is allocated 15 minutes.
2. Five minutes are reserved for audience questions and comment.

Suggestions for the Author

1. Assume that the audience is composed of interested physical therapists.
2. Do not spend time on the elementary aspects of the subject, and do not "speak down" to your colleagues.
3. Convey ideas in short, clear statements, using understandable terms.
4. Relate only the main points by restricting the amount of material presented. Leave the details for answers to questions the discussant or the audience may ask.
5. Speak at a relaxed pace so that the audience comprehends what you say.
6. Rehearse your talk before one or more experienced speakers and invite constructive criticism. Remember that the chairman of the session will allow you to speak for *only* 15 minutes.
7. Do not burden the listener with numerical data he cannot assimilate.
8. Allow sufficient time to summarize the main points established in your paper and explain how the findings can be applied to physical therapy.
9. Do not end your talk with a comment, such as, "That's all I have" (which is awkward and weak), or by saying "Are there any questions?" (which precludes applause and amounts to assuming the duties of the chairman of the sessions). Instead, make your final statement in a firm voice, and as a courtesy, you may thank the audience for their attention. The chairman will introduce the discussant.

[a] Adapted from Guidelines for Presenters and Discussants of Original Investigator Studies and Special Interest Papers. National Conference, APTA. Reprinted by permission of the American Physical Therapy Association.

Common Errors in Oral Reports

Some common errors in oral reporting have been noted by Johnson[33]: too extensive a review of literature, failure to identify the purpose of the study, too much material for the time allotted, failure to integrate literature with results, failure to rehearse the talk prior to the presentation, and poor slides.

"Reading" a paper at a professional meeting is commonplace among physical therapists, but the statement is misleading. Literally reading a paper is very poor style; it is boring to the audience. Speaking errors in oral reports can be reduced by using short sentences with correct grammar and clear pronunciation. Avoid structures that would require parentheticals if the sentences had been written.

Mistakes made when preparing slides can be disturbing to audiences. The amount of detail included on the slide should be clear and simple, like a figure in the written report. The audience is given limited time to view and obtain the information, so each slide should contain one thought; for example, no more than six lines of copy per slide. Tables should contain more data than figures, but care must be taken to avoid clutter on a slide. Generally, graphs have better audience appeal than tables. Closely printed slides should be avoided because reading them at distance can be difficult. Color slides are more attractive than black and white, but the amount of information contained in one slide is the most important concern. Black and white slides are effective if prepared properly. Color slides are more expensive but have great audience appeal, especially when colors are mixed and arranged differently in each slide. The change in color, design, and style can break the monotony and hold an audience's attention.

Previewing slides should be done under similar conditions as those anticipated for the oral presentation. Lighting and distance between screen and projector are important factors to consider when using slides. Varying the distances in projection can detract from the clarity. Large print on slides is helpful to avoid the problems encountered by distances.

Slides should be 5 × 5 cm (2 × 2 inches), clean, and marked for order of presentation and position of entry into the projector. Arrangements for the presentation of slides should be made in advance of the presentation so that proper equipment is available. When remote projection is not possible (from the speaker's platform), a copy of the presentation marked to show location of slides can be helpful to the speaker and the projectionist. Use duplicate slides for ease and efficiency when referring back. Unless experienced and skilled in preparing slides, the presenter should consult an expert.

SUMMARY

The culmination of investigative efforts is the report. Research is never complete until the results have been reported. Oral and published reports provide the researcher with an outlet for sharing the results of the investigation with colleagues.

Writing is not an easy task. It requires considerable effort and practice on the part of the researcher. The researcher is required to follow a certain format when preparing a manuscript for publication: The research report usually contains a title, an abstract, an introduction, a review of literature, the method, the results, a discussion, and a conclusion.

Editors prefer manuscripts that are informative, thought provoking, and interesting. All submitted manuscripts are reviewed thoroughly and evaluated for content, organization, contribution, grammar, and style.

The oral report, like the published report, is used to communicate the results of research. Although the oral report requires organization, it cannot be used for publication. The mode of the oral report differs from that of the published report and, therefore, requires different styles, format, and emphasis of content. The discussion of the results is the featured portion of the oral report.

The reader should now have an appreciation of the research process and be able to understand and interpret research literature better than before reading this book. Table 12.3 provides a summary of the research process as presented in this book.

The investigation of nature is an infinite pasture–ground, where all may graze, and where the more bite, the longer the grass grows, the sweeter is its flavor, and the more it nourishes.

T. H. Huxley
Administrative Nihilism

Table 12.3
Cumulative Summary of the Research Processes Presented

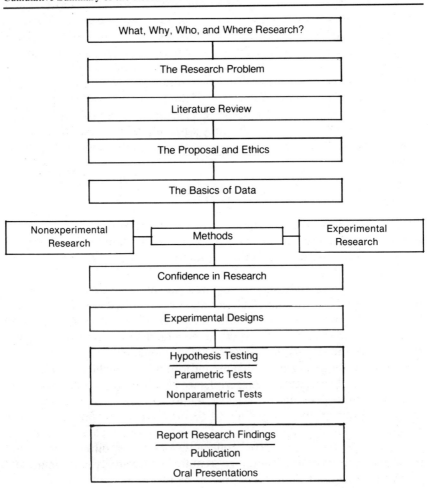

What, Why, Who, and Where Research?

The Research Problem

Literature Review

The Proposal and Ethics

The Basics of Data

Nonexperimental Research — Methods — Experimental Research

Confidence in Research

Experimental Designs

Hypothesis Testing
Parametric Tests
Nonparametric Tests

Report Research Findings
Publication
Oral Presentations

REFERENCES

1. McLaren HM: So you want to conduct a clinical study. Physiother Canada 25: 219–244, 1973
2. Mapwell C: Clinical Trials Protocol. Surrey, England, Stuart Phillips Publications, 1969
3. Worthingham C: The development of physical therapy as a profession through research and publication. Phys Ther Rev 40: 573–577, 1960
4. Boone D: A survey of the authorship of articles appearing in Physical Therapy during a five year period. Presented at a meeting of the Journal Committee of Phys Ther, 1975
5. Nelson C: Editorial readers and writers—help! Phys Ther 56: 807, 1976
6. Michels E: The 1970 presidential address. Phys Ther 50: 1579–1590, 1970
7. Ivy AC: The essentials for success in therapy. Phys Ther Rev 20: 259–260, 1940
8. Magistro CM: The 1976 presidential address. Phys Ther 56: 1227–1239, 1976
9. Lathrop RG: Introduction to Psychological Research. New York, Harper & Row, 1969
10. Ethridge DA, McSweeney M: Research in occupational therapy. Part VI. Research writing. Am J Occup Ther 25: 210–214, 1971
11. Fishbein M: Medical Writing: The Technic and the Art, ed 4. Springfield, IL, Charles C Thomas, 1978
12. Crocker LM: Let's reduce the communication gap: guidelines for preparing a research article. Phys Ther 54: 971–976, 1974
13. Meyers LS, Grossen NE: Behavioral Research Theory, Procedure and Design. ed 2. San Francisco, WH Freeman and Co, 1978
14. Style Manual, ed 5. Washington, Am Phys Ther Assoc, 1986
15. Hislop HJ: The rudiments of the scientific paper. J Am Phys Ther Assoc 44: 58–59, 1964
16. Gonnella C: Let's reduce the understanding gap. 4. Data presentation: guidelines for authors (and readers). Phys Ther 53: 871–875, 1973
17. Turabian KR: A Manual for Writers of Term Papers, Theses and Dissertations, ed 4. Chicago, the University of Chicago Press, 1973
18. Campbell WG: Form and Style, Theses, Reports, Term Papers, ed 6. Boston, Houghton Mifflin Co, 1982
19. List of Journals Indexed: Index Medicus, 1983, Bethesda, MD, Nat Lib Med, 1983, pp 11–75
20. Strunk W, Jr, White EB: The Elements of Style, ed 3. New York, The Macmillan Co, 1978
21. Trelease SF: How to Write Scientific and Technical Papers. Cambridge, MA, The MIT Press, 1969
22. Davies EJ: Let's reduce the communication gap: that's not what I meant! Phys Ther 54: 750–753, 1974
23. Sanger J: "Fog" in your pen? J Am Phys Ther Assoc 46: 512–515, 1966
24. Currier DP: Positioning for knee strengthening exercise. Phys Ther 57: 148–152, 1977
25. DeBakey L: Competent medical exposition: the need and the attainment. Bull Am Coll Surg 52: 85–92, 1967
26. DeBakey S: Basic principles of good writing. Am Op Room Nurse J 15: 69–72, 1972
27. Davies EJ: Let's reduce the communication gap: whatever happened to my paper? Phys Ther 54: 509–510, 1974
28. Strohm BR: Let's reduce the communication gap: what associate editors look at. Phys Ther 55: 266–267, 1975
29. Lister MJ: Manuscripts: what you always wanted to know. Phys Ther 57: 1007–1012, 1977
30. DeBakey L, Woodford FP: Extensive revision of scientific articles—whose job? Scholarly Publishing 4: 147–151, 1973
31. Michels E: Opinions and comments of readers: use of the *t* test. Phys Ther 50: 581–585, 1970

32. Small WP, Krause U: An Introduction to Clinical Research. Edinburgh, Churchill Livingston, 1972
33. Johnson PB: Oral Research Reports. In Hubbard AW (ed): Research Methods in Health, Physical Education, and Recreation, ed 3. Washington, Am Assoc Health Phys Educ Rec, 1973

SUGGESTED READINGS

George SA: Photographs that speak. Phys Ther 57: 1381–1382, 1977
Pal AC: Writing good abstracts: it's a tough job. Phys Ther 58: 175–177, 1978
Lister M (ed): Advice to authors: An Anthology. Washington (DC), APTA, 1982
Shilling LM: Twenty tips for conquering writing anxiety. Phys Ther 65: 1113–1116, 1985
Witt P: Research Writing Tips. Washington (DC), APTA, 1981

APPENDICES

Appendix A

EXAMPLE OF A RESEARCH PROPOSAL

A. Title of Study
Magnetic enhanced neuromuscular electrical stimulation after anterior cruciate ligament repair

B. Name of Investigator(s)
Dean P. Currier, Ph.D.
Professor, Physical Therapy
University of Kentucky
Tim Noteboom, PT, BS
Graduate student
University of Kentucky
Robert Kellogg, PT, BS
Graduate student
University of Kentucky

C. Specific Aim(s) of Study
To demonstrate effectiveness of combining magnetic and conventional neuromuscular electrical stimulation after anterior cruciate ligament surgery to:
A. prevent muscle wasting (H: knee extensor muscle girth, involved side, at 6 weeks postsurgery girth = presurgery)
B. maintain muscle torque performance (H: torque at 6 weeks postsurgery = presurgery)

D. Significance of Study and E. Related Research
Muscle wasting and weakness are recognized effects after anterior cruciate ligament repair and immobilization. Neuromuscular electrical stimulation (NMES) has been used to reduce these effects, but the result and levels of pulse charge have varied.[1-3] Our studies have shown that results are dependent on the levels of pulse charge; that is, the greater the pulse charge, the less muscle wasting and weakness.[4-6] Patient discomfort is, however, a limiting factor when using conventional neuromuscular electrical stimulation of great pulse charge; that is, induced current sufficient to produce the equivalent of 50% maximum voluntary contraction (MVC).[7,8]

Empirical observations in our laboratory indicate that magnetic electrical stimulation is only able to produce the equivalent of 20% to 51% MVC of the quadriceps femoris muscle in healthy volunteers. A stimulus capable of producing 50% MVC or more is critical in preventing muscle wasting and weakness[9] in healthy muscle tissue (muscle innervated by lower motoneuron). The combined use of magnetic and conventional neuromuscular electrical stimulation allows a decrease of pulse charge from conventional NMES, whereas the magnetic electrical stimulation supplements the stimulus sufficiently to produce muscle contractions of 50% or more MVC with reduced patient discomfort. Conventional neuromuscular electrical stimulation uses surface electrodes that concentrate the greatest charge density beneath each electrode, which activates sensory receptors. Magnetic electrical stimulation passes through high resistance (impedance) structures (like skin) where sensory receptors are located to activate muscle and nerve tissues; therefore there is minimum pain receptor activation.[10,11] The combined used of conventional and magnetic electrical stimulation provides the pulse charge necessary to prevent muscle wasting and weakness during the 6-week postsurgery period, with minimum patient discomfort.

F. Plan of Study
Subjects

This pilot study will examine 6 patients having anterior cruciate ligament repair. Each patient will be male, between the ages of 20 and 40 years, and otherwise healthy. Each subject will receive full explanations about the protocol, risks, and benefits.

Subjects will be recruited during orthopedic clinics when they have elected to have knee surgery. Only those subjects who can report regularly to the University of Kentucky Medical Center for NMES/MES treatment are eligible for the study. Subject participation will have the approval of both the patient and the referring surgeon.

Potential risks are minimal and not expected; however, those risks possible are: discomfort (pain from pulse charge caused by electrical stimulation) and delayed onset of muscle soreness.

Subjects are under routine medical management. During the NMES/MES, subjects routinely wear braces and NMES amplitudes are determined daily by the subject. The risks are the same for this study as for any routine physical therapy involving similar regimens and devices.

The experimental approach is intended to become a conventional therapeutic intervention when validated and determined reliable. The NMES/MES method can have a potentially important impact on the management of orthopedic, neurological, and soft tissue disease rehabilitation because of the minimum discomfort expected, as well as input to advance electrical engineering design where only MES would otherwise be used.

Subjects will represent a sample of convenience to be measured (girth, torque) prior to surgery, receive 6 weeks of physical therapy intervention (including the electrical stimulation), and be remeasured (girth, torque) at the end of 6 weeks. At the end of the proposed study, the subjects will continue physical therapy with personnel other than the investigators named in this study.

Procedure

A. Presurgery—Subjects will receive full explanation of study, risks, benefits, and plan and then will sign consent forms. Prior to surgery the thigh girth will be measured (4, 6, 8, 10 inches proximal to superior border of patella, bilaterally) using a tape measure. Muscle torque will be measured by a Biodex dynamometer system with the knee flexed at about 5°. The best of 3 torque scores performed with maximum voluntary contractions (MVC) will be selected as MVC and recorded, bilaterally. On the involved leg, the equivalent of 50% MVC will be determined with (1) conventional neuromuscular electrical stimulation (NMES), and (2) combined conventional and magnetic stimulation (MES). These data will serve as the training dosages.

B. Postsurgery—One day after surgery and daily until hospital discharge, the involved thigh muscles will be electrically stimulated with conventional NMES only (because MES cannot be made available for hospital use/storage; it is being used concurrently for other studies). On the first day after hospital discharge subjects will report to the physical therapy research laboratory for combined conventional ES and MES; they will continue this NMES/MES regimen (50% MVC) three times per week through the 6th week. Concurrent with the experimental electrical stimulation, each subject will receive conventional physical therapy consisting of: muscle setting exercises, straight leg raises, continuous passive motion (CPM) with a Sutter CPM device, and other exercises and treatment (for example, ice, compression, Bedsloe brace, ambulation). At the end of 6 weeks, the MES will be discontinued and measurements similar to presurgery will be recorded (additionally, a 10 cm visual analog pain scale will be administered to determine each subject's response to the NMES/MES). The patient will then continue physical therapy with personnel other than the investigators.

G. Time, Space, Equipment
  1. Time.
     The study will require 6 months to complete from the approval date.

During this period of time, volunteers will be obtained, data collected and analyzed, and the results prepared for oral and written presentations.
2. Space.
Laboratory space is available.
3. Equipment.
All necessary equipment and supplies are available. Instrumentation will consist of a modified Cadwell (MES–10) magnetic electrical stimulator to elicit muscular contractions, a Biodex dynamometer system, and a nonelastic tape measure.

H. Cost Analysis
1. MEDLINE search of literature $_____
2. Art work (graphs, illustrations, slides) for oral and written presentation $_____
3. Computer use, personnel $_____
4. Travel to and from _____ to present findings $_____

_____

Signature of Principal Investigator   Date

REFERENCES

1. Gould N, Donnermeyer D, Pope M, et al: Transcutaneous muscle stimulation as a method to retard disuse atrophy. Clin Orthop 164: 215–220, 1982
2. Gould N, Donnermeyer D, Gammon G, et al: Transcutaneous muscle stimulation to retard disuse atrophy after open meniscectomy. Clin Orthop 178: 190–197, 1983
3. Morrisey MC, Brewster CE, Shields CL, et al: The effect of electrical stimulation on the quadriceps during postoperative immobilization. Am J Sports Med 13: 40–45, 1985
4. Currier DP, Mann R: Muscular strength development by electrical stimulation in healthy individuals. Phys Ther 63: 915–921, 1983
5. Soo CL, Currier DP, Threlkeld AJ: Augmenting voluntary torque of healthy muscle by optimization of electrical stimulation. Phys Ther 68: 333–337, 1988
6. Currier DP, Noteboom T, Rooney J: Prevention of disuse atrophy by electrical stimulation after anterior cruciate repair. (Unpublished study), University of Kentucky, 1988
7. Basmajian JV, Milner M, Quanbury AQ: Force, pain, and electrode size in the electrical stimulation of leg muscles. Nature 223: 645, 1969
8. Currier DP, Mann R: Pain complaint: comparison of electrical stimulation with conventional isometric exercise. J Orthop Sports Phys Ther 5: 318–323, 1984.
9. Knuttgen HG (ed): Neuromuscular Mechanisms for Therapeutic and Conditioning Exercise. Baltimore, MD, University Park Press, 1976, p 107
10. Barker AT, Eng B, Freeston IL, et al: Magnetic stimulation of the human brain and peripheral nervous system: an introduction and the results of an initial clinical evaluation. Neurosurg 20: 100–109, 1987
11. Bickford RG, Guidi M, Fortesque P, et al: Magnetic stimulation of human peripheral nerve and brain: response enhancement by combined magnetoelectrical technique. Neurosurg 20: 110–116, 1987

Appendix B

SAMPLE CONSENT FORM

Magnetic enhanced electrical stimulation after anterior cruciate ligament repair

I, _____, freely and voluntarily agree to participate in a research project under the direction of Dr. Dean Currier, Robert Kellogg, and Tim Noteboom, to be conducted at the University of Kentucky (Hospital & PT lab).

I understand that prevention of muscle wasting and weakness is beneficial to me after anterior cruciate ligament surgery and may enhance my rehabilitation. The purpose of this study is to prevent muscle wasting and weakness by neuromuscular electrical stimulation with minimum discomfort.

In agreeing to participate in this study, I understand that I will be treated with neuromuscular electrical stimulation (conventional & magnetic) while in the hospital, then thereafter 3 times per week for a total of 6 weeks. Each treatment session of neuromuscular electrical stimulation will last about 15 minutes. I understand that the stimulation may be uncomfortable, and that the stimulation will be adjusted to my tolerance. I understand that I will be measured for strength, leg size, and level of stimulation comfort. I also understand that if I do not wish to participate in this study that alternate forms of treatment may be available through my physician or physical therapist.

I understand that review of the literature and experience of the researchers indicate no risks except possibly discomfort and muscle soreness.

I understand that participation is voluntary; refusal to participate will involve no penalty or loss of benefits to which I am otherwise entitled. I understand that no compensation is being offered or is available for my participation.

I understand that in the event of physical injury resulting from this research in which I am participating, no form of compensation is available. Medical treatment may be provided at my own expense or it may be at the expense of my health care insurer (i.e., Medicare, Medicaid, BC/BS, etc.), which may or may not provide coverage. I also understand that if I desire further information about this matter, I should contact Dr. Currier at 233-5941.

I authorize Dr. Currier and the Division of Physical Therapy to keep, preserve, use and dispose of the findings from this research with the provision that my name will not be associated with any of the results.

I have been given the right to ask, and have answered, any questions concerning the procedures to be used during this research. Questions have been answered to my satisfaction. I understand that my confidentiality and anonymity will be protected. I further understand that I have the right to terminate my involvement in this project at any time, without sustaining any form of penalty. I have read and understand the contents of this form and have received a copy.

_____   _____

Participant   Date   Witness   Date

I have explained and defined in detail the research procedure to which the subject has consented to participate.

_____

                    Researcher   Date

Appendix C

t DISTRIBUTION (VALUES OF t_α)*

Two–Tailed

df	$t_{.200}$	$t_{.100}$	$t_{.050}$	$t_{.020}$	$t_{.010}$	df

One–Tailed

df	$t_{.100}$	$t_{.050}$	$t_{.025}$	$t_{.010}$	$t_{.005}$	df
1	3.078	6.314	12.706	31.821	63.657	1
2	1.886	2.920	4.303	6.965	9.925	2
3	1.638	2.353	3.182	4.541	5.841	3
4	1.533	2.132	2.776	3.747	4.604	4
5	1.476	2.015	2.571	3.365	4.032	5
6	1.440	1.943	2.447	3.143	3.707	6
7	1.415	1.895	2.365	2.998	3.499	7
8	1.397	1.860	2.306	2.896	3.355	8
9	1.383	1.833	2.262	2.821	3.250	9
10	1.372	1.812	2.228	2.764	3.169	10
11	1.363	1.796	2.201	2.718	3.106	11
12	1.356	1.782	2.179	2.681	3.055	12
13	1.350	1.771	2.160	2.650	3.012	13
14	1.345	1.761	2.145	2.624	2.977	14
15	1.341	1.753	2.131	2.602	2.947	15
16	1.337	1.746	2.120	2.583	2.921	16
17	1.333	1.740	2.110	2.567	2.898	17
18	1.330	1.734	2.101	2.552	2.878	18
19	1.328	1.729	2.093	2.539	2.861	19
20	1.325	1.725	2.086	2.528	2.845	20
21	1.323	1.721	2.080	2.518	2.831	21
22	1.321	1.717	2.074	2.508	2.819	22
23	1.319	1.714	2.069	2.500	2.807	23
24	1.318	1.711	2.064	2.492	2.797	24
25	1.316	1.708	2.060	2.485	2.787	25
26	1.315	1.706	2.056	2.479	2.779	26
27	1.314	1.703	2.052	2.473	2.771	27
28	1.313	1.701	2.048	2.467	2.763	28
29	1.311	1.699	2.045	2.462	2.756	29
inf.	1.282	1.645	1.960	2.326	2.576	inf.

* Table C is taken from Table III of Fisher and Yates: *Statistical Tables for Biological, Agricultural and Medical Research*, published by Longman Group Ltd., London (previously published by Oliver & Boyd, Edinburgh), by permission of the authors and publishers.

Appendix D

F DISTRIBUTION (VALUES OF $F_{.05}$)*

	\multicolumn{19}{c|}{Degrees of freedom for numerator}

	1	2	3	4	5	6	7	8	9	10	12	15	20	24	30	40	60	120	∞
1	161	200	216	225	230	234	237	239	241	242	244	246	248	249	250	251	252	253	254
2	18.5	19.0	19.2	19.2	19.3	19.3	19.4	19.4	19.4	19.4	19.4	19.4	19.4	19.5	19.5	19.5	19.5	19.5	19.5
3	10.1	9.55	9.28	9.12	9.01	8.94	8.89	8.85	8.81	8.79	8.74	8.70	8.66	8.64	8.62	8.59	8.57	8.55	8.53
4	7.71	6.94	6.59	6.39	6.26	6.16	6.09	6.04	6.00	5.96	5.91	5.86	5.80	5.77	5.75	5.72	5.69	5.66	5.63
5	6.61	5.79	5.41	5.19	5.05	4.95	4.88	4.82	4.77	4.74	4.68	4.62	4.56	4.53	4.50	4.46	4.43	4.40	4.37
6	5.99	5.14	4.76	4.53	4.39	4.28	4.21	4.15	4.10	4.06	4.00	3.94	3.87	3.84	3.81	3.77	3.74	3.70	3.67
7	5.59	4.74	4.35	4.12	3.97	3.87	3.79	3.73	3.68	3.64	3.57	3.51	3.44	3.41	3.38	3.34	3.30	3.27	3.23
8	5.32	4.46	4.07	3.84	3.69	3.58	3.50	3.44	3.39	3.35	3.28	3.22	3.15	3.12	3.08	3.04	3.01	2.97	2.93
9	5.12	4.26	3.86	3.63	3.48	3.37	3.29	3.23	3.18	3.14	3.07	3.01	2.94	2.90	2.86	2.83	2.79	2.75	2.71
10	4.96	4.10	3.71	3.48	3.33	3.22	3.14	3.07	3.02	2.98	2.91	2.85	2.77	2.74	2.70	2.66	2.62	2.58	2.54
11	4.84	3.98	3.59	3.36	3.20	3.09	3.01	2.95	2.90	2.85	2.79	2.72	2.65	2.61	2.57	2.53	2.49	2.45	2.40
12	4.75	3.89	3.49	3.26	3.11	3.00	2.91	2.85	2.80	2.75	2.69	2.62	2.54	2.51	2.47	2.43	2.38	2.34	2.30
13	4.67	3.81	3.41	3.18	3.03	2.92	2.83	2.77	2.71	2.67	2.60	2.53	2.46	2.42	2.38	2.34	2.30	2.25	2.21
14	4.60	3.74	3.34	3.11	2.96	2.85	2.76	2.70	2.65	2.60	2.53	2.46	2.39	2.35	2.31	2.27	2.22	2.18	2.13
15	4.54	3.68	3.29	3.06	2.90	2.79	2.71	2.64	2.59	2.54	2.48	2.40	2.33	2.29	2.25	2.20	2.16	2.11	2.07
16	4.49	3.63	3.24	3.01	2.85	2.74	2.66	2.59	2.54	2.49	2.42	2.35	2.28	2.24	2.19	2.15	2.11	2.06	2.01
17	4.45	3.59	3.20	2.96	2.81	2.70	2.61	2.55	2.49	2.45	2.38	2.31	2.23	2.19	2.15	2.10	2.06	2.01	1.96
18	4.41	3.55	3.16	2.93	2.77	2.66	2.58	2.51	2.46	2.41	2.34	2.27	2.19	2.15	2.11	2.06	2.02	1.97	1.92
19	4.38	3.52	3.13	2.90	2.74	2.63	2.54	2.48	2.42	2.38	2.31	2.23	2.16	2.11	2.07	2.03	1.98	1.93	1.88
20	4.35	3.49	3.10	2.87	2.71	2.60	2.51	2.45	2.39	2.35	2.28	2.20	2.12	2.08	2.04	1.99	1.95	1.90	1.84
21	4.32	3.47	3.07	2.84	2.68	2.57	2.49	2.42	2.37	2.32	2.25	2.18	2.10	2.05	2.01	1.96	1.92	1.87	1.81
22	4.30	3.44	3.05	2.82	2.66	2.55	2.46	2.40	2.34	2.30	2.23	2.15	2.07	2.03	1.98	1.94	1.89	1.84	1.78
23	4.28	3.42	3.03	2.80	2.64	2.53	2.44	2.37	2.32	2.27	2.20	2.13	2.05	2.01	1.96	1.91	1.86	1.81	1.76
24	4.26	3.40	3.01	2.78	2.62	2.51	2.42	2.36	2.30	2.25	2.18	2.11	2.03	1.98	1.94	1.89	1.84	1.79	1.73
25	4.24	3.39	2.99	2.76	2.60	2.49	2.40	2.34	2.28	2.24	2.16	2.09	2.01	1.96	1.92	1.87	1.82	1.77	1.71
30	4.17	3.32	2.92	2.69	2.53	2.42	2.33	2.27	2.21	2.16	2.09	2.01	1.93	1.89	1.84	1.79	1.74	1.68	1.62
40	4.08	3.23	2.84	2.61	2.45	2.34	2.25	2.18	2.12	2.08	2.00	1.92	1.84	1.79	1.74	1.69	1.64	1.58	1.51
60	4.00	3.15	2.76	2.53	2.37	2.25	2.17	2.10	2.04	1.99	1.92	1.84	1.75	1.70	1.65	1.59	1.53	1.47	1.39
120	3.92	3.07	2.68	2.45	2.29	2.18	2.09	2.02	1.96	1.91	1.83	1.75	1.66	1.61	1.55	1.50	1.43	1.35	1.25
∞	3.84	3.00	2.60	2.37	2.21	2.10	2.01	1.94	1.88	1.83	1.75	1.67	1.57	1.52	1.46	1.39	1.32	1.22	1.00

Degrees of freedom for denominator

F DISTRIBUTION (VALUES OF F.01)*

Degrees of freedom for denominator	Degrees of freedom for numerator																		
	1	2	3	4	5	6	7	8	9	10	12	15	20	24	30	40	60	120	∞
1	4,052	5,000	5,403	5,625	5,764	5,859	5,928	5,982	6,023	6,056	6,106	6,157	6,209	6,235	6,261	6,287	6,313	6,339	6,366
2	98.5	99.0	99.2	99.2	99.3	99.3	99.4	99.4	99.4	99.4	99.4	99.4	99.4	99.5	99.5	99.5	99.5	99.5	99.5
3	34.1	30.8	29.5	28.7	28.2	27.9	27.7	27.5	27.3	27.2	27.1	26.9	26.7	26.6	26.5	26.4	26.3	26.2	26.1
4	21.2	18.0	16.7	16.0	15.5	15.2	15.0	14.8	14.7	14.5	14.4	14.2	14.0	13.9	13.8	13.7	13.7	13.6	13.5
5	16.3	13.3	12.1	11.4	11.0	10.7	10.5	10.3	10.2	10.1	9.89	9.72	9.55	9.47	9.38	9.29	9.20	9.11	9.02
6	13.7	10.9	9.78	9.15	8.75	8.47	8.26	8.10	7.98	7.87	7.72	7.56	7.40	7.31	7.23	7.14	7.06	6.97	6.83
7	12.2	9.55	8.45	7.85	7.46	7.19	6.99	6.84	6.72	6.62	6.47	6.31	6.16	6.07	5.99	5.91	5.82	5.74	5.65
8	11.3	8.65	7.59	7.01	6.63	6.37	6.18	6.03	5.91	5.81	5.67	5.52	5.36	5.28	5.20	5.12	5.03	4.95	4.86
9	10.6	8.02	6.99	6.42	6.06	5.80	5.61	5.47	5.35	5.26	5.11	4.96	4.81	4.73	4.65	4.57	4.48	4.40	4.31
10	10.0	7.56	6.55	5.99	5.64	5.39	5.20	5.06	4.94	4.85	4.71	4.56	4.41	4.33	4.25	4.17	4.08	4.00	3.91
11	9.65	7.21	6.22	5.67	5.32	5.07	4.89	4.74	4.63	4.54	4.40	4.25	4.10	4.02	3.94	3.86	3.78	3.69	3.60
12	9.33	6.93	5.95	5.41	5.06	4.82	4.64	4.50	4.39	4.30	4.16	4.01	3.86	3.78	3.70	3.62	3.54	3.45	3.36
13	9.07	6.70	5.74	5.21	4.86	4.62	4.44	4.30	4.19	4.10	3.96	3.82	3.66	3.59	3.51	3.43	3.34	3.25	3.17
14	8.86	6.51	5.56	5.04	4.70	4.46	4.28	4.14	4.03	3.94	3.80	3.66	3.51	3.43	3.35	3.27	3.18	3.09	3.00
15	8.68	6.36	5.42	4.89	4.56	4.32	4.14	4.00	3.89	3.80	3.67	3.52	3.37	3.29	3.21	3.13	3.05	2.96	2.87
16	8.53	6.23	5.29	4.77	4.44	4.20	4.03	3.89	3.78	3.69	3.55	3.41	3.26	3.18	3.10	3.02	2.93	2.84	2.75
17	8.40	6.11	5.19	4.67	4.34	4.10	3.93	3.79	3.68	3.59	3.46	3.31	3.16	3.08	3.00	2.92	2.83	2.75	2.65
18	8.29	6.01	5.09	4.58	4.25	4.01	3.84	3.71	3.60	3.51	3.37	3.23	3.08	3.00	2.92	2.84	2.75	2.66	2.57
19	8.19	5.93	5.01	4.50	4.17	3.94	3.77	3.63	3.52	3.43	3.30	3.15	3.00	2.92	2.84	2.76	2.67	2.58	2.49
20	8.10	5.85	4.94	4.43	4.10	3.87	3.70	3.56	3.46	3.37	3.23	3.09	2.94	2.86	2.78	2.69	2.61	2.52	2.42
21	8.02	5.78	4.87	4.37	4.04	3.81	3.64	3.51	3.40	3.31	3.17	3.03	2.88	2.80	2.72	2.64	2.55	2.46	2.36
22	7.95	5.72	4.82	4.31	3.99	3.76	3.59	3.45	3.35	3.26	3.12	2.98	2.83	2.75	2.67	2.58	2.50	2.40	2.31
23	7.88	5.66	4.76	4.26	3.94	3.71	3.54	3.41	3.30	3.21	3.07	2.93	2.78	2.70	2.62	2.54	2.45	2.35	2.26
24	7.82	5.61	4.72	4.22	3.90	3.67	3.50	3.36	3.26	3.17	3.03	2.89	2.74	2.66	2.58	2.49	2.40	2.31	2.21
25	7.77	5.57	4.68	4.18	3.86	3.63	3.46	3.32	3.22	3.13	2.99	2.85	2.70	2.62	2.54	2.45	2.36	2.27	2.17
30	7.56	5.39	4.51	4.02	3.70	3.47	3.30	3.17	3.07	2.98	2.84	2.70	2.55	2.47	2.39	2.30	2.21	2.11	2.01
40	7.31	5.18	4.31	3.83	3.51	3.29	3.12	2.99	2.89	2.80	2.66	2.52	2.37	2.29	2.20	2.11	2.02	1.92	1.80
60	7.08	4.98	4.13	3.65	3.34	3.12	2.95	2.82	2.72	2.63	2.50	2.35	2.20	2.12	2.03	1.94	1.84	1.73	1.60
120	6.85	4.79	3.95	3.48	3.17	2.96	2.79	2.66	2.56	2.47	2.34	2.19	2.03	1.95	1.86	1.76	1.66	1.53	1.38
∞	6.63	4.61	3.78	3.32	3.02	2.80	2.64	2.51	2.41	2.32	2.18	2.04	1.88	1.79	1.70	1.59	1.47	1.32	1.00

*These tables were reproduced from M. Merrington and C. M. Thompson, "Tables of percentage points of the inverted beta (F) distribution." Biometrika, vol. 33 (1943), by permission of the Biometrika trustees.

Appendix E

CHI SQUARE DISTRIBUTION (VALUES OF χ^2_α)*

d.f.	$\chi^2_{.995}$	$\chi^2_{.99}$	$\chi^2_{.975}$	$\chi^2_{.95}$	$\chi^2_{.05}$	$\chi^2_{.025}$	$\chi^2_{.01}$	$\chi^2_{.005}$	d.f.
1	.0000393	.000157	.000982	.00393	3.841	5.024	6.635	7.879	1
2	.0100	.0201	.0506	.103	5.991	7.378	9.210	10.597	2
3	.0717	.115	.216	.352	7.815	9.348	11.345	12.838	3
4	.207	.297	.484	.711	9.488	11.143	13.277	14.860	4
5	.412	.554	.831	1.145	11.070	12.832	15.086	16.750	5
6	.676	.872	1.237	1.635	12.592	14.449	16.812	18.548	6
7	.989	1.239	1.690	2.167	14.067	16.013	18.475	20.278	7
8	1.344	1.646	2.180	2.733	15.507	17.535	20.090	21.955	8
9	1.735	2.088	2.700	3.325	16.919	19.023	21.666	23.589	9
10	2.156	2.558	3.247	3.940	18.307	20.483	23.209	25.188	10
11	2.603	3.053	3.816	4.575	19.675	21.920	24.725	26.757	11
12	3.074	3.571	4.404	5.226	21.026	23.337	26.217	28.300	12
13	3.565	4.107	5.009	5.892	22.362	24.736	27.688	29.819	13
14	4.075	4.660	5.629	6.571	23.685	26.119	29.141	31.319	14
15	4.601	5.229	6.262	7.261	24.996	27.488	30.578	32.801	15
16	5.142	5.812	6.908	7.962	26.296	28.845	32.000	34.267	16
17	5.697	6.408	7.564	8.672	27.587	30.191	33.409	35.718	17
18	6.265	7.015	8.231	9.390	28.869	31.526	34.805	37.156	18
19	6.844	7.633	8.907	10.117	30.144	32.852	36.191	38.582	19
20	7.434	8.260	9.591	10.851	31.410	34.170	37.566	39.997	20
21	8.034	8.897	10.283	11.591	32.671	35.479	38.932	41.401	21
22	8.643	9.542	10.982	12.338	33.924	36.781	40.289	42.796	22
23	9.260	10.196	11.689	13.091	35.172	38.076	41.638	44.181	23
24	9.886	10.856	12.401	13.848	36.415	39.364	42.980	45.558	24
25	10.520	11.524	13.120	14.611	37.652	40.646	44.314	46.928	25
26	11.160	12.198	13.844	15.379	38.885	41.923	45.642	48.290	26
27	11.808	12.879	14.573	16.151	40.113	43.194	46.963	49.645	27
28	12.461	13.565	15.308	16.928	41.337	44.461	48.278	50.993	28
29	13.121	14.256	16.047	17.708	42.557	45.722	49.588	52.336	29
30	13.787	14.953	16.791	18.493	43.773	46.979	50.892	53.672	30

Index